LUMBAR DISCECTOMY AND LAMINECTOMY

Robert G. Watkins, M.D.
Series Editor

Principles and Techniques in Spine Surgery

LUMBAR DISCECTOMY AND LAMINECTOMY

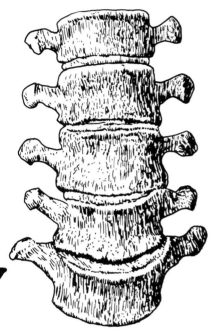

Edited by

Robert G. Watkins, M.D.
Kerlan-Jobe Orthopaedic Clinic
Inglewood, California

John S. Collis, Jr., M.D.
St. Vincent's Charity Hospital
Cleveland, Ohio

AN ASPEN PUBLICATION
Aspen Publishers, Inc.
Rockville, Maryland
Royal Tunbridge Wells
1987

Library of Congress Cataloging-in-Publication Data

Lumbar discectomy and laminectomy.

(Principles and techniques of spine surgery)
"An Aspen publication."
Includes bibliographies and index.
1. Vertebrae, Lumbar—Surgery. 2. Discectomy. 3. Laminectomy.
I. Watkins, Robert G. II. Series. [DNLM: 1. Intervertebral Disk—surgery.
2. Lumbar Vertebrae—surgery. WE 750 L9565]
RD768.L84   1987   617'.375   86-28674
ISBN: 0-87189-617-6

Editorial Services: Jane Coyle and Marsha Davies

Library of Congress Catalog Card Number: 86-28674
ISBN: 0-87189-617-6

Printed in the United States of America

1 2 3 4 5

Table of Contents

Contributors

Michael L.J. Apuzzo, M.D.
Neurological Surgery
University of Southern California School of Medicine
Los Angeles, CA

Charles Burton, M.D.
Neurosurgery
Institute for Low Back Care
Minneapolis, MN

John S. Collis, M.D.
Neurosurgery
St. Vincent's Charity Hospital
Cleveland, OH

William H. Dillin, M.D.
Spine Surgery
Kerlan-Jobe Orthopaedic Clinic
Inglewood, CA

Paul Duchesneau, M.D.
Cleveland Clinic
Cleveland, OH

Pierre-R. Dupuis, M.D.
Department of Orthopedics
University Hospital
University of Saskatchewan
Saskatoon, Canada

Peter Dyck, M.D.
Neurosurgery
University of Southern California
Los Angeles, CA

Harry Farfan, M.D.
St. Mary's Hospital Center
Montreal, Canada

Bonnie Flannigan, M.D.
Valley Presbyterian Hospital
Van Nuys, CA

William V. Glenn, Jr., M.D.
Radiology
Long Beach Medical Imaging Center
Long Beach, CA

Joseph Hahn, M.D.
Department of Neurological Surgery
Cleveland Clinic Foundation
Cleveland, OH

Kenneth Heithoff, M.D.
Center for Diagnostic Imaging
St. Louis Park, MN

Scott Kingston, M.D.
Centinela Hospital
Inglewood, CA

William Kirkaldy-Willis, M.D.
University Hospital
University of Saskatchewan
Saskatoon, Canada

Irv Klein, M.D.
Department of Anesthesiology
Centinela Hospital Medical Center
Inglewood, CA

Donlin Long, M.D.
Department of Neurosurgery
The Johns Hopkins Hospital
Baltimore, MD

John O'Brien, M.D.
The London Clinic
London, England

Charles D. Ray, M.D.
Sister Kinney Institute
Minneapolis, MN

Stephen L.G. Rothman, M.D.
Neural Radiology
MPDI, Inc.
Torrance, CA

Gary Schneiderman, M.D.
Orthopedic Surgery
University of California, Davis
Sacramento, CA

James Thomas, M.D.
Attending Surgeon
Memorial Medical Center Long Beach
Co-Chief Spinal Cord Injury Service
Rancho Los Amigos
Downey, CA
California Spine Surgery Medical Group, Inc.
Long Beach, CA

Robert G. Watkins, M.D.
Kerlan-Jobe Orthopaedic Clinic
Inglewood, CA

Arthur H. White, M.D.
Orthopedic Spine Surgery
St. Mary's Hospital Spine Center
San Francisco, CA

Robert Warren Williams, M.D.
Neurological Surgery
University of Nevada School of Medicine
Humana Hospital Sunrise
Las Vegas, NV

Leon L. Wiltse, M.D.
Attending Surgeon
Memorial Medical Center Long Beach
California Spine Surgery Medical Group, Inc.
Long Beach, CA

Foreword

Lumbar Discectomy and Laminectomy is not a textbook in the usual sense. It is an advanced and very detailed work on a small but most important segment of the lumbar spine. Surgical anatomy and surgical technique are stressed. Although there are chapters dealing with pathological anatomy and theories as to the cause of pain and so forth, this is fundamentally a "how to" book, and scant space is devoted to reporting subjective clinical results.

The major thrust of the book is how to deal with sciatica. Consequently, many of the chapters describe methods of decompressing the spinal nerves from their point of exit from dura to the far lateral zone.

For centuries, the word "sciatica" was used to describe the leg pain with which we are all so familiar, but no one had a notion of the real cause. Domenico Cotugno, in 1764, stated that the pain was attributable to "an acrid and irritating matter which, lying on the nerve, preys on the stamina and gives rise to the pain."[1] In 1917 Bertollati incriminated enlarged transverse processes.[2] Danforth and Wilson, in the 1920s, recognized hard discs bulging into the lateral canals along with osteoarthritic spurring and disc space narrowing as the causes of pain down the course of the sciatic nerve.[3] They even

thought tight ligaments in the far lateral zone caused the pain. But it was Mixter and Barr, who, in 1932, fired the shot heard 'round the world with their description of the ruptured disc in the central canal.[4] Thus began the "dynasty of the disc," as Farfan has so eloquently stated it.[5] Strangely, the lateral canals were to a large extent ignored until attention was again called to them in the early 1970s by Kirkaldy-Willis.[6]

In reading this work, I was struck by how absolutely current it is. Because of the advanced nature of much of the material, this book will appeal especially to the spine surgeon. Neurological and orthopaedic surgeons preparing for their boards will also find it most valuable. However, anyone doing lumbar spine surgery should read it.

Very recent developments are presented. Dr. Watkins has succeeded in compiling a book representing the state of the art in a most difficult and controversial area.

Leon L. Wiltse, M.D.
California Spine Surgery
Medical Group
Long Beach, California

NOTES

1. Cortugno D: *De Ischiade Nervose Canmentarius.* Naples, Simoncos Brothers, 1764.

2. Bertolotti. *Radiol Med* 1917.

3. Danforth M, Wilson P: The anatomy of the lumbosacral region in relation to sciatic pain. *J Bone Joint Surg* 1925;7:109.

4. Mixter WJ, Barr JS: Rupture of the intervertebral disc with involvement of the spinal canal. *N Engl J Med* 1934;211:210.

5. Farfan HF: *Mechanical Disorders of the low back.* Lea & Febinger, Philadelphia, 1973.

6. Kirkaldy-Willis WH, Paine KWE, Cauchoix J, et al: Lumbar spinal stenosis. *Clin Orthop* 1974;99:30.

Chapter 1

The Natural History of Degenerative Changes in the Lumbar Spine

Pierre-R. Dupuis, M.D.

INTRODUCTION

The number of patients seeking treatment for low back pain is steadily increasing. The prevalence of back pain has been reported to be anywhere from 5 to 25 percent and the incidence from 30 to 90 percent.[1,2,3,7,11,13,16,28] A study shows that 85 to 90 percent of patients with attacks of low back pain will have recovered within 8 to 10 weeks.[27] Even if most pathologies causing low back pain and sciatica are minor in nature and self-limiting in time, the cost of treatment, the impact on health care delivery, and the effects on industry are becoming a terrible burden for society.[18,19,23,26,31] Those 10 to 15 percent of back pain patients out of work for more than 8 weeks account for about 80 percent of the cost.[5,22,23]

For treatment to be successful, an early and accurate diagnosis is imperative. This diagnosis can be secured only if the physician has a thorough understanding of the disease process. The following discussion puts into perspective what is known or suspected about the degenerative process in the lumbar spine. We will see that there are natural phenomena occurring during the life of the individual which may have an effect on the degenerative process. We will also see that, although the lumbar spine has its own "degenerative personality," most events that occur in its degenerative process are not unlike the ones occurring in other joints.

CHANGES WITH AGE

The Bone of the Vertebra

One of the more important aspects of the skeletal aging process is bone loss. For both sexes, a gradual decrease in cortical bone of 3 percent per decade can be expected. In postmenopausal women, a 9 percent rate of decrease in cortical bone per decade has been demonstrated. Trabecular bone also decreases. A 6 to 8 percent decrease per decade can be expected for both sexes from between 20 to 40 years of age onward.[17]

These changes modify the load-bearing capacity of the vertebra. Studies show that after age 40 the load-bearing capacity of cortical and cancellous bone in vertebrae changes dramatically.[25] Before age 40 the cancellous portion contributes about 55 percent of the load-bearing capacity. This decreases to about 35 percent from age 40 onward. Furthermore, bone strength decreases more rapidly than bone quantity.[4] Such decrease is thought to be secondary to a decrease in the cross-sectional area of the vertically oriented trabeculae and to the loss of the horizontal trabecular cross-linkage systems. This accounts for the end plates bending away from the disc, end plate fractures, and wedge fractures of vertebral bodies that are so common in osteoporotic spines.

The End Plates

Between 23 to 40 years of age, there is a gradual mineralization of end plate cartilage. By the age of 60 only a thin layer of bone separates the disc from the vascular channels that were previously in direct contact with the cartilage. Moreover, these nutrient channels are slowly obliterated, either partially or completely, by amorphous intensely PAS-positive material. In addition, the walls of the arterioles and venules progressively thicken.[6] Such changes can have a deleterious effect on disc nutrition. The adult disc has no blood supply[9] and must rely on diffusion for nutrition.[18] Glucose and oxygen penetrate the disc mainly via the end plates. Any disturbance of this major nutritional pathway may play an important role in the pathogenesis of lumbar disc disease. This seems to be confirmed by the observation, in the experimental animal, of a progressive decrease in the permeability of the intervertebral disc in relation to aging.[8]

The Disc

At birth the nucleus pulposus of the disc is a gel-like substance in which notochordal type cells are suspended in a ground substance made up of 88 percent water and a meshwork of collagen fibrils and protein polysaccharide complexes.[21] From birth to old age, a gradual dessication occurs. The original water content will decrease from 88 percent to about 70 percent. This loss of water content is less important in the annulus fibrosus. Here, the original content of about 78 percent will decrease to about 70 percent. Beginning at the third decade, there will also be a 55 percent decrease in the glycosaminoglycans content of the nucleus pulposus.[12] There is also a gradual increase in glycoproteins (noncollagen),[15] particularly in the cross-beta form.[20] Although the collagen content in the annulus fibrosus changes little with age, there is a slight increase in the collagen content of the nucleus pulposus, from 15 percent in the first decade to about 20 percent in the remaining years.

DEGENERATIVE CHANGES

The Three-Joint Complex

At any one level, the motion segment is made up of three distinct parts: the two zygapophyseal joints and the intervertebral joint (the disc). In the normal motion segment, the three joints are anatomically linked and mechanically balanced. Any trauma or pathological changes in one part of the complex will, in time, ultimately spread to the two others through changes in the mechanical behavior of the construct. The changes may be symmetrical if the injury was to all three parts, but more often they are asymmetrical, being predominant either in the disc or facet joints.

Phases of Degeneration

To understand the phases of motion segment degeneration, one must understand that degenerative changes in general are the human body's attempt to heal itself. Every tissue carries its own potential for healing. Thus, the human body will tend to stabilize an unstable joint by increasing the surface area of a joint where damage to the cartilage surface interferes with optimal function or by immobilizing the joint by the natural splintage of muscle spasm. It is, therefore, understandable that degenerative changes will develop only if the extent of tissue damage exceeds local healing potential. The spectrum of

degenerative changes in the motion segment can be divided into three phases that widely overlap.[14,30]

The first phase is the one of dysfunction in which there is interruption in normal function of the three-joint complex either by acute trauma or repeated microtrauma to a primary restraint structure. In this phase, if the repair of the traumatized tissue is competent and the complex exhibits mechanical behavior similar to the one before the traumatic episode, return to normal function is likely. If, on the other hand, damage exceeds local healing potential, permanent injury and sequelae are likely. Repeated trauma will push the motion segment slowly toward the second phase—instability.

Normal biomechanical function requires tissue restraints to prevent abnormal motion. Supporting structures are organized into primary, secondary, and tertiary restraints. In the phase of instability, the primary restraints have become incompetent because of inadequate or incomplete healing. Increased loads are put on the secondary restraints and, in turn, these restraints slowly fail, which produces a hypermobile motion segment. Since the human body cannot tolerate this laxity, which concentrates too much load on the tertiary restraints (muscles), it directs its efforts toward the restabilization of the loose motion segment.

The motion segment thus enters the final phase, that of restabilization, where osteophyte formation around the three joints increases the load-bearing surface and decreases motion, resulting in a stiff and less painful motion segment. As we will see later, each of the three phases carries its own potential for incidental complications.

Phase of Dysfunction

Changes that occur in the facet joints during the phase of dysfunction (Figure 1–1a) are the same as those that occur in any other synovial joints. Trauma can involve the capsule, the synovium, the cartilage surface, or supporting bone. More often it primarily involves the capsule and synovium. The early joint response to trauma is synovitis. Chronic synovitis and joint effusion can stretch a traumatized capsule. The

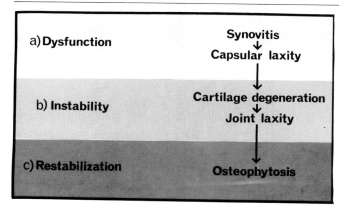

Figure 1–1 The progressive degenerative changes in the facet joint overlaid by the three phases of the degenerative process.

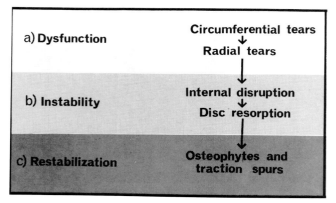

Figure 1–2 The progressive degenerative changes in the annulo-nuclear complex of the intervertebral disc overlaid by the three phases of the degenerative process.

inflamed synovium may, in turn, project folds, which may become entrapped in the joint between the cartilage surfaces, and may in turn initiate cartilage damage.

The exact nature of disc dysfunction (Figure 1–2a) is not as clear as with facet joint dysfunction. It is likely that early changes involve the appearance of circumferential tears in the annulus fibrosus. If these tears are situated in the outer layer where some vascular supply is available, healing is possible. In the deeper layers where no blood supply is available, the healing process is at best difficult. Slowly, there is progressive enlargement of the circumferential tears, which tend to coalesce into radial tears. These tears may extend into the nucleus pulposus. In turn, the nucleus will begin to exhibit changes by losing water and proteoglycan content.

Phase of Instability

As the changes continue in the facet joint (Figure 1–1b), capsular stretching and progressive loss of joint cartilage will progress to the point where permanent laxity exists. This increasing laxity will allow joint subluxation. Continuing changes in the nucleus (Figure 1–2b) will result in internal disruption with concomitant loss of disc height and annular radial bulge. This, in turn, causes the anterior longitudinal ligament and posterior longitudinal ligament to become relatively longer and looser, and disc instability follows.

Phase of Restabilization

As either or both facet joint and disc become increasingly unstable, attempts at restabilization (Figures 1–1c and 1–2c) will take the form of subperiosteal bone formation or bone formation along ligaments and capsule fibers resulting in perifacetal and peridiscal osteophytes and traction spurs. The

facet joint enlarges both in its ventral and dorsal aspects. This, along with similar changes in the disc, will progressively reduce movement and so produce a stable motion segment.

Incidental Complication Syndromes

In some patients, the degenerative process affects mainly the posterior joints. In others, it affects mainly the disc. In the majority of patients, the three joints are affected with some predominance in the disc or in the facet joint. Clinical experience has shown that it is indeed possible for the three-joint complex to go through these changes with very few symptoms. Pain is only a signal of impending or actual tissue damage and will manifest itself only if the tissue failure threshold, the transition from plastic deformation to permanent deformation, is reached or transgressed. Thus, patients with minimal degenerative changes may present with chronic recurrent symptoms, while others may exhibit severe radiological changes and present with few or no symptoms. There is no correlation between the incidence of low back pain and degenerative changes on x-rays of the lumbar spine.

Each phase carries a specific set of incidental complications which find their expression in painful clinical syndromes (Figure 1–3). In the phase of dysfunction, facet pathology will manifest itself in the facet syndrome. In the same phase, disc pathology will manifest itself in the annular tear syndrome. It is not unusual to find both in the same patient, nor is it unusual to find that they carry over in other phases.

Disc herniation is found in the phase of instability. Later in the same phase, dynamic degenerative spondylolisthesis is found when laxity predominates in the posterior restraining structures and dynamic degenerative retro-olisthesis is found when laxity predominates in the disc.[10] Both can produce dynamic lateral or central nerve entrapment. This has been confirmed experimentally.[24,29]

In the phase of restabilization, both dynamic degenerative spondylolisthesis and/or retro-olisthesis become fixed and can produce symptomatic single-level spinal stenosis. Enlargement of facet joints and circumferential osteophytes around the disc space can also produce symptomatic single-level central and/or lateral stenosis. Sometimes, this stenotic process will spread to several other contiguous levels. How this happens is not well understood but it is probable that arthritic stabilization of one level causes the stresses and loads to be redistributed to adjacent levels.

This dynamic approach to looking at the degenerative process in the lumbar spine should give the reader perspective when diagnosis, conservative care, and surgical care are discussed in the next chapters.

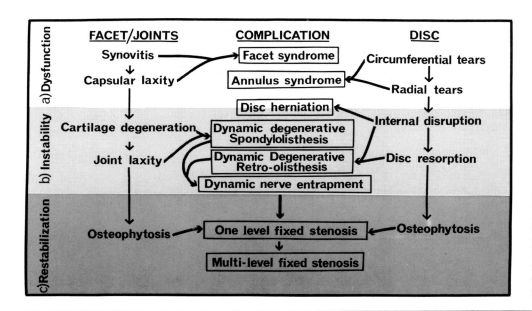

Figure 1–3 The incidental complication syndromes: each phase of the degenerative process carries the potential for complications that are related to specific pathologies encountered in the facet and/or disc. If none of these materialize, it is possible to go through life with few symptoms.

REFERENCES

1. Anderson JAD: Back pain and occupation, in Jayson M (ed): *The Lumbar Spine and Back Pain*. London, 1980, Pitman Medical, pp 57–82.

2. Anderson JAD: Low back pain—Cause and prevention of long term handicap (A critical review). *Int J Rehabil Res* 1981;3:89–93.

3. Andersson GBJ: Epidemiologic aspects on low-back pain in industry. *Spine* 1981;6:53–60.

4. Bell GH, Dunbar O, Beck SJ, Gibb A: Variation in strength of vertebrae with age and their relation to osteoporosis. *Calcif Tissue Res* 1967;1:75–86.

5. Benn RT, Wood PHN: Pain in the back; An attempt to estimate the size of the problem. *Rheumatol Rehabil* 1975;14:121–128.

6. Bernick S, Caillet R: Vertebral end-plate changes with aging of human vertebrae. *Spine* 1982;7:97–102.

7. Bigos SJ, Spengler DM, Nachemson AL, Fisher LD, Wortey MD: Back injuries in industry. *Abstracts of The International Society for the Study of the Lumbar Spine*, 1982.

8. Brown MD, Tsaltas TT: Studies on the permeability of the intervertebral disc during skeletal maturation. *Spine* 1976;1:240–245.

9. Coventry MB, Ghormley RK, Kernohan JW: The intervertebral disc: Its microscopic anatomy and pathology. Part I: Anatomy, Development and Physiology. *J Bone Joint Surg* 1945;27-A:105–112.

10. Dupuis PR, Yong-Hing K, Cassidy JD, Kirkaldy-Willis WH: Radiological diagnosis of degenerative lumbar spinal instability. Accepted for publication in *Spine* 1984.

11. Glover J: Low back pain, the 120 million ache. *Medical Tribune* 1972;10:6–7.

12. Happey F, Weissman A, Naylor A: Polysaccharide content of the prolapsed nucleus pulposus of the human intervertebral disc. *Nature* 1961;192:868.

13. Hirsh C, Jonsson B, Lewin T: Low back symptoms in a Swedish female population. *Clin Orthop* 1969;63:171–176.

14. Kirkaldy-Willis WH: The pathology and pathogenesis of low back pain, in Kirkaldy-Willis (ed): *Managing Low Back Pain*. New York, Churchill Livingstone, 1983, pp 23–44.

15. Lyons H, Jones E, Quinn FE, Sprunt DH: Changes in the protein polysaccharide fraction of the nucleus pulposus from human intervertebral disc with age and disc herniation. *J Lab Clin Med* 1966;68:930–939.

16. Magora A: An investigation of the problem of sick leave in the patient suffering from low back pain. *Indust Med Surg* 1969;38:398–408.

17. Mazess RB: On aging bone lost. *Clin Orthop* 1982;165:239–252.

18. Nachemson AL: The lumbar spine: An orthopaedic challenge. *Spine* 1976;1:59–71.

19. Nagi SZ, Riley LR, Newby LG: A social epidemiology of back pain in a general population. *J Chronic Dis* 1973;26:769–779.

20. Naylor A: The biochemical changes in the human intervertebral disc in degeneration and nuclear prolapse. *Orthop Clin North Am* 1971;2:343–358.

21. Naylor A, Shentall R: Biochemical aspects of intervertebral discs in aging and disease, in Jayson M (ed): *The Lumbar Spine and Back Pain*, New York, Grune & Stratton Inc, 1976, pp 317–326.

22. Pheasant HC: The problem back. *Curr Pract Orthop Surg* 1977;7:89–115.

23. Pheasant HC: Backache—Its nature, incidence and cost. *West J Med* 1977;126:330–332.

24. Posner I, White AA, Edwards WT, Hayes WC: A biomechanical analysis of the clinical stability of the lumbar and lumbosacral spine. *Spine* 1982;7:374–389.

25. Rockoff SD, Sweet E, Bluestein J: The relative contribution of trabecular and cortical bone to the strength of human lumbar vertebrae. *Calcif Tissue Res* 1969;3:163–175.

26. Rowe ML: Low back pain in industry. A position paper. *J Occup Med* 1969;11:161–169.

27. St. J. Dixon A: Diagnosis of low back pain—Sorting the complainers, in Jayson M (ed): *The Lumbar Spine and Back Pain*, New York, Grune & Stratton, Inc, 1976, pp 77–92.

28. Valkenburg HA, Haanen HCN: The epidemiology of low back pain, in White AA and Gordon SL (eds): *Symposium on Idiopathic Low Back Pain*. St. Louis, C.V. Mosby, 1982, pp 9–82.

29. Van Akkerveeken PF, O'Brien JP, Park WM: Experimentally induced hypermobility in the lumbar spine. *Spine* 1979;4:236–241.

30. Wedge JH: The natural history of spinal degeneration, in Kirkaldy-Willis (ed): *Managing Low Back Pain*. New York, Churchill Livingstone, 1983, pp 3–8.

31. Wood PHN: Epidemiology of back pain, in Jayson M (ed): *The Lumbar Spine and Back Pain*. New York, Grune & Stratton, Inc, 1976, pp 13–27.

Chapter 2

Sciatic Pain

Peter Dyck, *M.D.*

INTRODUCTION

"Es schmerzt aber es tut nicht weh."

A leukotomy patient, 1970

This chapter addresses the topic of sciatic pain. A discussion of specific sources of pain is probably better understood if some of the general principles that govern pain perception are reviewed. Pain is not just another sensory impulse that is governed by a certain neurophysiologic threshold. It is, instead, a complex human reaction that takes into account past experience, ethnic background, and emotional state when interpreting a noxious stimulus.

"Es schmerzt aber es tut nicht weh" (It pains but it does not hurt). This was a statement made by a patient who was dying from terminal malignancy and suffering from disabling pain resulting from metastatic disease of the spine. What the patient meant was that she was consciously aware of the painful stimuli but the psychic torment associated with the stimuli after a frontal leukotomy had been performed was gone. This is not to say there had been a diminution in primary pain perception, but only a salutary modification of its affective elaboration. Such asymbolia for pain is accompanied by a lack of anxiety, depression, and fear, even following unilateral frontal leukotomy. There is also an attendant euphoria, pervaded by an inability to judge the gravity of the situation at hand, which might in part explain the clinical reaction to pain.

Almost all neurosurgical intracranial ablative procedures have endeavored to modify this psychic response to pain, rather than interrupt the primary painful impulse from reaching the somatosensory cortex. It is even more disconcerting to note that, in some instances, topectomy of sensory cortex does not ameliorate pain, although retrograde degeneration occurs in the appropriate sensory thalamic nuclei. Hence, primary cerebralization of pain might actually occur in the thalamus and not the cerebral cortex after all. Thalamic pain lends credence to this hypothesis.

These brief comments should indicate the complexity of the topic before we discuss, in a broader sense, the better known facts that govern perception of pain.

THE SOMATIC AFFERENT SYSTEM

Sensory receptors are generally divided into endings that are encapsulated by non-neuronal tissue and free nerve endings. There is general agreement that free-lying nonmyelinated nerve endings react to noxious stimulation of their receptive fields. Within this group of "nociceptive" afferents are subclasses of nonmyelinated (C) and thinly myelinated (A-delta) afferents that respond to noxious stimulation. Some of these respond to mechanical trauma such as pinching and prodding, others to only noxious heat or cold. In fact, one of the most common of these is the C-polymodal nociceptor. This class of C-fibers is responsive to mechanical, thermal, and chemical stimulations that are noxious.[6,44,56] Then there are afferent fibers, which respond to both innocuous as well as noxious stimuli.

Our interest will be focused primarily on the general somatic afferents that are present in the skin, the muscles, ligaments, joints, and fascia. Then we will follow these exteroceptive and some proprioceptive pathways through the spinal cord to their sensory cortical terminals.

The dorsal root ganglion harbors the perikarya of all somatic (and visceral) afferents. The dorsal root fibers are known to be arranged somatotopically. As a rule, laterally located ganglion cells send their central processes into the rostral aspect of the dorsal root, while those lying medially occupy the caudal region of the dorsal root. The ganglion cells are large and small. The large cells give rise to myelinated fibers, the small dark cells to the unmyelinated afferents. It is also probable that different neurotransmitters are employed.[22]

The dorsal root ganglion is a unipolar cell, which gives off a single process (dendraxon) that divides dichotomously into a central and peripheral branch. The peripheral afferent branch has been discussed above. The central branches enter the spinal cord via the dorsal root, where they comprise part of Lissauer's tract. Within this tract, these nociceptive fibers run rostrocaudal for one to two segments before entering the dorsal horn.

The dorsal gray of the spinal cord is arranged in dorsoventral laminae. Lamina I (marginal layer) has been shown to contain perikarya that synapse primarily with first-order thinly myelinated (A-delta) afferents, although nonmyelinated (C) fibers also terminate here.[27] Laminae II and III comprise the substantia gelatinosa. The cells in this area are small and they serve primarily as terminations for the small (C) afferents.

The neuropil within the substantia gelatinosa manifests a special arrangement, called glomeruli, which may well serve as integrating circuits for afferent input within the dorsal horn.[20,45] Such glomeruli appear microscopically as an outer ring of small diameter fibers (dendrites) and probably axonal endings that encompass a large central axon. Within the glomerulus, an axonal ending of a C-fiber afferent synapses on several different dendrites. Synapses between dendrites and axoaxonic connection probably also exist. It is at this level that inhibition or excitation of interneurons possibly plays a role in the final expression of what we call "pain."

It is known that second-order neurons project axons from the dorsal gray laminae IV, V, and VI to the brain stem reticular formation as well as the thalamus. Traditional teaching says that fibers arising in the substantia gelatinosa (laminae II, III) cross over in the white commissure and ascend within the lateral spinothalamic tract to the ventroposterolateral nucleus of the thalamus. The ventroposteromedial nucleus receives trigeminal somatosensory projections.

From here, to use somewhat simplistic terms, the third-order neuron projects to the postcentral parietal sensory cortex.[24] Electrical stimulation of the primary sensory cortex in man produces well localized sensations of tingling, pressure, heat, and sometimes pain.[31] Yet topectomy of somatosensory cortex results only in lessened sensory discrimination, only occasionally in relief or amelioration of pain followed by hyperpathia in some instances.[61]

Thus we end our journey, which began as a nociferous stimulus to a naked nerve ending, and we arrive at the primary somatosensory cortex; but have we solved the riddle of pain? The answer is *no.*

THE GATE CONTROL THEORY OF PAIN

A "gate control" theory of pain was proposed by Melzak and Wall in 1965.[35] It correlated with Sir Charles Sherrington's notion that "physical pain was not a simple fact of nervous impulses traveling over a nerve at a predetermined gait. It is the resultant of the conflict between the stimulus and the individual."[49] Based on the suggestion that neurons within the substantia gelatinosa could modify the activity of dorsal root afferents by way of presynaptic inhibition, Melzak and Wall proposed a skiagram (Figure 2–1) to explain the neurophysiological events we interpret as pain. This hypothesis postulates a differential effect of thin and thicker somatosensory afferents on the substantia gelatinosa (laminae II and III). Hence, a summation of impulses from both the large (A-delta) and thin (C) fibers activates the transmission (T) cells in lamina IV of the dorsal horn. This begins impulses that are relayed centrally and that culminate as a perception of pain. Thus, excitation in thick afferent somatosensory fibers closes the gate, by inhibition of the neuropil of the substantia gelatinosa, which in turn inhibits the T-cell in lamina IV. The end result is: no pain. In contrast, the unmyelinated (C) fibers facilitate excitation in the substantia gelatinosa and, hence, within the T-cells. This produces pain.

This notion of pain is simple and hence, attractive, but taking into consideration the complexity of the nervous sys-

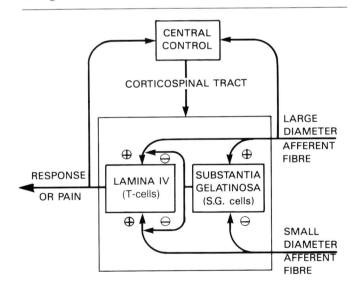

Figure 2–1 The gate control theory (after Melzak and Wall). It is stated that the larger (A-delta) fibers and smaller C-fibers act by summation on the transmitter cells (T-cells) in the dorsal gray. The substantia gelatinosa acts as a modulating gate on the afferent impulses. When the impulses from the large fibers stimulate the substantia gelatinosa, the latter inhibits the T-cell and hence there is a closed gate: no pain, if impulses in small fibers predominate, they inhibit the substantia gelatinosa; it then allows more activity at the T-cell level and the gate is open: pain is the result. *Source:* Reprinted with permission from *Science* (1965;150:971–979), Copyright © 1965, American Association for the Advancement of Science.

tem, even from the standpoint of a neuroanatomic novice, the gate hypothesis of pain is probably not the complete answer. Nathan and Wall also conclude that some of the assumptions made in the gate control theory may well be incorrect.[39,59]

NEUROTRANSMITTERS OF PAIN

A discussion of pain would be incomplete without a brief mention of the neuropeptides, which are believed to have a neurophysiologic effect on perception of pain.[33]

Two types of neuropeptides have been histochemically identified in the small dorsal root ganglion cells.[22] One is substance P, the other is somatostatin. Substance P is also found in both laminae I and II of the dorsal horn; somatostatin is most abundant in lamina II. Deafferentiation of the dorsal horn depletes its substance P stores. Substance P (P for powder) was discovered by Von Euler and Gaddum in 1931.[16] Since then it has been isolated from the sites within the central and peripheral nervous system. Its function is believed to be excitation of fine dorsal root afferents, hence, the fasciculation of pain. Iontophoretic application of substance P to a neuron in the dorsal gray causes protracted depolarization and increased neuronal firing. Could this be the neurophysiologic event that produces hyperpathia? Although somatostatin reduces spontaneous neuronal firing, its exact function appears unclear.

In 1975, Hughes reported isolating a peptide that had properties similar to morphine.[23] Other pentapeptides were soon found in different parts of the brain. They were called enkephalins. Specifically, opiates block contraction of the vas deferens. This biologic test was then used as the benchmark of the extract's purity and function.[52] It was found that the large, 91 amino acid peptide β-lipotropin (LPH) contained many of these opioid peptides, depending on where the chain is broken, beginning with the sixty-first amino acid, tyrosine. Hence, we have methionine-enkephalin (α-LPH 61-65), α-endorphin (β-LPH 61-66), β-endorphin (β-LPH 61-91), and finally γ-endorphin (β-LPH-61-77).[50]

When an enkephalin is applied to a neuron in the rat, it depresses neuronal activity by 70 percent. This is reversed by the application of naloxone, an opiate antagonist.[4] The β-endorphins depress nociceptive units in the spinal cord but other cells are not affected. When β-endorphin is injected into brain parenchyma its analgesic effect is 18 to 33 times more potent than that of morphine.[34] Similarly, intravenous β-endorphin is a better analgesic agent than morphine. When injected into the third ventricle of a cat, β-endorphin was 100 times as potent an analgesic agent as morphine itself.[3] The β-endorphin produces transient analgesia and the γ-endorphin only a seizure discharge. All of these effects could be reversed by intravenous injection of naloxone. Curiously, however, if a second dose of β-endorphin is injected within 72 hours, no analgesia ensues.

It seems clear that the nervous system is capable of producing opioids that play a role in how we handle pain. Yet the last chapter on this topic has by no means been written, because human responses to endorphins fall short of the animal model.

INNERVATION OF THE SPINAL CANAL

In 1932, Jung and Brunschwig reported finding fine nerve fibers in the anterior and posterior longitudinal ligaments of the spinal cord.[25] In 1940, Roofe,[47] employing the Bodian stain[2] demonstrated an abundance of nerve endings within the annulus fibrosus and the posterior longitudinal ligament. He presumed these to be pain fibers. He also dissected out the sinuvertebral nerve of Luschka. Luschka's original description could not be located, but there is general agreement that this recurrent nerve arises from the dorsal root, distal to its sensory ganglion. The nerve then enters the spinal canal in the ventral aspect of the intervertebral foramina to innervate contiguous structures including the common dural sac, the annulus fibrosus, and the posterior longitudinal ligament and blood vessels, possibly also the superior articular facet of the lower vertebra and the periosteum.[42] Thus, an anastamotic network of fibers is created that spans over one to two spinal segments. Plexi of nerve fibers are particularly abundant in the posterior longitudinal ligament, and encapsulated nerve endings have been found in the joint capsule. The ligamentum flavum however, is only sparsely innervated and the nucleus pulposus and vertebral trabecular bone is totally devoid of nerve endings.

The posterior rami of the posterior primary division of the spinal nerve roots innervate the paraspinal muscles, fascia, ligaments, and most of the posterior arthrodial joints and the overlying skin.

CLINICAL PATTERNS OF BACK PAIN

Above, the central relays and the regional peripheral neuroanatomy of pain were reviewed, by no means exhaustively, but hopefully sufficiently enough to allow one to concede the complexity of the topic. Now, some clinical correlates will be discussed.

Francis Murphy relates the case of a soldier who was admitted to a military field hospital complaining of severe low back and leg pain, without neurologic deficits. A myelogram was normal. The patient died of unrelated complications. At autopsy an annular tear was found with a fragment of nucleus wedged into the rend but no evidence of root compression.[37] Since limb pain was such a significant component, Murphy questions whether this is not true referred pain, not unlike angina pectoris in myocardial ischemia.

Possibly much of the groin pain seen associated with L4-5 disc herniation might be similarly explained. Murphy goes on to explain that when operating under local anesthesia, compression of a normal disc causes no pain. If a normal nerve root is manipulated, a slight shock might be experienced but no pain. When a nerve root is traumatized, although it becomes exquisitely sensitive and extremely painful, manipulation causes back, buttock, and leg pain. When the root is infiltrated with procaine, it can be manipulated without discomfort to the patient.

Annular compression of a herniated disc produces deep aching back pain. The pain is midline if the compression is in the middle and lateralized if the compression is to one side. This, too, is reminiscent of referred pain. It is of interest to note that although compression or deformation of these structures causes pain, sharp incision does not. It is believed that most of the pain produced by the ligamentum flavum is due to its mechanical irritation directly on the root rather than stimulation of its own nociceptive nerve endings.

Recent interest in facet joint pain also shows that aside from midlumbar pain, the patient may experience lateralizing pain that can be abolished by facet injection.[32] This has led to a number of deafferentation procedures directed at the facet joints. These procedures have had variable clinical success from the standpoint of pain amelioration. Partially, this may be accounted for by the fact that the sources of pain in disc degeneration are more often than not multifactorial rather than the result of a single cause.[61]

LOW BACK PAIN

Studies show that 90 percent of people experience enough low back pain at some time in their lives to warrant medical attention. Yet most pain is probably musculofascial rather than discogenic in origin. Men are afflicted more often than women and the incidence is highest in middle age.

It is a general illusion that a specific injury precipitates most back pain; yet in more than half of the patients the pain evolves insidiously. In the remainder, a lifting, bending, or twisting episode, be it at work or play, brings on the pain.

Discogenic pain is often accompanied by a dull, aching discomfort, which is frequently more severe on one side. It should be remembered that pain arising from the sacroiliac joint may be quite similar to discogenic pain and is often referred to the ipsilateral buttock and thigh as well.

Muscle spasm, presumably a protective response, may be so disabling that patients cannot bend to brush their teeth or put on their shoes. The epitome of muscle spasm is seen in patients suffering from lumbar discitis. Even sitting down next to them on their bed can cause agony. This pain is a clinical sign not unlike the "railroad track" sign of appendicitis. Analgesics will not control this pain unless it is combined with some form of lumbar immobilization in a corset or cast, even at bed rest.

Straightening of the lumbosacral angle is a consequence of muscle spasm. It is evident enough to allow its clinical grading by severity, normally graded from 1 to 4.

SCIATIC PAIN

The ancient physicians referred to all pain in the region of the hip and back as ischia. In 1764, Cotugno, a young Neapoli-

tan surgeon, divided the ischias into two main types: "ischias arthritica" (hip disease) and "ischias nervosa" (sciatica).[8] The latter were subdivided further into "ischias nervosa postica," with pain radiating down the back of the thigh, and "ischias nervosa antica," with pain radiating down in front. Cotugno attributed the pain to a distention of the neurilemma. His monograph describes the clinical presentation of sciatica but no diagnostic test is proposed.

This period in history was marked by a considerable discourse on the etiology of sciatica. Danforth and Wilson were among the first to believe that sciatica was the result of a root rather than a plexus lesion.[11] Since Mixter and Barr's hallmark paper, the etiology of sciatica is no longer contested.[36] We know that sciatic pain is the end result of radicular trauma, and disc protrusion is the commonest cause for it.

Coughing and sneezing increase intraspinal pressure and aggravate radicular pain. Valsalva maneuver or jugular compression, be it manual or by pressure cuff applied around the neck, also aggravate sciatic pain.[58] Aside from straightening of the lumbosacral angle brought on by muscle spasm, sciatica almost invariably produces scoliosis.

Disc protrusion, lateral to the root, causes medial displacement of the neural structures. To avoid pain, the patient leans away from the lesion. In contrast, if the disc herniation is more medial and it impales the root at the level of the axilla of the root sleeve, the scoliosis is toward the lesion.

Percussion or firm palpation of the midline spine almost invariably aggravates sciatica, and aside from the sharp lancinating pain into the affected dermatome, a deep aching pain is produced in the affected limb.

Sciatic notch tenderness, in fact, along the entire sciatic trunk, is invariably present when a nerve root is traumatized.

NERVE ROOT TRACTION TESTS

A discussion of the literature on the various traction tests is not trivial if one wants to remain historically accurate. The most controversial is Ernest Charles Laségue's contribution to this topic. In 1864, Laségue published a paper in which he reviewed Cotugno's observations and discussed three cases of sciatica.[28] No provocative test is mentioned in the manuscript, yet Oppenheim appears to be the principal offender in this faux pas by stating in a very convincing manner that Laségue described a stretch test. He cites Laségue's 1864 article and mentions De Beurmann's 1884 publication in support.[41] DeBeurmann states expressly that Laségue's 1864 article contained no clinical stretch sign.[12]

In 1881, J.J. Forst presented his doctoral dissertation with Charles Laségue, his mentor, sitting in the front row.[19] In his dissertation, Forst described a test to separate hip from sciatic pain. Figure 2–2, a-d illustrate the components of maneuvers proposed by Forst. Although Laségue was aware of these

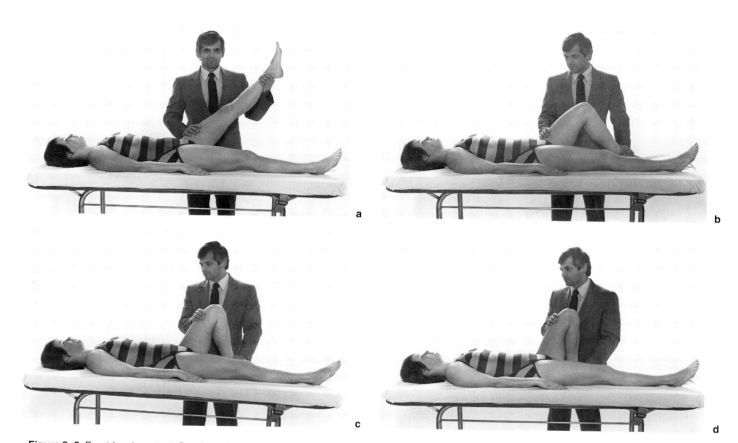

Figure 2–2 Forst-Laségue test. Consists of straight-leg raising and if pain is produced, the knee is flexed, the foot placed on the bed sheet, and the knee and hip flexion is then continued. In hip disease the pain will persist through both maneuvers while in sciatica the pain is abolished at the time of the second phase of the test.

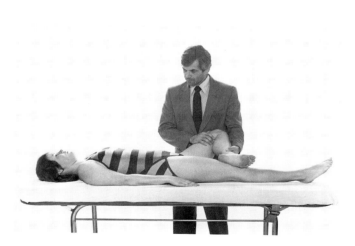

Figure 2–3 Patrick's sign was described by Hugh Patrick. The letters in the acronym, "fabere" refer to motions made by the hip in performance of the test, namely "f" for flexion, "ab" for abduction, "er" for external rotation and "e" for extension.

observations, he did not describe a sciatic stretch sign, but it carries his eponym in endless neurology texts.

Be that as it may, the test described in Forst's thesis, which consists of straight-leg raising followed by knee flexion and continued hip flexion, provides a simple clinical method of separating pain resulting from hip disease from that of sciatica (Figure 2–2).

In present clinical practice, probably the best-known test for hip disease is Patrick's F-AB-E-R-E test. The acronym stands for flexion, abduction, external rotation, and extension of the hip (Figure 2–3), a maneuver often limited and painful in hip disease but seldom seen in patients with sciatica.

Lazar Lazarevic was a Serb, hence, he published in his native tongue his first observations on the role sciatic tension played in the differential diagnosis of sciatica.[29] Four years later, in 1884, he reiterated his observation in German.[30] This is the first available description of the straight-leg raising test as we know it (Figure 2–4, a-b). Cotugno had attributed sciatica to "hydrops of the nerve," and Forst[19] and Laségue[28] to nerve compression by the hamstring muscles. Lazarevic concluded that pain in straight-leg raising was due to sciatic

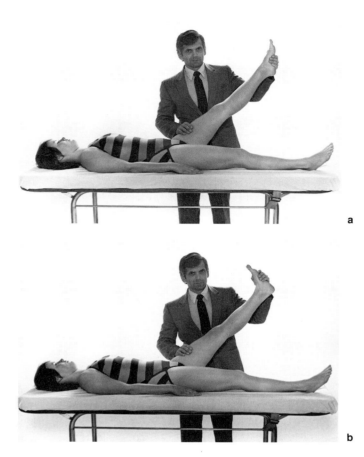

Figure 2–4 Straight-leg raising as originally described by Lazarevic. Passive straight-leg raising followed by dorsiflexion of the foot.

stretch. He supported his clinical observations by anatomic dissection. Therefore, if the test needs an eponym, it might be called the "Lazarevic's sign." He also demonstrated that dorsiflexion of the foot augmented sciatic tension in a cadaver.[30] It should be noted that one of Lasègue's patients described an increase in sciatic pain on active dorsiflexion of the foot.[28]

DeBeurmann corroborated Lazarevic's conclusions by resecting a piece of sciatic nerve and interposing an elastic band, to show that it stretched when the leg was raised.[12]

The straight-leg raising test was modified by Hermann Oppenheim in 1908[41] so it could be performed with a patient sitting instead of lying down. One year later Karl Petrén restated Oppenheim's observations that the straight-leg raising test might be performed with a patient sitting, by simply extending the knee.[43]

Finally, one might mention another commonly used provocative maneuver to elicit sciatic pain. It is commonly known as the "Cram test"[9] (Figure 2–5, a-b). With the patient lying supine, the painful limb is raised with the knee only partially extended. Compression of the sciatic trunk in the popliteal space produces or augments radicular pain in patients with sciatica. It is interesting to note that this identical maneuver was described by Gower in 1902 in his classic text *Diseases of the Nervous System*.

Internal rotation during straight-leg raising is also provocative of sciatic pain, as observed by Deutsch in 1924[13] and reaffirmed by Breig and Troup in 1978.[5]

Irrespective of how the straight-leg raising test is carried out, sciatic tension produces, at first, a deep aching pain in the affected limb, which begins in the buttocks and radiates down the leg. Where severe root compression exists, lancinating pain may shoot into the affected dermatome followed by an increased sensory disturbance. Protective paraspinal muscle spasm then triggers back pain.

A discussion of sciatic traction tests would be incomplete without mention of what Woodhall called the well-leg raising test of Fajerszajn.[62] Fajerszajn, in 1981, observed that when the painless leg in a patient with unilateral sciatica is raised, it

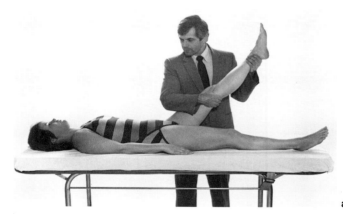

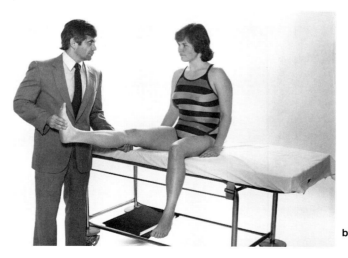

Figure 2–5 The Cram test is also known as the bow-string sign. With the leg slightly elevated, be it seated or supine, the sciatic nerve trunk in the popliteal space is briskly compressed or strung. This causes neuritic pain in the presence of sciatica.

is followed by increased pain in the contralateral limb. Wood-hall supported his historic observations with anatomic dissection. This test is also known as the "crossed-leg" sign. It has a high correlation with large central disc protrusions that impale on the root in its axilla.

Since about 80 percent of all disc protrusions occur at L4–5 or L5–S1, it is not surprising that most nerve tension tests have dealt with production of traction on the sciatic nerve and, hence, its principal components, the L5 and/or S1 nerve roots. Yet, as far back as 1764, Cotugno recognized that not all "ischiade nervosa" radiated to the back of the thigh and then into the leg; in some instances, the pain extended down the front of the thigh.[8] In 1918, Wassermann described femoral nerve trunk tenderness when the L3 or L4 nerve roots were involved in an irritative process.[60] He also observed that by placing a patient prone and flexing the knees, pain was increased. Nachlas described this identical maneuver and proposed it as a stress test of the lumbosacral and the sacroiliac joints 18 years later, in 1936.[38]

There is ample anatomic data to support the premise that traction on the femoral nerve causes increased tension on the third and fourth lumbar nerve roots. Production of such radicular tension on the upper lumbar nerve roots is the basis of the femoral nerve traction test.[14] The patient lies on his painless side with the lower limb flexed at both hip and knee joints in order to stabilize the trunk. The head is flexed slightly to increase tension on the cauda equina. In the first maneuver, the uppermost (painful) limb then is passively extended at the hip but short of provoking lumbar spine extension. As a second maneuver, the knee is then progressively flexed to increase femoral nerve tension by stretching the quadriceps femoris muscle (Figure 2–6, a-b). Depending upon the severity of the radicular irritation, pain that radiates down the front of the thigh may be brought on initially, or only after the second maneuver is performed. When the L3 root is involved, the pain stops at the knee; where an L4 radiculopathy is present, it extends to the midtibial area of the leg. Femoral nerve trunk tenderness is a frequent concomitant finding.

Once again, in the presence of unilateral disc extrusion or large central protrusions with compression of a root at its root sleeve axilla, a "crossed-leg" phenomenon may be seen similar to that described by Fajerszajn during straight-leg raising of the painless contralateral leg in the presence of sciatica.

THE PATELLAR AND ACHILLES REFLEXES

According to Helweg, the first reported association of sciatica and an absent ankle jerk was described by Sternberg in 1893.[21] In time, this observation became widely accepted, but its occurrence and its segmental level of involvement continued to produce a great deal of dialogue even into the first half of this century.

In 1940, Love and Walsh reported a depressed or absent ankle jerk in 60 percent of their cases.[34] Barr and Mixter cited 70 percent.[1] Dandy believed that a diminished Achilles reflex was brought on by disc protrusion at L4–5.[10] Spurling and Grantham incriminated the level below.[54] As we now know, it is Spurling's observations that have stood the test of time. An elegant review of this topic is offered in Norlén's monograph on sciatica.[40] In Norlén's series, the ankle jerk was absent in one-third of his cases of disc protrusion at L5–S1.

Since this work in the 1940s, numerous reports have appeared supporting the clinical observation that the Achilles reflex is suppressed or abolished by an S1 root lesion, but it must be remembered that the S1 root might be injured at the L4–5 level, if disc herniation is extensive.

Testing for reflexes requires a patient who is cooperative and relaxed. When a reflex is hypoactive, it may be enhanced by the Jendrassik maneuver or, in the case of the ankle jerk, by having the patient kneel on a chair.

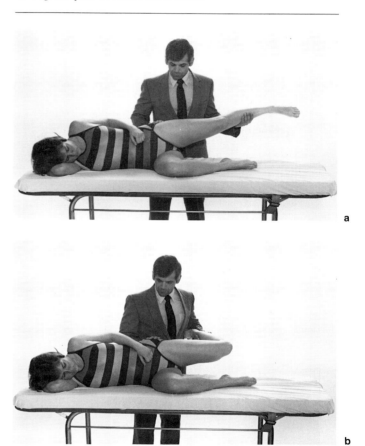

a

b

Figure 2–6 The femoral nerve traction test has two components. With the patient lying on the well side, the hip is first extended, thus creating tension in the ileopsoas and hence traction on the upper lumbar nerve roots. The second maneuver adds tension on the femoral nerve and hence its component roots. In the presence of an L3 radiculitis, pain radiates down the medial thigh to the knee. When the L4 root is involved, the pain is more anterior on the thigh and extends to the midtibial portion of the leg.

It should also be remembered that if one encounters an absent ankle jerk and a settled disc space in a patient with acute sciatica, these findings may be a residue of a previous problem and the current symptoms are due to disease at the lumbar segment above.

It is generally accepted that the reflex arc of the knee jerk runs primarily through the third and fourth lumbar nerve roots.[13,18,26]

Von Reis' observations in a case report shed some interesting light on this topic.[46] At operation under local anesthesia, both the L4 and L5 roots were exposed at L4–5. A disc protrusion, compressing primarily the L4 root, was found. Manipulation of the L5 root caused pain in the posterior thigh, but did not abolish the patient's limb pain. The root was blocked but the discomfort persisted. Then the L4 root was blocked with novocaine and the pain disappeared. A dorsal rhizotomy was performed. Postoperatively, the patellar reflex was absent. Although Foerster had also performed rhizotomies in spastic patients, this is the most graphic depiction of the role the L4 root plays in relation to the patellar reflex.

Norlén sectioned the dorsal roots of L4 in 10 cases; in five cases the knee jerk was abolished; in the remainder it persisted. In six cases both the dorsal roots of L3 and L4 were cut; the patellar reflex was abolished in all.[40] This suggests that the reflex arc may reside in L4 alone or be carried in both the L3 and L4 root pathways. There is clinical support for this theory in that L4 root compression is frequently associated with an abnormal knee jerk, but it should not be considered pathognomonic of it. An L2–3 disc can also diminish this reflex, although it can seldom abolish it.

Finally, we might note that though neither of the above reflexes are generally associated with an L5 root lesion, there is a reflex abnormality for it. It is the posterior tibial tendon reflex. The problem with this reflex is that great difficulty might be encountered in eliciting it under normal circumstances; hence, it has never reached popular acclaim.

In conclusion, it might be said that the ankle jerk reflects injury to the S1 root; the knee reflects injury to L4 and probably L3 in some cases.

SENSORY DISTURBANCES

Rousset, in 1804, appears to have been the first to describe sensory disturbance in sciatica;[48] but it appears that various peripheral nerves were usually incriminated.[21] In 1931, Stenström demonstrated dermatomal abnormalities in 26 of 110 patients.[55] Many other reports followed, but it was Spurling and Bradford who emphasized that the type of sensory disturbance present is an accurate clue to the level of disc herniation.[53]

The problem arises when we try to match the sensory dysfunction of root lesions to the various dermatome charts. Generally speaking, Foerster's dermatome charts seem to fit

best[17,18] in that the dorsum of the foot falls into the L5 dermatome, and the small toes and lateral ankle are innervated by S1; L4 innervates the anteromedial leg to the ankle and L3 the anteromedial thigh to just below the knee.

Norlén found that section of the fifth lumbar root produced numbness in the dorsum of the foot and great toe. Section of the fourth lumbar root brought with it hypalgesia on the inner anterior side of the lower leg and also down the medial side of the foot. When the S1 root is cut, numbness is produced on the lateral side of the foot, especially the little toe.[40] Section of the S1 or the L4 roots never produced sensory disturbance in the great toe or the contiguous dorsum of the foot.

It should be noted that the subjective hypalgesia is often greater than the actual hypalgesia and that one must concede that there is probably a great deal of overlap between dermatomes. Hence, an area of sensory disturbance may decrease in time. A single root lesion may not involve an entire dermatome, but its distal involvement has more precise localizing value, neuroanatomically speaking. Keegan, whose dermatome chart clashes with much clinical observation and investigation, believes that distal segmentation is more discrete because there is less dermatomal overlapping.[26]

In conclusion, sensory disturbance below the knee, but not in the great toe, probably incriminates the L4 root. Hypalgesia of the great toe is an L5 root lesion. Numbness on the outside of the foot, and especially the little toe, signals S1 involvements. The more proximal sensory disturbances would fit better into a Keegan than a Foerster dermatome, in that S1 root lesions often show hypalgesia on the posterior thigh and the L5 root lesion manifests this abnormality more anterolaterally.

A sensory examination is as good as the clinician's perspicacity in assessing the available facts.

MOTOR DEFICITS

Vallaix observed atrophy in the limb musculature of patients with sciatica. He attributed the atrophy to disuse.[57] Similarly, Cotugno was aware of atrophy.[8] He attributed it to perineural edema (hydrops). In 1864, exactly one century after Cotugno's observations, Laségue also mentions that some sciatica is followed by atrophy, which he proposed be called "sciatique grave," and if there was no atrophy, "sciatique benigne."[28] It was not until the twentieth century that endeavors were made to sort out the motor deficits into dysfunctions of specific myotomes. In 1942, Sjöqvist reported dorsiflexion weakness of the foot and great toe in L4–5 disc protrusion.[51] Norlén's data supported the contention that a foot drop was, for all practical purposes, the end result of an L4–5 disc protrusion.[40]

Looking at this topic from a current perspective, there is general agreement that specific roots innervate designated motor groups or myotomes. The problem arises in that each specific muscle has a myotomic overlap not unlike cutaneous sensation. Hence, from a clinical standpoint, some general ground rules are in order. Hip flexion weakness is most likely an L4 root lesion. Leg extension invokes quadriceps femoris function; weakness in this muscle suggests an L4 root lesion. The extensor hallucis longus muscle is innervated by three myotomes, but clinically paresis in great toe extension should suggest an L5 root lesion until proven otherwise. Dorsiflexion of the remaining toes of the foot is less specific. Plantar flexion of the foot and toes is a function of the S1 myotome and, particularly when coupled with inversion weakness, suggests an S1 root lesion. This is not to say that the L5 dermatome does not contribute, but its contribution would have been attended by a foot drop and dorsiflexion weakness of the great toe.

When severe motor deficits are prolonged, atrophy ensues. Atrophy can be recorded by comparative circumferential measurements of the calves and thighs.

Finally, there are probably anatomic variations in sensorimotor innervation of the limbs. Hence, as for the pre- and postfixed optic chiasm, Eisler has proposed that pre- and postfixation of the cauda equina also occurs.[15] This approach has particular merit when lumbosacral anomalies are present, but it should not detract from common everyday clinical observation.

CONCLUSION

The purpose of this chapter has been to take the reader along a path that shows the complexity that underlies a full understanding of pain, even if it limits itself to a discussion of sciatica. Most readers of this text are seasoned clinicians; hence, a historical perspective is justified. Yet latitude in conclusion and deductions is inevitable since there are no absolutes when dealing with a neuroanatomic substrate that has no absolutes. Pain remains a clinical enigma.

REFERENCES

1. Barr JS, Mixter WJ: Posterior protrusion of lumbar intervertebral discs. *J Bone Joint Surg* 1941;23:444–456.

2. Bodian D: A new method for staining nerve fibers and nerve endings in mounted paraffin sections. *Anat Rec* 1936;65:89–97.

3. Bradbury AF, Feldberg WF, Smyth DG, Snell CR: Lipotropin C-fragment: an endogenous peptide with potent analgesic activity, in Kosterlitz HW (ed): *Opiates and Endogenous Opioid Peptides.* Amsterdam, North Holland Publishing Co, 1976, pp 9–17.

4. Bradley PB, Briggs L, Gayton RJ, Lambert LA: Effects of microiontophoretically applied methionine-enkephalin on single neurons in the rat brain stem. *Nature* 1976;261:425–426.

5. Breig A, Troup JDG: Biomechanic considerations in the straight-leg raising test: Cadaveric and clinical studies of the effects of medial rotation of the hip. Personal Communication, June 1978.

6. Bradal A: *Neurological Anatomy, In Relation to Clinical Medicine,* ed 3. NY, Oxford Univ Press, 1981, pp 46–55.

7. Chusid JG: *Correlative Neuroanatomy and Functional Neurology,* ed 17. Los Altos, Lange, 1979.

8. Cotugno D: *De Ischiade Nervosa, Commentarios,* Napoli, Apud Frat, Simonios, 1764.

9. Cram RH: A sign of nerve root pressure. *J Bone Joint Surg* 1953;35–B:192–195.

10. Dandy WE: Concealed ruptured intervertebral discs. *JAMA* 1941; 117:821–823.

11. Danforth MS, Wilson PD: The anatomy of the lumbosacral region in relation to sciatic pain. *J Bone Joint Surg* 1925;23:109–160.

12. DeBeurmann: Note sur un signe peu connu de la sciatique. Reserches experimentales. *Arch de Physiol, norm et pathol* 1984;16:375–380.

13. Deutsch F: *Neurologie and Neuritis; Specielle Pathologie und Therapie.* Band I: Nervenkrankheiten, Alexander W (ed). Berlin, Urban und Schwarzenberg, 1924, pp 341–608.

14. Dyck P: The femoral nerve traction test in lumbar disc protrusion. *Surg Neurol* 1976;6:163–166.

15. Eisler P: Der Plexus Lumbosacralis des Menschen. *Abh d narufor-schenden Gesellsch z Halle* 1982;17:279–364.

16. Euler (von) US, Gaddum JH: An unidentified depressor substance in certain tissue extracts. *J Physiol* (London) 1931;72:74–87.

17. Foerster O: Zur Kemtnis der spinalen Segment-innervation der Muskeln. *Neurol* 1913;261:32:1202–1214.

18. Foerster O: Symptomatologie der Erkrankungen des Rückenmarks und seine Wurzeln, in Bumke, Foerster (eds): *Handbuch des Neurologie.* 1936; 2:1–403.

19. Forst JJ: *Contribution a l'etude clinique de la sciatique.* Paris, These 33, 1881.

20. Goebel S: Synaptic organization of the substantia gelatinosa glomeruli in the spinal trigeminal nucleus of the adult cat. *J Neurocytol* 1974;3: 219–243.

21. Helweg J: *Ischias, en clinik studie.* Koebenhavn, Henrik Koppel, 1920, p 272.

22. Hökfelt T, Elde R, Johansson O, Luft R, Nielsson G, Arimera A: Immunohistochemical evidence for separate populations of somatostatin containing and P-substance containing afferent neurons in the rat. *Neuroscience* 1976;1:131–136.

23. Hughes J: Isolation of an endogenous compound from the brain with pharmacological properties similar to Morphine. *Brain Res* 1975;88: 295–308.

24. Jones EG, Powell TPS: Connections of the somatic sensory cortex of the rhesus monkey: Thalamic connections (III). *Brain* 1970;93:37–46.

25. Jung A, Brunschwig A: Researches histologiques sur l'innervation des articulations des corps vertebraux. *Presse Med* 1932;40:316–317.

26. Keegan JJ: Dermatome hypalgesia associated with herniation of intervertebral disc. *Arch Neurol Psychiat* 1943;50:67–83.

27. La Motte C: Distribution of the tract of Lissauer and the dorsal root fibers in the primate spinal cord. *J Comp Neurol* 1977;172:229–261.

28. Laségue EC: Consideration aure la sciatique. *Arch Gen de Med* 1864; 6:558–580.

29. Lazarevic LK: Ischias postica Cotunni. *Sypski Arch* 1980;7:23.

30. Lazarevic LK: Ischias postien Cotunni. Ein Beitrag zu deren Differential-Diagnose. *Allg Wien Med Ztg* 1884;29:425–429.

31. Libet B: Electrical stimulation of cortex in human subjects and conscious sensory aspects, in A Iggo (ed): *Handbook of Sensory Physiology.* NY, Springer-Verlag, 1973, vol II. *Somatosensory System,* pp 743–790.

32. Lippill AB: The facet joint and its role in spine pain. Management with facet injections. *Spine* 1984;9:746–750.

33. Loh HH, Tseng LF, Wei E, Lich SE: Endorphin is a potent analgesic agent. *Proc Natl Acad Sc USA* 1976;73:2895–2898.

34. Love JG, Walsh MN: Intraspinal protrusions of intervertebral discs. *Arch Surg* 1940;40:454–484.

35. Melzak R, Wall PD: Pain mechanisms; A new theory. *Science* 1965; 150:971–979.

36. Mixter WJ, Barr JS: Rupture of the intervertebral disc with involvement of the spinal canal. *New Engl J Med* 1934;211:210–215.

37. Murphy F: Experience with lumbar disc surgery. *Clin Neurosurg* 1973; 20:1–8.

38. Nachlas W: The knee flexion test for pathology in the lumbosacral and sacroiliac joint. *J Bone Joint Surg* 1936;18:724–725.

39. Nathan PW: The gate control theory of pain, A critical review. *Brain* 1976;99:123–158.

40. Norlén G: On the value of the neurological symptoms in sciatica for the localization of a lumbar disc herniation, *Acta Chir Scand XCI* 1944; (suppl 96):1–96.

41. Oppenheim H: *Textbook of Nervous Diseases*, ed 3. Bruce A (trans). London, TN Foulis, 1911, vol I, p 583.

42. Pederson HE, Blunk CFV, Gardner E: The anatomy of the lumbosacral posterior rami and meningeal branches of the spinal nerves (sinuvertebral nerves). *J Bone Joint Surg* 1956;38A:377–391.

43. Petrén K: Remarks on sciatica and morbis coxal senilis. *Rev Neurol Psychiatr* 1909;7:305–345.

44. Price DD, Dubner R: Neurons that subserve the sensory discriminative aspects of pain. *Pain* 1977;3:3–2–338.

45. Rallston HG (III): The organization of substantia gelatinosa Rolundi in the cat lumbosacral spinal cord. *Z Zellforsch* 1965;67:1–23.

46. Von Reis G: Om smärttillstand inom IV lumbalrotens om räde. *Nord Med* 1944;21:344–346.

47. Roofe PG: Innervation of annulus fibrosus and posterior longitudinal ligament, fourth and fifth lumbar level. *Arch Neurol Psychiat* 1940;rr: 100–103.

48. Rousset: quoted by Norlen (Ref. 40).

49. Sherrington C: Cited by Nashold BS, in *Clinical Neurosurgery*. Baltimore, Williams & Wilkins Co, 1974, vol 21, p 311.

50. Simon EJ: Current concepts on pain and analgesia. 1977;4:1.

51. Sjöqvist O. De lumbala disk bräckens klinik, diagnos samt extipation utan laminectomi. *Nord Med* 1942;13:687–690.

52. Smith TW, Hughes J, Kusterlitz HW, Sosa RP: Enkephalins: isolation, distribution and function, in Kosterlitz HW (ed): *Opiates and Endogenous Opioid Peptides*. Amsterdam, North Holland Press, 1976, pp 57–62.

53. Spurling GR, Bradford FK: Neurologic aspects of herniated nucleus pulposus at fourth and fifth lumbar interspace. *JAMA* 1939;113:2019–2022.

54. Spurling GR, Grantham EG: Neurologic picture of herniations of nucleus pulposus in lower parts of lumbar regions. *Arch Surg* 1940;40: 375–388.

55. Stenström T: Eine klinische Studie über Neuritis—Symptome bei Ischias. *Acta Psychiatr et Neurol* 1931;6:593–644.

56. Tobejörk HE: Afferent C-units responding to mechanical, thermal and chemical stimuli in human non-glabrous skin. *Act Physiol Scand* 1974;92: 374–390.

57. Vallaix FLI: *Traite des neuralgies*. Paris, JB Baillere, 1841, pp 480–647.

58. Viets HR: Two new signs suggestive of cauda equina tumor: root pain on jugular compression and shifting of the lipoidal shadow on change in posture. *N Engl J Med* 1928;198:671–674.

59. Wall PD: The gate control theory of pain mechanisms; a re-examination and restatement. *Brain* 1978;101:1–18.

60. Wassermann S: Ueber ein neues Schenkel-nervsymptom nebst Bemerkung auf Diagnostik der Schenkelnerver krankung. *Dtsch Zschft Nervenhk* 1918;63:140–143.

61. White JC, Sweet WH: *Pain and the Neurosurgeon: A Forty Year Experience*. Springfield, Ill, Charles C Thomas Publisher, 1969.

62. Woodhall B, Hayes GJ: The well-leg-raising test of Fajerszajn in the diagnosis of ruptured lumbar intervertebral disc, *J Bone Joint Surg* 1980; 32A:786–792.

Chapter 3

Neurogenic Claudication

Peter Dyck , M.D.

INTRODUCTION

The purpose of these introductory comments is to familiarize the reader with the nosologic diversity by which neurogenic claudication is addressed. A sufficient body of literature exists to have made this neurologic syndrome a well-known clinical fact some time ago. Yet, that has not been the case. In part this is due to the endless titles the syndrome holds. Following is a review of some of the titles to help the reader understand the problem.

The word "claudication" is derived from the Latin *claudicatio* meaning to limp and be lame. Bouley, in 1831, noted that trotting carriage horses would limp, then stop, but after a short interval were able to trot again.[8] At autopsy, it was discovered that these horses had suffered from obliterative disease of their hind-limb vessels. The term "intermittent claudication" was thus introduced into medical jargon for the first time.

In 1858, the eminent Parisian physician, Jean Martin Charcot, observed what Bouley had described in carriage horses (Figure 3–1). As chief of the "clinique á la Charité," Charcot was presented with the case of a 54-year-old French legionnaire. While on duty in Africa, the legionnaire had sustained a missile injury to one lower quadrant and flank. In time he developed pain and weakness in the leg on the injured side whenever he walked. Yet strength would return and the pain abate after a short period of rest. Activity brought it on again. This pain-rest-relief cycle had a fairly constant distance range, and hence, was predictably reproducible.

The patient became progressively more anemic and one day lost consciousness and died. At autopsy, a traumatic aneurysm of the common iliac artery was found. It had eroded into the

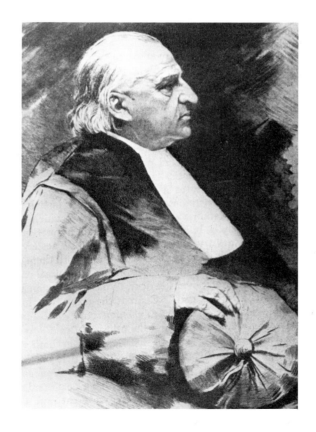

Figure 3–1 Jean Martin Charcot (1825–1893). He was born the son of a carriage builder and became a giant of medicine in the 19th century. Aside from his major contributions in neurology, he also discovered intermittent claudication in man. *Source:* Portrait, courtesy of Dr. Maurice Genty, Académie de Médecine, Paris, France.

intestinal tract, producing massive hematemesis. Distal to the aneurysm, the vessel was completely occluded. This is the first description of intermittent claudication in man.[10] If muscle ischemia could produce limping and pain, why not vascular insufficiency of the neural structures that innervate the limb?

Pursuant with this line of reasoning, Joseph Jules Déjèrine, in 1911, introduced the concept of intermittent spinal claudication.[13] He described three cases in which activity was followed by limb weakness and appearance of pyramidal signs. These deficits disappeared with rest. Although the underlying disease was probably syphilis, spinal cord ischemia was believed to be the cause of the exercise-related weakness.

In 1950, Bergmark addressed this topic once again by reporting an additional two cases.[6] His second case was that of a 76-year-old woman who noted a "bursting sensation" while trying to move a heavy cupboard. Her legs became instantly paralyzed and she fell to her knees. Propelled by her arms, she got into bed. Several days later leg strength improved but was never quite normal. Six months later she could walk 200 meters before the legs would fail her. Yet after a short period of rest, she was able to walk once again. One sad day, paraplegia ensued from which she never recovered and she soon died. At autopsy it was observed that:

> there was a softened area in the lumbar part of the spinal cord caused by a transverse lesion. The anterior fibers were totally demyelinated. The anterior horn was destroyed.

This is the only known autopsy verification of "spinal claudication." One concludes that Déjèrine had established the neurologic entity and had proven it by neuropathologic examination. This spawned speculation about the existence of "claudication" of the pons, mesencephalon, and cerebral cortex, among others. Hermann Oppenheim denied ever seeing such a case.

Yet the notion of spinal cord ischemia was widely accepted, hence, it was logical for Blau and Logue, in 1961, to introduce the term "intermittent claudication of the cauda equina."[7] Because walking brought on pain in their patients and standing abolished it, they reasoned that it was caudal ischemia rather than mechanical compression that brought on the symptoms. They reasoned that Déjèrine had discovered ischemia of the spinal cord; they applied it to the cauda equina, not unlike what Bergmark had done in 1950.[6]

In 1964, Evans added an additional four cases but entitled them "neurogenic intermittent claudication."[29] Supporting the notion of caudal ischemia causing pain as proposed by Blau and Logue, Evans devised a foot ergometer to measure the amount of exercise done. This device was employed in only one case of four.

Although it is doubtful that under normal circumstances spinal cord ischemia can be induced, under extraordinary conditions it certainly can. This was well documented by

Kendall and Andrew, where coarctation of the aorta produced a hemodynamic "steal" with adverse effects on the spinal cord blood supply.[40] Kendall and Andrew's case is that of an 11-year-old boy who experienced leg weakness whenever he exercised. Repair of the coarctation and diversion of the main collateral vessels from the anterior spinal artery relieved the extremity weakness brought on by the "steal-induced" spinal cord ischemia. A Brown-Séquard syndrome, based on similar hemodynamics, has also been reported in a patient with aortic coarctation.[36] However, it should be underlined that in all these instances it was neurologic dysfunction, not pain, that heralded attention. This is quite different from caudal compression, where pain is the overriding complaint.

Cooke and Lehmann chose the title "neurogenic intermittent claudication," thus veering away somewhat from an endorsement of a neural ischemic hypothesis.[11] Looking at it from an even more mechanical pathophysiologic perspective, the title "intermittent ischemia of the cauda equina due to stenosis of the lumbar spine" has been proposed. Yamada et al chose "intermittent cauda equina compression due to narrow spinal canal" to describe their five cases.[70] They differed very little from those of Joffe, Appleby, and Arjona, who titled it "claudication caused by compression of the cauda equina."[38]

To throw a further monkey wrench into this nosologic jungle, Kavanaugh et al coined the term "pseudoclaudication."[39] It was based on the premise that if true claudication produced limping because of muscle ischemia, lameness for other reasons should be a "pseudo-form" of the major clinical entity, intermittent claudication.

Most orthopedists refer to neurogenic claudication as simply "spinal stenosis."[4,32,35,49,65,68]

In 1977, I had proposed the title "intermittent cauda equina compression syndromes" so as to encompass all etiologic aspects of caudal compression.[17] Since this title is unwieldy and long, it would promote better understanding of this syndrome if it were known as "neurogenic claudication." This by no means simplifies the issue, but from a clinical standpoint at least, it is concise and more accurate than "spinal stenosis," which is a neuroradiologic term.

Finally, if this disorder is ever in need of a name, it might be justifiably called "Verbiest's disease" (Figure 3–2).

HISTORICAL DATA

"Neurogenic claudication" will be the term applied to the disorders discussed here. They all have common symptoms and signs that are produced by intermittent cauda equina compression. Such compression may affect all the caudal roots or manifest itself as specific root lesions.

William A. Lane was probably the first to relate this clinical entity in 1893.[42] He described a 34-year-old woman who became progressively paraparetic. His operative report describes an instance of degenerative lumbar vertebral subluxation, com-

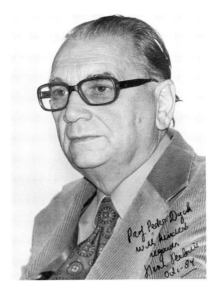

Figure 3–2 Prof. Henk Verbiest. Chairman of the Department of Neurosurgery, Academic Hospital, University of Utrecht, Holland. The father of neurogenic claudication.

monly referred to as "pseudospondylolisthesis," which in this case produced caudal compression, as it so often does.

In 1900, Sach's and Fraenkel's Case 3 may be the next historical link.[53] A 48-year-old tailor developed progressive lower limb weakness over a period of two and a half years. This weakness was associated with pain on lumbar extension. The patient was operated on by Dr. Arpad Gerster of New York, an eminent surgeon in his time. To his chagrin, no tumor was encountered but only "unusual thickness of the laminae." Postoperatively, the patient improved. The authors believed they were dealing with a case of Marie-Strümpell spondylitis rather than lumbar spondylosis.

In 1911, Bailey and Casamajor presented five cases with neurologic symptoms that they attributed to lumbar and lower thoracic degenerative disease of the spine.[5] In two instances, a thoracolumbar decompressive laminectomy was performed by Elsberg. Both patients improved. Degenerative changes and bony thickening was the principal finding in each case, but this was not emphasized by the authors as the etiologic cause of neurogenic claudication in the patients they described.

Probably more important than Bailey and Casamajor's paper was the publication of Goldthwait's case report in the same year.[34] It was prompted as a result of

> an experience . . . with the treatment of a patient with a spinal lesion [that] was so disastrous to the patient and so distressing to the writer that a series of investigations were started in the hope of bringing some relief to the patient and at the same time of preventing such happenings in the future.

The case is that of a 39-year-old man who was treated for a slipped sacroiliac joint. As part of treatment the spine was hyperextended and then held in place by a plaster of Paris jacket. As the cast was applied, there was sharp limb pain followed by numbness in both legs. Several moments later all sensation was lost in the legs; this was followed shortly by paraplegia and loss of sphincter control. The patient was returned to the ward. When he was log-rolled on his left side, neurologic function returned; yet during the night when the patient rolled on his back the paraplegia returned. By next morning he was paraplegic. Intense saddle pain was present. After six weeks of deliberation, Dr. Harvey Cushing performed a decompressive laminectomy of the entire lumbar spinal canal but found no neoplasm or hemorrhage. A grossly normal cauda equina was encountered. Yet the patient improved in time and became ambulant with a cane in eight months. Cushing had mentioned that the spinal canal at the lumbosacral junction was narrowed. Goldthwait concluded that this arthrosis may have been sufficient enough to cause paraplegia in this case. He also mentioned, in passing, that disc protrusion could play a role in the production of neurologic deficits.

This case is presented in some detail because it vividly illustrates the relationship of lumbar extension to caudal compression.

In 1913, Elsberg joined with Kennedy of the New York Neurological Institute to publish, once again, on the "peculiar and undescribed disease of cauda equina."[41] The common denominator was progressive neurologic deficits attended by limb pain that was relieved by lumbar laminectomy, although no apparent cause was found. At lumbar puncture no manometric block was encountered, and the spinal fluid protein was within normal limits. In his monograph on spinal tumors, Elsberg mentions again the similarity of this clinical presentation with that of intraspinal neoplasm.[25] In time, Elsberg microscopically examined the caudal roots in this disorder but found only inflammatory changes.[24]

By 1916, Elsberg refers to a nonsyphilitic neuritis of the cauda equina that was treated by intradural exploration and by application of mercuric bichloride to the caudal roots.[25] Once again he makes passing mention of lumbar spondylosis as it relates to neurologic dysfunction.

In 1925, Parker and Adson from the Mayo Clinic contributed to the dialogue of spinal cord and caudal compression in their report of eight cases. Case 3 presented with longstanding intermittent left lower limb pain and weakness. At operation (T12–L5), only an edematous cauda and conus medullaris were found after removal of laminae that "were three times as thick as normal."[50] Two years later Putti observed that sciatica, in many instances, was due to arthritic changes of the lumbar spine, particularly of the facet joints, thus accounting for the radicular symptoms.[52] Although Towne and Reichert, in 1931, attributed the cauda equina lesions with myelographic blocks at L2 and the next at L4 to hypertrophy of the ligamentum flavum, they were probably dealing with congenital spinal canal stenosis with superimposed degenerative changes. In both instances, the patient improved after decompressive laminectomy and excision of the intervening ligamentum flavum.

In 1934, Fritz Cramer, also of the New York Neurological Institute, reviewed Elsberg's cases, which had been labeled as the "peculiar disease" or later idiopathic "cauda equina radiculitis."[12] There were 26 cases in the group; 15 were operated, 11 were treated conservatively. In those that were operated, congested caudal roots were found. In all instances where arthritic changes were prominent, neurologic recovery followed decompression.

With the introduction of lumbar disc protrusion as a clinical entity by Mixter and Barr in 1934, all other diagnostic options for sciatica were put on a shelf for a decade or so.[46] The surgical preoccupation centered instead on how best to remove a disc.[43,44]

In 1954, Sir Russell Brain outlined the challenge to the medical community with regard to the known and unknown facts about spinal stenosis by saying:[9]

> Our problem then is to correlate the patient's symptoms and signs both with the radiological appearance of the affected portion of the spine and with the pathological changes responsible for the symptoms.

Henk Verbiest, professor of neurosurgery at Utrecht, Netherlands, has dedicated a significant portion of his professional life to the elucidation of the relationship between lumbar arthrosis and the neurologic manifestations it produced.[62,64] In 1949 he described three instances of lumbar spinal stenosis whose symptoms were relieved by lumbar decompressive laminectomy.[58] Impressed with the fact that a congenitally shallow canal can produce neurologic symptoms, he devised calipers to measure its dimensions.[59,60,61] These were later compared with normal values obtained by Huizinga, Heiden, and Vinken.[37]

There is only one article published by Verbiest in American neurosurgical literature. It appeared in 1973 at special request.[63] The remainder of his contributions have appeared in the orthopedic literature.[60,61] Verbiest's two English-language papers were rejected by the editorial board of an American neurosurgical journal on the grounds that congenital lumbar canal narrowing was clinically unimportant. The British neurosurgical editors have made the same faux pas. Yet these same papers established Henk Verbiest as the father of neurogenic claudication, though ironically they appeared in the orthopedic literature.

Thereafter, a number of reports appeared that dealt with neurogenic claudication.[54,56,70] Some of these reports will be discussed in other contexts in this chapter.

What Verbiest was unable to do was accomplished by George Ehni; he published most of his observations in neurological literature[19,20,23,47] and elsewhere.[18,21,22] Aside from what now may be accepted as a known fact, Ehni contributed several singularly important observations. In

1970, Ehni, Moiel, and Bragg described the so-called "redundant" or knotted nerve root, not as a sign of an arteriovenous malformation of the cauda equina, but rather a simple kinking of its roots by a narrowed spondylotic spine.[23]

Even more important is Wilson and Ehni's contribution of the potential detriment of lumbar extension at time of surgery.[69] The report deals with six cases. In four of these six cases, previously undescribed spondylotic caudal radiculopathy produced by lumbar lordosis prompted neurologic dysfunction. In all instances, some neurologic improvement ensued after appropriate lumbar decompression.

In America, Ehni remains the preeminent contributor to this field as of this date (Figure 3–3).

PATHOPHYSIOLOGY OF CAUDA EQUINA PAIN

Supported by a large body of literature, one can safely say that lumbar radicular pain is either produced by ischemia or mechanical compression of caudal nerve roots. In order to discuss this topic, it is imperative that one understands the blood supply and innervation of the spinal canal and its contents.

The principal blood supply to the upper spinal cord is derived from the anterior spinal artery, with its recognized radicular contribution. The lower spinal cord similarly depends on the artery of Adamkiewicz and its segmental contributions.[1–3,33]

In the lumbar region, four segmental arteries arise from the aorta, the fifth one often arises from the middle sacral artery. These segmental vessels give rise to radicular vessels that enter the spinal canal and provide its blood supply.[33] Each radicular artery divides into an anterior and posterior branch. This provides the blood supply to the cauda equina and the remaining spinal contents. According to Gillilan,[33] in the

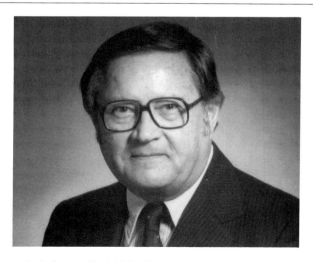

Figure 3–3 George Ehni, M.D., Chairman, Division of Neurosurgery, Baylor University, College of Medicine, Houston, Texas.

sacral region, these radicular vessels ascend along the sacral nerve roots.

The artery of Adamkiewicz arises usually on the left side at L1 or L2. Interference with its blood supply in monkeys caused a neurologic picture similar to that with cauda equina lesions in man.[71] Yet radicular vessel interference presented no neurologic impairment. Based on the data that sacral nerve roots receive both antigrade and retrograde blood supply, it is difficult to postulate root compression syndromes as proposed in the past.

The preeminent proponents of such a notion were Blau and Logue, and their logic is summarized as follows[7]:

> the syndrome [of intermittent claudication] seems to be due to a temporary and recurring disturbance of the blood supply to parts of the cauda equina which improves after rest. Although we appreciate that the cauda equina cannot itself ''limp'' we suggest that the term ''intermittent claudication'' is suitable and compares with that of intermittent claudication of the spinal cord given by Déjèrine.

This is hardly a sound basis, much less scientific proof, of an ischemic theory of lumbar radicular pain. The same authors do not explain the stabbing knifelike low back pain in one of their patients. Evans bases his conclusions on the pathophysiology of pain once again on caudal ischemia with a flippant statement that it is the ''likeliest explanation'' of the symptoms in their patients.[29] Joffe, Appleby, and Arjona supply two cases of spinal stenosis and lay it on the pathophysiologic pyre of Blau and Logue without even a question.[38] Based on this data, the premise that lumbar radicular pain is due to ischemia remains an unsubstantiated fact.

A discussion on mechanical compression theories of nerve roots follows but first it is imperative that one understands the innervation of the spinal canal and its contents.

Von Luschka (1850) described the sinu-vertebral nerve.[45] The nerve filaments were seen as arising from the post-ganglionic dorsal root, destined to supply the spinal canal and its contents. In 1939, Spurling and Bradford showed that the sinu-vertebral nerve may span several lumbar segments.[55]

Neuroanatomically speaking, to date Pedersen et al have the hallmark paper on this topic.[51] These authors state that the sinu-vertebral nerve innervates the intraspinal vessels, the posterior longitudinal ligamentum, and annulus fibrosus as well as the periosteum. The zygapophyseal joints are innervated by the sensory branches arising from the posterior ramus. (A more complete discussion of pain is offered in Chapter 2.)

It is a well accepted fact that an injured nerve root is extremely sensitive to manipulation. Pressure on the annulus fibrosus or posterior longitudinal ligament also causes pain. Deformation of the ligamentum flavum may also play a role,

although most authors believe this causes pain simply by root compression.

In spinal stenosis, the volume of the spinal content and its exit foramina is reduced. Under such circumstances neural compression is quite likely, but also compression of such structures as the annulus fibrosus and the posterior longitudinal ligament may produce some of the back pain. This notion is subscribed to by most authorities in the field without much reservation.

Hence, it may well be said that pain and neurologic dysfunction is probably due to mechanical compression of the nerve roots in the spinal canal or their respective exit foramina and to radicular ischemia.

SYMPTOMS

William Osler taught that a carefully taken patient history should allow one to make a diagnosis and that the physical examination often served only to corroborate one's clinical suspicion. This is probably more true of neurogenic claudication than many other human maladies.

Pain

Severe back pain, a pervading complaint in patients with lumbar disc protrusion, is not a common concomitant of neurogenic claudication. Since the pain of neurogenic claudication is primarily radicular in nature, it often radiates up and down the affected limbs. Patients describe the pain as a deep aching discomfort that, as a rule, begins not in the midback but rather in the buttocks and then descends down the thighs, often going below the knee. Walking aggravates this pain, and standing often does not relieve it. Most patients learn in time that bending forward or sitting down where possible usually abrogates their misery. When caudal compression is severe, even lying supine in bed is impossible because of ''restless legs'' or frank sclerotomal pain in the limbs. Tingling in the toes may progress to numbness. Saddle pain, which often involves the perineum or genitalia, is quite intense in some instances. Patients learn that the only way to survive the night is to remain in a fetal position and never to sleep on the abdomen.

In less than one-third of patients, low back pain is a significant complaint; a lesser degree of pain may be present in about one-half the patients, but it is overshadowed by the limb pain and extremity neurologic deficits.

Sensory Dysfunction

The sensory symptoms reflect both the severity and duration of neural compression. Limb pain frequently gives way to various gradations of sensory dysfunction. Words such as ''poor circulation,'' ''cold feet,'' ''tingling,'' ''burning,'' or "frank numbness" are generally used. As with pain, so with sensory disturbance; posture and activity play an important provocative role. Hence, patients often express that sharp jabbing limb pain gives way to hyperesthesia, which is followed by major sensory disturbance. If a monoradicular syndrome caused by foraminal root compression is the culprit, the symptoms will affect the respective dermatome. The L5 and then L4 roots are most commonly involved. When saddle pain is intense, genital sensory dysfunction as a result of transverse caudal compression is a frequent sequel.

Stooping forward while walking, or preferably sitting down, promptly returns normal sensation to the limbs in many instances. As shown by Goldthwait in 1911,[34] prolonged caudal compression will compound the agony by profound neurologic damage.

MOTOR FUNCTION

When one speaks of disc herniation, lesions that affect the L5 and S1 roots account for about 85 percent of neurologic dysfunction. Hence "foot-drop" and "plantar flexion weakness" pervade the clinical dialogue. This is not so with neurogenic claudication. Compression of L4 is probably more common than L5. Such higher cauda equina injury results in hip flexion weakness or loss of knee extension. The consequence is sudden proximal limb weakness that results in falls, particularly if both limbs are affected.

Once again weakness is often posture related in that extension of the lumbar spine compresses the caudal roots whereas forward flexion ameliorates it. A patient who repeatedly fell was investigated extensively to exclude a cardiac arrhythmia. During one fall he fractured his right humerus. Neurologic consultation lead to a diagnosis of neurogenic claudication with a myelographic block at L3–4. Appropriate lumbar decompression resolved this patient's problem.

SPHINCTER DYSFUNCTION

Impairment of bowel and bladder control is a persistent possibility. In one instance, a patient developed neurogenic bladder dysfunction after lying prone for myelography with lumbar spine in lordosis for only the duration of the study. On another occasion a patient could only void if he leaned forward to the right side. In a male, when genital numbness ensues or sphincter impairment sets in, sexual potency also suffers.

Finally, it must be underscored that it is the duration and severity of caudal compression that eventually determines the prognostic outcome. Table 3–1 shows a breakdown of the various symptoms and signs.

SIGNS OF NEUROGENIC CLAUDICATION

From the onset, one must emphasize that the classical root signs associated with lumbar disc protrusion are frequently absent in patients with neurogenic claudication. Back pain does not play an important role, although it is present in about one-half the patients to some degree. Such back pain is often posture related, with lumbar extension aggravating it, while stooping usually ameliorates or completely abolishes it.

The following are some neurologic signs and tests that help one arrive at a diagnosis of neurogenic claudication.

Spine Percussion Test

With the spine in lumbar extension, the volume of the spinal canal decreases, which produces caudal entrapment. Hence, percussion of the lumbar spine in extension often produces radiating pain down the legs, but when percussion is performed with the lumbar spine in flexion, radicular pain disappears (Figure 3–4, a–b).

Stoop Test

Patients will often complain that walking aggravates their limb pain and neurologic deficits, while stooping forward or sitting improves them. For want of a better term, we will call this the "stoop test." The test can be performed by having the patient walk upright down a corridor. As the pain increases or numbness ensues, the patient walks with a progressively increasing stoop, thus relieving caudal compression and its concomitant pain. Yet, when the walking stops and the patient

Table 3–1 Symptoms and Signs Analysis of 50 Cases

Symptoms	No. Cases.	%
Severe back pain	10	20
Some back pain	27	54
Radicular pain	48	96
Sensory impairment	45	90
Saddle numbness	4	8
Limb weakness	25	50
Sexual impotence	4	8
Neurogenic incontinence	6	12

Signs	No. Cases	%
Sensory deficits	30	60
Motor weakness	28	56
Muscle atrophy	8	16
Impaired knee jerks	15	30
Impaired ankle jerks	22	44
Neurogenic bladder	4	8
Positive straight-leg raising	15	30
Positive femoral (nerve stretch test)	30	60
Positive stoop test	40	80
Positive straight-leg raising	10	20

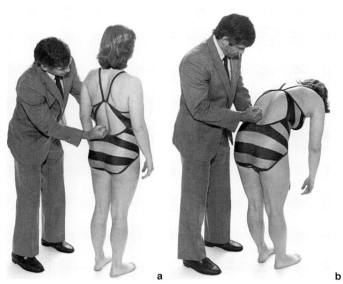

Figure 3–4 Percussion test. (a) When the spine is extended and lumbar percussion is performed, radicular limb pain is elicited. (b) This radicular pain disappears on forward flexion.

simply stands upright again, the pain promptly returns. Forward flexion, by stooping forward or sitting down, again abolishes it (Figure 3–5, a–d). This test is less reliable when high-grade stenosis exists or major vertebral subluxation is present, in other words, when the spinal canal volume does not change with posture.

Bicycle Test

In 1948, van Gelderen described two male patients whose legs became painful and numb and gradually weak as they walked for 10 to 15 minutes. Both also experienced the same pain when they stood erect. The pain was relieved when they sat down. One of the men played tennis and rode his bicycle without pain, yet he could not walk upright without discomfort. Hence, van Gelderen reasoned that the pain was not due to muscle ischemia but rather to the lordotic posture of the lumbar spine.[31]

The first patient van Gelderen dismissed somewhat lightly; the second he took more seriously. He noted cycling without pain was possible only if the patient bent over the handle bars of the bicycle. Yet the same man could not kneel erect or lie prone on a hammock without heralding numbness and weakness in the legs. A laminectomy was performed at L3–4 with excision of the intervening thickened ligamentum flavum. Postoperatively the patient could walk for hours without discomfort. It was this observation that earned van Gelderen historical mention whenever neurogenic claudication is discussed. His observations were summarized in the "Bicycle test of van Gelderen. . . ."[16]

To perform the test, the patient is asked to sit upright on an exercise cycle and begin pedaling the bike until limb pain or neurologic symptoms ensue (Figure 3–6, a–c). The pedaling is continued but the patient leans forward to see if it ameliorates the symptoms. If symptoms persist, the patient leans over the handle bars to see if it abolishes his or her pain or sensorimotor complaints. If it does, the limb symptoms were probably neurogenic; if not, more likely than not they are due to ischemia of the limb musculature. In the latter instance, careful plethysmographic and physical examination of the limbs' arterial circulation will often supply additional corroborative evidence of arterial insufficiency of the lower limbs. Over the past decade, this has been a simple and reliable test.[15,57]

Femoral Nerve Traction Test

Although Epstein, in 1960, stated that positive straight-leg raising was commonly encountered in patients with neurogenic claudication, this is contrary to the experience of most other authors.[26,27,28] Teng reported positive straight-leg raising in 16 of 30 cases.[57] The incidence is probably even less than that, particularly if the test is performed with the patient sitting.[15,57]

The lumbar spinal stenosis that heralds neurogenic claudication occurs most commonly at L4–5. The next most common level of involvement is the one above. Even L2–3 is more commonly affected than the lumbosacral level.[57] The straight-leg raising test puts traction on the L5 and S1 roots but not on the two roots above. In order to produce tension on the upper lumbar roots, the femoral nerve traction test was devised.[14] In 1918 and 1919, Wassermann observed that femoral nerve tension might be augmented by placing the patient prone and then flexing the patient's knees.[66,67] Nachlas described the identical maneuver as a stress test of the lumbosacral and sacroiliac joints.[48] In order to avoid lumbar extension, the femoral nerve traction test is performed with the patient lying on the side.

To carry out the test, the patient is placed on the painless side. The knee is bent to offer stability. The head is flexed to increase tension on the cauda equina. Motion of the low back, particularly hyperextension, is avoided. The painful limb is grasped with the knee remaining straight. The hip is passively extended to its limit. This maneuver exerts tension on the L3 and L4 lumbar roots; pain will radiate down the front of the thigh when either root is compressed. The second maneuver consists of passive flexion of the knee, thus causing additional femoral nerve tension resulting from quadriceps femoris muscle stretch. In the presence of an L4 radiculitis, pain will often radiate to the midtibial area of the leg. In most instances of L3 root involvement, the pain stops at the knee. As with the well-leg raising sign of Fajerszajn, the same may be observed when the femoral nerve traction test is performed on the unaffected limb, whenever major root compression is present.[14,15,30] It should be underscored that this sign is more commonly

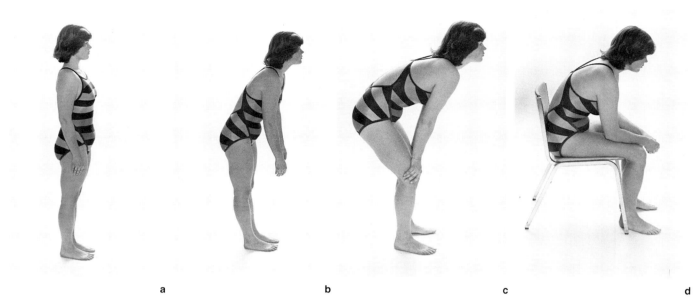

a   b   c   d

Figure 3–5 The stoop-test, for want of a better term, relates pain to posture. Hence, lumbar extension (a) with most likely caudal compression, but as forward flexion is assumed pain may lessen (b). Stooping forward sometimes further ameliorates the discomfort (c). In some instances the patient needs to sit down in order to decompress the caudal roots (d).

observed with soft disc protrusion and axillary root compression rather than with spinal stenosis.

Retroperitoneal injury to the lumbar plexus or the peripheral femoral nerve produces a diffuse dysesthetic discomfort, which is less intense, although it affects the anterior thigh and the medial leg below the knee as well.

Figure 3–7, a–b illustrates the femoral nerve traction test as originally described and a modification of it.

Straight-Leg Raising Test

This test is seldom of value in the diagnosis of spinal stenosis causing neurogenic claudication, particularly if the patient is sitting and the lumbar spine is slightly flexed. Hence, it will not be discussed here any further. For details the reader is referred to the chapter on sciatic pain.

SUMMARY

The purpose of this chapter was to introduce the reader to the historical literature that deals with neurogenic claudication and to sort out the confusion that reigns in this field. Pathophysiologically, it is a generally accepted premise that

caudal pain and deficits are the end result of mechanical compression of neural structures, although the ischemic theory held its own for a while.

The symptoms of neurogenic claudication are quite different from those of lumbar radiculopathy resulting from disc protrusion. Signs that are often applicable to one are not to the other. Hence, only those tests and signs applicable to neurogenic claudication were emphasized here.

Neuroradiologic investigation will be discussed elsewhere. Briefly, computed tomography of the lumbar spine has its "Achilles heel" in the diagnosis of spinal stenosis because the test is performed in lumbar flexion, whereas neurogenic claudication is produced by lumbar extension. This also applies to lumbar myelography. If during myelography only partially tilted prone roentgenograms are obtained, the diagnosis may be missed. Upright films must be obtained with the patient standing and these should include neutral, flexion, and extension views. Lumbar puncture should never be performed at L4–5, the most common level of involvement.

There is no conservative treatment; hence, surgical decompression of the appropriate neural elements is the only avenue of recourse. Resolution of pain and stabilization or neurologic improvement are the usual outcome in the vast majority of patients.

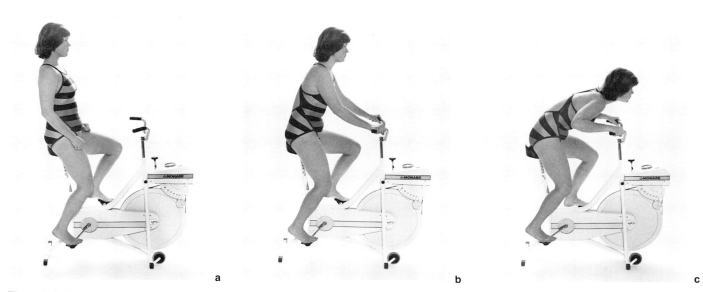

Figure 3–6 The bicycle test separates ischemic pain from that due to caudal compressive radiculopathy. (a) cycling is begun with the lumbar spine in extension. Should pain persist, forward flexion (b) is assumed, but the pedaling never stops. As pain increases (c) the patient leans over the handlebars. In spinal stenosis, pain decreases with the extent of spinal flexion. When pain is due to muscle ischemia, posture will not alter the increasing limb discomfort.

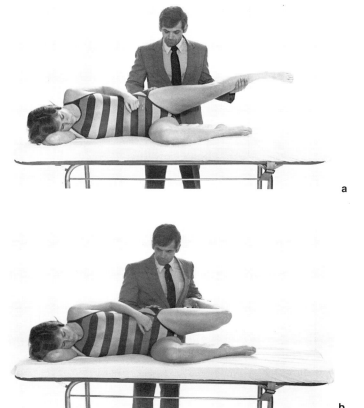

Figure 3–7 The femoral nerve traction test is positive more often than the straight-leg raising test in patients with neurogenic claudication. (a) tension is placed on the iliopsoas muscle when the hip is extended; (b) this is augmented when the quadriceps femoris muscle is stretched. L3 root lesions radiate to the knee, L4 root lesions to the midtibial portion of the leg. The lumbar spine is not extended as in previously described tests.

REFERENCES

1. Adamkiewicz A: Über die Gefässe des menschlichen Rückenmarks. *Trans Int Med Cong* (London) 1881;1:155–157.

2. Adamkiewicz A: Die Blutgefässe des menschlichen Rückenmarks (I). Die Gefässe der Rückenmarksubstanz. Sitzung. *d k Akad d Wissensch in Wien Math Naturw* 1882;84:469–502.

3. Adamkiewicz A: Die Blutgefässe des menschlichen Rückenmarks (II). Die Gefässe der Rückenmarksoberfläche. *d k Akad d Wissensch in Wien Math Naturw* 1882;85:101–130.

4. Anoldi CC, et al: Lumbar spinal stenosis and nerve root entrapment syndromes. Definition and classification. *Clin Orthop* 1976;115:4–5.

5. Bailey P, Casamajor L: Osteoarthritis of the spine as a cause of compression of the spinal cord and its roots. *Nerv Ment Dis* 1911;38:588–609.

6. Bergmark G: Intermittent spinal claudication. *Acta Med Scand Suppl* 1950;246:30–36.

7. Blau JN, Logue V: Intermittent claudication of the cauda equina. An unusual syndrome resulting from central disc protrusion of the lumbar intervertebral disc. *Lancet* 1961;24:1081–1086.

8. Bouley M: Claudication intermitténte par oblitération arterielle. *Arch Gen d Med* 1831;27:425.

9. Brain R: Spondylosis, the known and unknown. *Lancet* 1954;3:689–693.

10. Charcot JM: Sur la claudication intermitténte; dans un cas d'oblitération complete de lune des artéres iliaques primitives. *Compt Rend Soc Biol* 1858;5:225–237.

11. Cooke TDV, Lehmann PO: Intermittent claudication of neurogenic origin. *Can J Surg* 1968;11:151–159.

12. Cramer F: A note concerning the syndrome of cauda equina radiculitis. *Bull Neurol Inst NY* 1934;3:501–505.

13. Déjèrine JJ: La claudication intermitténte de la moelle epiniere. *Presse mèd* 1911;19:981–984.

14. Dyck P: The femoral nerve traction test with lumbar disc protrusions. *Surg Neurol* 1976;6:163–166.

15. Dyck P: Lumbar nerve roots. The enigmatic eponyms. *Spine* 1984;9:3–6.

16. Dyck P, Doyle JB Jr: Bicycle test of van Gelderen in diagnosis of intermittent cauda equina compression syndrome: Case report. *J Neurosurg* 1977;46:667–670.

17. Dyck P, Pheasant H, et al: Intermittent cauda equina compression syndrome. Its recognition and treatment. *Spine* 1977;2:75–81.

18. Ehni G: Spondylotic cauda equina radiculopathy. *Tex State J Med* 1965;61:746–752.

19. Ehni G: Acute compressions artificially induced during operation. *J Neurosurg* 1969;31:507–512.

20. Ehni G: *Neurologic Disorders Associated with Skeletal Changes*. Miami, Symposia Specialists, 1975, pp 33–50.

21. Ehni G: Effects of certain degenerative diseases of the spine, especially spondylosis and disc protrusion on the neural content, particularly in the lumbar region. *Mayo Clin Proc* 1975;50:327–337.

22. Ehni G: Lumbar compressive radiculopathy in diagnosis and surgical management. *Orthop Rev* 1977;2:41–47.

23. Ehni G, Moiel RH, Bragg TG: The redundant or knotted nerve root; A clue to spondylotic cauda equina radiculopathy. Case report. *J Neurosurg* 1970;32:252–254.

24. Elsberg CA: Experiences in spinal surgery: Observation upon 60 laminectomies for spinal disease. *Surg Gynecol Obstet* 1913;16:117–132.

25. Elsberg CA: *Diagnosis and Treatment of Surgical Diseases of the Spinal Cord and Its Membranes*. Philadelphia, WB Saunders Co, 1916.

26. Epstein JA: Diagnosis and treatment of painful neurological disorders caused by spondylosis of the lumbar spine. *J Neurosurg* 1960;17:991–1001.

27. Epstein JA, Epstein BS, Levine SL: Nerve root compression associated with narrowing of the lumbar spinal canal. *J Neurol Neurosurg Psychiatry* 1962;25:165–176.

28. Epstein JA, Epstein BS, Rosenthal RC, et al: Sciatica caused by nerve root entrapment in the lateral recess; The superior facet syndrome. *J Neurosurg* 1972;36:584–589.

29. Evans JG: Neurogenic intermittent claudication. *Br Med J* 1964;2:985–987.

30. Fajerszajn J: Über das gekreuzte Phenomen Wien Klin Wochschr 1901;14:41–47.

31. (van) Gelderen C: Ein orthotisches (lordotisches) Kaudasyndrom. *Acta Psychiatr Neurol Scand* 1948;23:57–68.

32. Getty CJM: Lumbar spinal stenosis. *J Bone Joint Surg* 1980;64(B):481–485.

33. Gillilan LA: The arterial blood supply of the spinal cord. *J Comp Neurol* 1958;110:75–103.

34. Goldthwait JE: The lumbosacral articulation. An explanation of many cases of lumbago, sciatica, and paraplegia. *Boston Med Surg J* 1911;164:365–372.

35. Helfet AJ, Gruebel-Lee DM: *Disorders of the Lumbar Spine*. Philadelphia, JB Lippincott Co, 1980, pp 51–68.

36. Herron PW, Foltz EL, et al: Partial Brown-Séquard Syndrome associated with coarctation of the aorta: Review of the literature and report of a surgically treated case. *Am Heart J* 1958;55:129–134.

37. Huizinga J, Heiden JA, Vinken PJ: The human lumbar vertebral canal; A biometric study. *Proc R Acad Sci* (Amst) 1952;C55:22–23.

38. Joffe R, Appleby A, Arjona V: Intermittent ischemia of the cauda equina due to stenosis of the lumbar canal. *J Neurol Neurosurg Psychiat* 1966;29:315–318.

39. Kavanaugh GJ et al: "Pseudoclaudication" syndrome produced by compression of the cauda equina. *JAMA* 1968;206:2477–2481.

40. Kendall BE, Andrew J: Neurogenic intermittent claudication associated with aortic steal from the anterior spinal artery complicating coarctation of the aorta. *J Neurosurg* 1972;37:89–94.

41. Kennedy F, Elsberg CA: A peculiar and undescribed disease of the nerves of the cauda equina. *Trans Am Neurol Assoc* 1913;39:51–65.

42. Lane WA: Spondylolisthesis associated with progressive paraplegia: Laminectomy. *Lancet* 1893;1:991–992.

43. Love JG: Protrusion of the intervertebral disc (fibrocartilage) into the spinal canal. *Proc Mayo Clin* 1936;11:529–535.

44. Love JG: Removal of protruded intervertebral discs without laminectomy. *Proc Mayo Clin* 1939;14:800–806.

45. (von) Luschka H: *Die Nerven des menschlichen Wirbelkanals*. Tübingen, H. Laup, 1850.

46. Mixter WJ, Barr JS: Rupture of the intervertebral disc with involvement of the spinal canal. *N Engl J Med* 1934;211:210–215.

47. Moiel RH, Ehni G: Cauda equina compression due to spondylolisthesis with intact neural arch. Report of 2 cases. *J Neurosurg* 1968;28:262–265.

48. Nachlas W: The knee-flexion test for pathology in the lumbosacral and sacroiliac joints. *J Bone Joint Surg* 1936;18:714–725.

49. Nelson MA: Lumbar spinal stenosis. *J Bone Joint Surg* 1973;55(B):506–512.

50. Parker HL, Adson AW: Compression of the spinal cord and its roots by hypertrophic arthritis. *Surg Gynecol Obstet* 1925;41:1–14.

51. Pedersen HE et al: The anatomy of the lumbosacral posterior rami and meningeal branches of the spinal nerves (sinu-vertebral nerves). *J Bone Joint Surg* 1956;38(A):377–391.

52. Putti V: New conceptions in the pathogenesis of sciatic pain. *Lancet* 1927;2:53–60.

53. Sachs B, Fraenkel J: Progressive ankylotic rigidity of the spine (spondylose rhizomelique). *J Nerve Ment Dis* 1900;27:1–15.

54. Snyder EN, Mulfinger GL, et al: Claudication caused by compression of the cauda equina. *Am J Surg* 1975;130:172–177.

55. Spurling RG, Bradford FK: Neurological aspects of herniated nucleus pulposus of the fourth and fifth lumbar interspaces. *JAMA* 1939; 113:2019–2022.

56. Steenwinkel FLM: Dysbasia cum dysstasia een compressiesyndrom van de lumbosacrale wortels. *Nederlands Tijdsch Geneesk* 1959; 103:2005–2009.

57. Teng P, Papatheodorou C: Lumbar spondylosis with compression of cauda equina. *Arch Neurol* 1963;8:221–229.

58. Verbiest H: *Sur certáines formes rares de compression de la queue de cheval: Hommage à Clovis Vincent.* Paris, Maloine, 1949, pp 161–174.

59. Verbiest H: Primaire stenose van het lumbale wervelkanaal bij volwassenen. Een nieuw ziektebeeld. *Ned Tijdsch Geneesk* 1950;94:2415–2433.

60. Verbiest H: A radicular syndrome from developmental narrowing of the lumbar vertebral canal. *J Bone Joint Surg* 1954;36(B):230–237.

61. Verbiest H: Further experiences on the pathological influence of a developmental narrowness of the bony lumbar vertebral canal. *J Bone Joint Surg* 1955;37(B):576–583.

62. Verbiest H: Spondylolisthesis: The value of radicular signs and symptoms. A study based on surgical experience and treatment. *J Int Coll Surg* 1963;39:461–481.

63. Verbiest H: Neurogenic intermittent claudication in cases with absolute and relative stenosis of the lumbar vertebral canal (ASLC and RSLC) in cases with narrow lumbar intervertebral foramina and in cases with both entities. *Clin Neurosurg* 1973;20:204–214.

64. Verbiest H: Results of surgical treatment of idiopathic developmental stenosis of the lumbar vertebral canal. *J Bone Joint Surg* 1977; 59(B):181–188.

65. Wackenheim A, Babin E: *The Narrow Lumbar Canal.* New York, Springer-Verlag, 1980.

66. Wassermann S: Über ein neues Schenkelnervsymptom nebst Bemerkungen auf Diagnostik der Schenkelnerverkrankungen. *Dtsch Zschr Nervenhk* 1918;63:146–143.

67. Wassermann S: Die Schenkelnervneuritis und ihre Kombination mit Ischias. *Dtsch Zschr Nervenhk* 1919;64:162–182.

68. Wedge JH, Kinnard P, Foley RK, Kirkaldy-Willis WH: The management of spinal stenosis. *Orthop Rev* 1977;6:89–93.

69. Wilson CB, Ehni G, et al: Neurogenic intermittent claudication. *Clin Neurosurg* 1971;18:62–85.

70. Yamada H et al: Intermittent cauda equina compression due to narrow spinal canal. *J Neurosurg* 1972;37:83–88.

71. Yoss RE: Vascular supply of the spinal cord: The production of vascular syndromes. *U Mich Med Bull* 1950;16:333–345.

Chapter 4

Basis for a Diagnostic and Therapeutic Plan for Lumbar Disc Disease

Robert G. Watkins, M.D.

This chapter describes posterior decompressive surgery for symptoms resulting from noxious stimuli to the spinal nerve. The usual source of such stimuli lies in the structure and biomechanics of the intervertebral disc and its neuromotion segment. A neuromotion segment is defined as an intervertebral disc; its adjacent vertebral body end plates; two facet joints; and the nerves, vessels, ligaments, and muscles functioning with those structures.

Every spinal motion segment undergoes certain morphological changes as the result of acute or chronic injury or age.[3] There are nociceptors present in the spine that translate pathophysiologic and biomechanical abnormalities related to these morphologic changes into pain.[4] Critical for the transition from morphology to pain is function. Function is expressed by motion and activity in a living human. Function studied scientifically is the biomechanics of spinal motion. From a person bending over, to straight-leg raising, to abnormal motion present in a damaged disc, it is this functional biomechanics that connects morphology to pain. Current understanding of the normal motion and stress in a living spinal motion segment is rudimentary. The concept of dysfunction, instability, and restabilization is a reasonable view of the sequence of events that translates morphology into pain,[8] but a biomechanical definition of dysfunction, instability, and stabilization is vague.

Spinal instability in spinal injuries is different. That instability is best defined as the inability of the structural integrity of the spinal column to prevent neurological deficit.[8] This instability is usually caused by one major injury.

Spinal instability in spinal pain should be defined as a defect in the biomechanical functioning of a neuromotion segment that results in pain. The segmental motion present in spinal instability is not necessarily excessive motion but rather abnormal motion. This biomechanical abnormality in the intervertebral disc and its neuromotion segment can be caused by a single, acute injury or repeated, multiple traumas.

An intervertebral disc may be damaged by a variety of combined stresses and loads.[16] Rotational and axial loading is a common mechanism of injury to an intervertebral disc. The resulting damage may be circumferential or radial tears in the annulus fibrosus, fractures in the vertebral body end plate, or avulsion of the annulus from the end plate. A single high-strain rate rotation of 15 to 20 degrees of body motion or 20 degrees of forced axial rotation in the neuromotion segment can produce annular injury in the disc.[5] The disc transforms compression into radial directed tensile forces in the annulus. Torsion, bending, and forced rotation can produce disc rupture and nuclear extrusion. The posterolateral corner is probably more vulnerable because of the shape of the disc, the axis of rotation, and the resultant force vectors. This is the usual location for the earliest changes of disc degenerations that result from repeated small annular tears and for eventual disc herniations.[5]

Change in the disc morphology does change joint kinematics.[2,6,12] A damaged disc does not exhibit the same mechanical behavior that it did before it was injured and the degenerative process began. A degenerative disc has less viscoelasticity, so it distributes stress less evenly. Motion, such as twisting or bending, may produce an axis change and an abnormal rotational pattern in the damaged neuromotion segment. That abnormal motion produces friction. Friction increases inflammation, producing pain from pain fibers in the annulus and the facet joints. In a similar fashion, a torn shoulder rotator cuff produces mechanical dysfunction, inflammation, and pain.

The total amount of motion is irrelevant to this pain-producing process. There is an alteration in the micromotion of the neuromotion segment, a mechanical dysfunction. Most investigators have found the correlation between disc degeneration and a specific amount of spinal motion to be poor.[11,13] As in a knee pyarthrosis, an inflamed joint moves very little, but what motion there is produces an extreme amount of pain. In cases of an acute isolated disc resorption or an infected disc, it is the stiff, poorly moving segment that is painful, not the hypermobile joints above that may be moving more to compensate for the inflamed joint. Measuring the total amount of flexion/extension in a damaged spinal segment should have very little correlation to the origin of the patient's pain[14] and little predictive value as to which level to fuse. Abnormal motion may be only a change in the axis of rotation, not an increase in flexion/extension range of motion.

There is no good way to measure pain-producing micromotion. A logical sequence is that damage gives rise to abnormal motion that leads to inflammation that leads to pain with any motion in the segment. Pain with any motion leads to stiffness. Abnormal motion resulting from damaged articular structures produces post-traumatic scar, stiffness, and osteophytic changes of localized generative arthritis. The eventual loss of range of motion accompanying the osteophytic changes allows the painful motion to dissipate and the neuromotion segment to stabilize. The concept of dysfunction, instability, and stabilization as a chronological sequence applies very well to this sequence of events.[8]

Disc degeneration is associated with biochemical changes in the tissue of the disc, vascular changes in the subchondral bone of the vertebral end plate, and changes in the type of mechanical stresses endured by that motion segment. There is difficulty in relating disc degeneration to any one specific injury, any certain testable mechanical alteration, and any specific amount of pain.

Understanding the relation of morphological changes, such as disc degeneration, to pain is limited by our means of diagnosing disc degeneration. A degenerated disc may or may not bulge more on the computed tomography (CT) scan.[16] There are many bulging discs on CT scans that are asymptomatic. Disc narrowing and osteopathic changes are generally accepted as changes of disc degeneration and may be the result of injury.[9] But many degenerated discs are not narrowed[11] and 53 percent of a group of pain-free people had degenerated changes on x-ray.[7]

The nerve root sleeves, the dural sac, the annulus of the disc, the posterior longitudinal ligament, and the facet joint capsules are richly innervated with sensory nerves. The biomechanical environment of the spinal column—i.e., the discs, bones, joints, and ligaments—is a major determinant of whether there will be spinal pain. Biomechanical stresses on the neurological structure, such as the dural sac and nerve roots, also determine a major component of spinal pain.[1] This is especially true in the increase of leg pain associated with sciatica. Nerve root inflammation may result from compres-

sion, tension, or other noxious stimuli.[1] The sudden appearance of a disc herniation into the spinal canal initially compresses and contuses the nerve root. The herniation becomes a space-occupying lesion around which the nerve root is stretched. The root and dural root sleeve are under tension; stretching the nerve—putting it under more tension—by straight-leg raises, foot dorsiflexion, or neck flexion increases the pain from the inflamed, tense nerve.

Trunk extension produces smaller spinal canal and intervertebral foramina diameters. The disc bulges posteriorly or in the direction of the motion. But the neurological structures, the dura, and the nerve roots slacken and experience less tension upon extension. Disc space collapse is usually accompanied by annular bulge into the canal, but it relieves root tension. Trunk flexion has the opposite effect, causing larger canal diameters but greater root tension. With flexion there is an increase in intradiscal pressure, but the disc bulges anteriorly.

If neurogenic claudication is caused by microvascular shunting from compressed nerve roots, the larger canal and foramina diameters may help explain why flexion relieves neurogenic claudication from spinal stenosis. The relief of root tension concomitant with these increased diameters may explain why sciatica caused by acute disc herniation or rapid loss of disc height after chemonucleolysis is alleviated by properly done extension exercises. The criterion for a successful intraoperative decompression is the relief of root tension, tested by retractability. Understanding the biomechanical functioning of the neurological column is critical to understanding the diagnosis and treatment of back and leg pain.[1]

Chapter 1 presents the changes that result from age and injury as they relate to periods of dysfunction, instability, and restabilization—general biomechanical concepts. This biomechanical basis for evolutional anatomic change is important in relating diagnostic studies to clinical symptoms. Chapters 2 and 3 present the anatomy of pain perception, identify potentially painful spinal structures, and discuss their relationship to the physical examination of a patient.

With an understanding of the morphological changes in the spine and the potential sources of pain, the history and physical examination is the key to relating the science of spinal pain to the patient. The commonly used diagnostic tests such as plain x-ray, CT scan, and myelogram demonstrate the morphology of the spine. These tests can show pathological anatomy capable of pain. An operation on a structure with the potential for pain does not accomplish the ultimate objective of producing a happy, healthy patient. Invariably, the key to successful surgery is direct correlation of the anatomic changes to the patient's complaints and findings and only operating when the patient's morbidity is sufficient to justify the risk of potential complications and failure.

The key to a proper history and physical examination is to have a standardized form that accomplishes the needed specific objectives. (See Exhibits 4–1 and 4–2.)

Exhibit 4–1 Patient History Form

PLEASE TAKE TIME TO FILL OUT THE APPROPRIATE SPACES.

Name _____ Date _____

Age _____ Present Job _____

Type of work done _____

When did your back or neck pain originally start? _____

When did your arm or leg pain originally start? _____

When did your current episode begin? _____

Did your pain start gradually _____ Suddenly _____ Injury _____

What type of injury _____

What time of day is your pain worse: Morning _____ Later in the day _____

Middle of the night _____

Do you have numbness or tingling in an arm or leg? Please describe.

_____

Are there any recent changes in bowel or bladder habits? Please describe.

_____

Do you feel stiffness in the morning? _____

My pain is: check the appropriate box.	BETTER	WORSE	NO DIFFERENT
With cough or sneeze	_____	_____	_____
With straining	_____	_____	_____
Sitting in straight chair	_____	_____	_____
Sitting in soft easy chair	_____	_____	_____
Bending forward to brush teeth	_____	_____	_____
Walking up stairs	_____	_____	_____
Walking down stairs	_____	_____	_____
Lying flat on stomach	_____	_____	_____
On side with knees bent	_____	_____	_____
When bending	_____	_____	_____
When lifting	_____	_____	_____
When working overhead	_____	_____	_____
Lying on back	_____	_____	_____
Standing	_____	_____	_____

Source: Modified from the Greater Los Angeles Orthopedic Medical Group, Downey, CA.

Exhibit 4–1 continued

	YES	NO
My back sometimes gets stuck when I bend forward	——	——
After walking, bending forward relieves my pain	——	——
My back feels like giving way when I bend forward	——	——
Do you have headaches	——	——
Have you had a change in hearing, vision	——	——
Have you had dizzy spells	——	——
My pain stops me when I walk a certain distance	——	——
Have you been in a hospital for back, leg or neck pain	——	——

Number of times hospitalized _____. Please give dates.

How long can you sit? _____

How long can you walk? _____

If you have to stop walking, how long does the pain last? _____

Have you had myelograms? _____   Number of times _____

Have you had neck or back surgery _____

Number of times _____. Please give dates and types _____

Have you been in the hospital with other medical problems? _____

Number of times _____. Please describe.

What treatments have made your pain better? _____

What treatments have made your pain worse? _____

Who referred you to this office? _____

Do you have an attorney helping you? _____

Do other members of your family have significant back trouble? _____

Who? _____

Did you have to change jobs _____ To what? _____

Are you under any pressure at home? _____ At work? _____

Mild _____ Moderate _____ Severe _____.

What can you not do because of your pain that you want to do. _____

_____

What was the date of your last physical exam and the name of the M.D.

who did it? _____

Pelvic done? _____ Rectal done? _____

Exhibit 4–2 Outline for the History and Present Status of the Painful Back and Neck

Patient's Name _____ Date _____

CHIEF COMPLAINT (Major items only) _____

_____

_____

ONSET: Time – sudden or gradual – Date and time of day _____

*Cause-injury, sickness, etc. _____

_____

**Immediate Symptoms _____

_____

_____

_____

COURSE: Detailed chronological study of symptoms and medical care and reaction to each procedure.

_____

_____

_____

_____

_____

_____

_____

_____

PAST RELEVANT HISTORY: Previous and recent attacks, etc._____

_____

_____ Pain   1 2 3 4

_____ Function   1 2 3 4

_____ Occupation 1 2 3 4

*Describe carefully just how forces of the accident affected the patient, how he or she was thrown, fell, landed: twists to back or limbs. Just mechanical factors. (Don't include extraneous material as who was to blame.)

**How patient felt immediately: Unconscious—how long: catch, ache, severe pain, gradual increase, inability to walk or use certain joints, numbness, and/or paralysis.

Source: Modified from the Greater Los Angeles Orthopedic Medical Group, Downey, CA.

Exhibit 4–2 continued

PROGRESS: Better, worse, stationary _____

RELATION TO ACTIVITY:

Lying down – Position of greatest comfort: _____

Does rest or activity relieve? _____

Awakened often and why? _____

Sitting – one side, or shifts _____ How most comfortable? _____

Getting up from sitting – need assist? _____ Hard or soft _____ Driving _____

Standing – one side or shifts _____ Time, and what happens? _____

Walking-Distance _____ What happens? _____

Walking-Distance _____ What happens? _____

Stairs, inclines, irregular ground _____

Bending-Degree _____ Pain and assist returning to erect position _____

Lifting: Wt. _____ lbs. _____ Fatigue _____

Working _____ Type _____ Date discontinued _____ returned _____

Effect of manipulation _____ Support: type and effect _____

Effect of Exercise _____

NEUROLOGICAL EFFECTS:

Radiation of pain: Where? _____ When? _____

Effects of coughing, sneezing and straining during bowel movements: On back, where? _____

_____ On referred pain, how far? _____

Areas of skin tingling, numbness, coldness _____ Muscle weakness? _____

CHRONIC INFLAMMATORY FACTORS:

Stiffness after rest: Getting out of bed _____ after sitting _____

Effect of change of weather _____ Cold, damp weather _____ Hot _____

Effect of heat to part _____ Type of heat _____

(Women) Relation to menstrual periods _____

Remarks: _____

_____

(Secretary: Insert here items from Past History Check Face Sheet.)

Exhibit 4–2 continued

PHYSICAL EXAMINATION

Neck examination is as follows:

MUSCLE STRENGTH:	**RIGHT**	**LEFT**
Trapezius		
Cuff		
Deltoid		
Rhomboid		
Serrant		
Pectoralis		
Biceps		
Triceps		
Triceps supination		
Triceps pronation		
Wrist extension		
Wrist flexion		
Thumb		
Grip		
Intrinsics		

SENSORY FUNCTION:	**RIGHT**	**LEFT**
Light touch		
Pin prick		
Vibratory		

REVIEW OF SYSTEMS:
- PERRLA
- Gag
- Tongue
- Smile
- Hearing
- Sight
- Thyroid
- Neck mass
- Bruits
- Carotids
- Subclavicular
- Axillary

RANGE OF MOTION:
- Flexion
- Extension
- Left flexion
- Right flexion
- Left rotation
- Right rotation

TESTS:	**RIGHT**	**LEFT**
Spurling		
Adson		
Allen		
Tinel elbow		
Tinel wrist		

Exhibit 4–2 continued

TESTS:	RIGHT	LEFT
Phalen		
Referred biceps		
Hoffman		
Horner		
Vertebral artery		

POINT TENDERNESS:		
Occiput		
C1		
C2		
C3		
C4		
C5		
C6		
C7		
T1		
T2		

	RIGHT	LEFT
Paraspinous		
Sternocleidomastoid		
Scapula		
Bicipital groove		
Rotator cuff		
Trapezius		
Anterior spine		

REFLEX GRADES:	RIGHT	LEFT
Biceps		
Brachioradialis		
Triceps		
Patella		
Achilles		

TESTS:	RIGHT	LEFT
Babinski		
Clonus		
Chaddock		
Oppenheimer		

Exhibit 4–2 continued

REVIEW OF SYSTEMS:
  HEENT
  Chest
  Cardiovascular
  Abdomen
  Rectal
  Fundi
  Prostate

PULSES:	RIGHT	LEFT
Femoral		
Popliteal		
Pedal		

RANGE OF MOTION:
  Flexion
  Extension
  Left lateral flexion
  Right lateral flexion
  Tape flexion
  Chest expansion

MUSCLE STRENGTH:	RIGHT	LEFT
Hip abduction		
Hip adduction		
Hip flexion		
Hip extension		
Knee flexion		
Knee extension		
Ankle dorsiflexion		
Ankle plantar flexion		
Toes dorsiflexion		
Toes plantar flexion		

REFLEX GRADES:	RIGHT	LEFT
Patella		
Achilles		
Posterior tibia		

PAIN RADIATION:	RIGHT	LEFT
Thighs		
Calves		
Feet		
Big toe		
Little toe		

SENSORY FUNCTION:	RIGHT	LEFT
Light touch		
Pin prick		
Vibratory		

Exhibit 4–2 continued

	RIGHT	LEFT
LEG LENGTHS:		
Leg lengths		
Thighs		
Calves		
Muscle spasm		
Convexity scoliosis		
TESTS:	**RIGHT**	**LEFT**
Babinski		
Clonus		
Lasegue		
Flip		
Bowstring		
Foot dorsiflexion		
Neck flexion		
Fabere		
Hip range of motion		
Gaenslen		
Nafsinger		
Femoral stretch		
POINT TENDERNESS:		
Thoracic spine		
L1		
L2		
L3		
L4		
L5		
S1		
S2-5		
Coccyx		
Anterior spine		
	RIGHT	**LEFT**
Sacroiliac joint		
Sciatic notch		
Greater trochanter		
Ischial tuberosity		
Paraspinous		
STRAIGHT LEG RAISING:	**RIGHT**	**LEFT**
Supine		
Sitting		
Contralateral		
REFLEX GRADES	**RIGHT**	**LEFT**
Biceps		
Brachioradialis		
Triceps		
Patella		
Achilles		

1. Quantitate the morbidity. Use a scale value of pain, function, and occupation to understand how sick the patient is. Converse in detail with the patient to hear the inflections and manner of the pain description. Detail the time of disability and the time of origin of the pain.
2. Delineate the psychosocial factors. Know what psychological effect the pain has had on the patient. Know the social, economic, and legal results of the patient's disability. Understand what can be gained by his or her being sick or well. Derive an understanding of what role these factors are playing in the patient's complaints.
3. Eliminate the possibility of tumors, infections, and neurologic crisis—these diseases have a certain urgency that requires immediate attention and a diagnostic therapeutic regimen that is very different from disc disease.
4. Diagnose the clinical syndrome.
   a. Nonmechanical back and/or leg pain. Inflammatory, constant pain, minimally affected by activity, usually worse at night or early morning.
   b. Mechanical back and/or leg pain. Made worse by activity, valsalva, relieved by rest.
   c. Sciatica. Predominantly radicular leg pain, positive stretch signs, with or without neurological deficit.
   d. Neurogenic claudication. Radiating leg pain or calf pain, worse with ambulation, negative stretch signs, worse with spine extension, relief with flexion.

Pinpoint the pathophysiology causing the syndrome. Three important determinations are:

1. What level? Which neuromotion segment?
2. What nerve?
3. What pathology: What is the exact structure or disease process in that neuromotion segment that is causing the pain?

The history and physical examination is the first step in determining the clinical syndrome. Some key factors are:

1. The time of day during which pain is worse
2. A comparison of pain levels during walking, sitting, and standing
3. The effects of Valsalva, coughing, and sneezing on pain
4. The type of injury and duration of the problem
5. A percentage of back versus leg pain

The physical examination should address:

1. The presence of sciatic stretch signs
2. The neurological deficit
3. Back and lower extremity stiffness and loss of range of motion
4. The exact location of tenderness and radiation of pain or paresthesias
5. Maneuvers during the examination that reproduce the pain

The history determines whether it is an axial (back pain) or extremity (leg pain) problem. What is the exact percentage of back versus leg pain? Is the pain made worse by the mechanical activity or is it a constant resting pain? Is the pain worsened by maneuvers that increase intradiscal or intraspinal pressure?

Classic radiculopathy causes radicular pain radiating into a specific dermatomal pattern, with paresis, loss of sensation, and reflex loss. The radicular pattern of the pain and neurological examination determines the nerve involved (Exhibit 4–3).

The classic history for radiculopathy resulting from disc herniation is back pain that progresses to predominantly leg pain. It is made worse by increases in intraspinal pressure such as coughing, sneezing, and sitting. Leg pain predominates over back pain and mechanical factors increase the pain. Physical examination shows positive nerve stretch signs. A dermatomal distribution leg pain that is made worse by straight-leg raising, sitting or supine, leg-straight foot-dorsal flexion, neck flexion, juggler compression, and by direct palpation of the popliteal nerve or sciatic notch is characteristic of radiculopathy. A source of radicular pain not found in this description is that caused by spinal stenosis (Exhibit 4–4). Spinal stenosis usually lacks positive nerve stretch

Exhibit 4–3 Radicular Pain Checklist

Radicular pain is worse with:
1. Coughing, sneezing, straining
2. Sitting more than lying
3. Leg pain more than back pain
4. Pain radiation in a specific dermatomal pattern
5. Positive nerve stretch tests
   a. Straight-leg raise supine
   b. Straight-leg raise sitting
   c. Lasègue
   d. Straight-leg raise with foot dorsiflexion
   e. Straight-leg raise with neck flexion
   f. Contralateral straight-leg raise
   g. Bowstring test—deep palpation of the popliteal nerve with straight-leg raise
6. Sciatic notch tenderness
7. Pain, paresis, paresthesia, reflex loss, corresponding to a specific nerve root.

Exhibit 4–4 Neurogenic Claudication Checklist

1. Calf and leg pain that is produced by and limits walking.
2. Bending forward relieves the pain.
3. It progresses from proximal to distal in the leg.
4. Stopping walking does not produce immediate relief.
5. Pedal pulses are normal.

signs but has the characteristic history of neurogenic claudication (i.e., leg and calf pain produced by ambulation). Pain that does not go away immediately upon stopping is made worse with spinal extension and is relieved by flexion. The pain progresses from proximal to distal.

The pain drawing is a major help in accomplishing the objectives of the physical examination. Each patient completes the pain drawing using a rating system, which distinguishes organic from psychological pain fairly well.[10,15] It also helps localize the symptoms for future reference such as with discography and postoperative evaluations (Exhibit 4–5).

The initial history and physical examination (Exhibits 4–6 and 4–7) determines the aggressiveness of the diagnostic and therapeutic regimen. The morbidity rating (Exhibit 4–8) and the time the patient has had the problem are important parts of the history and physical examination that help determine the aggressiveness and invasiveness of the diagnostic plan. The leg pain versus back pain ratio is an important factor in determining which diagnostic tests are indicated. The clinical syndrome should be divided into predominantly mechanical pain, nonmechanical pain, axial pain, and leg pain. An appropriate treatment program can begin, based on the initial evaluation.

Our concern in this volume is decompression of a nerve root or excision of a portion of the spinal column to relieve an irritation to a nerve root. Successful results depend on starting with a patient who has radicular symptoms. From our four clinical syndromes it is obvious that syndromes 3 and 4 are more likely to have radicular symptoms and are most amenable to surgical decompression. Syndrome 2—a combination of back and leg pain—depends heavily on the percentage of back and leg pain (% back/leg) for determining suitability for decompression. The higher the percentage of leg pain, the more suitability for decompression. The lower the percentage of leg pain, the poorer the result from decompression. The history and physical examination should identify the proper symptom complex and radicular symptoms. Diagnostic tests should confirm which nerve is injured and what portion of the spinal column is causing the nerve injury. After identification of the pathology, any contemplated surgery must be specifically designed to correct that pathology with a minimum of risk.

REFERENCES

1. Brieg A: *Adverse Mechanical Tension in the Central Nervous System.* New York, John Wiley and Sons, Inc., 1978, pp 152–176.

2. Brown T, Hanson R, Yorra A: Some mechanical tests on the lumbosacral spine with particular reference to the intervertebral discs. *JBJS* 1957;39-A:1135.

3. DuPuis P: The natural history of degenerative changes in the lumbar spine, in Watkins RG (ed): *Lumbar Discectomy and Laminectomy*, Rockville, Md., Aspen Publishers, Inc., 1987, Chapter 1.

4. Dyck P: Sciatic pain, in Watkins RG (ed): *Lumbar Discectomy and Laminectomy*, Rockville, Md., Aspen Publishers, Inc., 1987, Chapter 2.

5. Farfan HF: *Mechanical Disorders of the Low Back.* Philadelphia, Lea & Febiger, 1973.

6. Hirsch C: The reaction of intervertebral discs to compression forces. *JBJS* 1955;37-A:1188.

7. Hult E: Cervical, dorsal and lumbar spinal syndromes. *Acta Orthop Scand* 1954;(suppl 17):5–102.

8. Kirkaldy-Willis WH (ed): *Pathology and Pathogenesis of Low Back Pain in Managing Low Back Pain.* New York, Churchill Livingstone, 1983.

9. McNab I: *Backache.* Baltimore, Williams & Wilkins Co., 1977.

10. Mooney V, Cairns D, Robertson J: A system for evaluating and treating chronic back disability. *West J Med* 1976;124:370–376.

11. Nachemson A, Schulz A, Berkson M: Mechanical properties of human lumbar spine motion segment: Influence of age, sex, disc level and degeneration. *Spine* 1979;4:1–8.

12. Pennal GF, Conn GS, McDonald G, Dale G, Garside H: Motion studies of the lumbar spine. *JBJS* 1972;54-B:442.

13. Posner I, White AA III, Edwards WT, Hayes WC: A biomechanical analysis of clinical stability of the lumbar and lumbo-sacral spine. *Spine*, to be published.

14. Sweetman BJ, Anderson JAD, Dalton ER: The relationship between little finger mobility, straight leg raising and low back pain. *Rheumatol Rehab* 1974;13:161.

15. Watkins R, O'Brien J, Drauglis R, Prickett C: Comparisons of preoperative and postoperative MMPI data in chronic back patients. *Spine*, to be published, 1986.

16. White AA, Panjabi MM: *Clinical Biomechanics of the Spine.* Philadelphia, JB Lippincott Co, 1978.

Exhibit 4–5 Pain Drawing

Date _____

PLEASE GIVE THIS PAPER TO THE DOCTOR AT THE TIME OF EXAMINATION

Mark the areas on your body where you feel the described sensations. Use the appropriate symbol. Mark areas of radiation. Include all affected areas. Just to complete the picture, please draw in your face.

NUMBNESS ----   PINS & NEEDLES oooo   BURNING xxxx   STABBING ////

BACK

FRONT

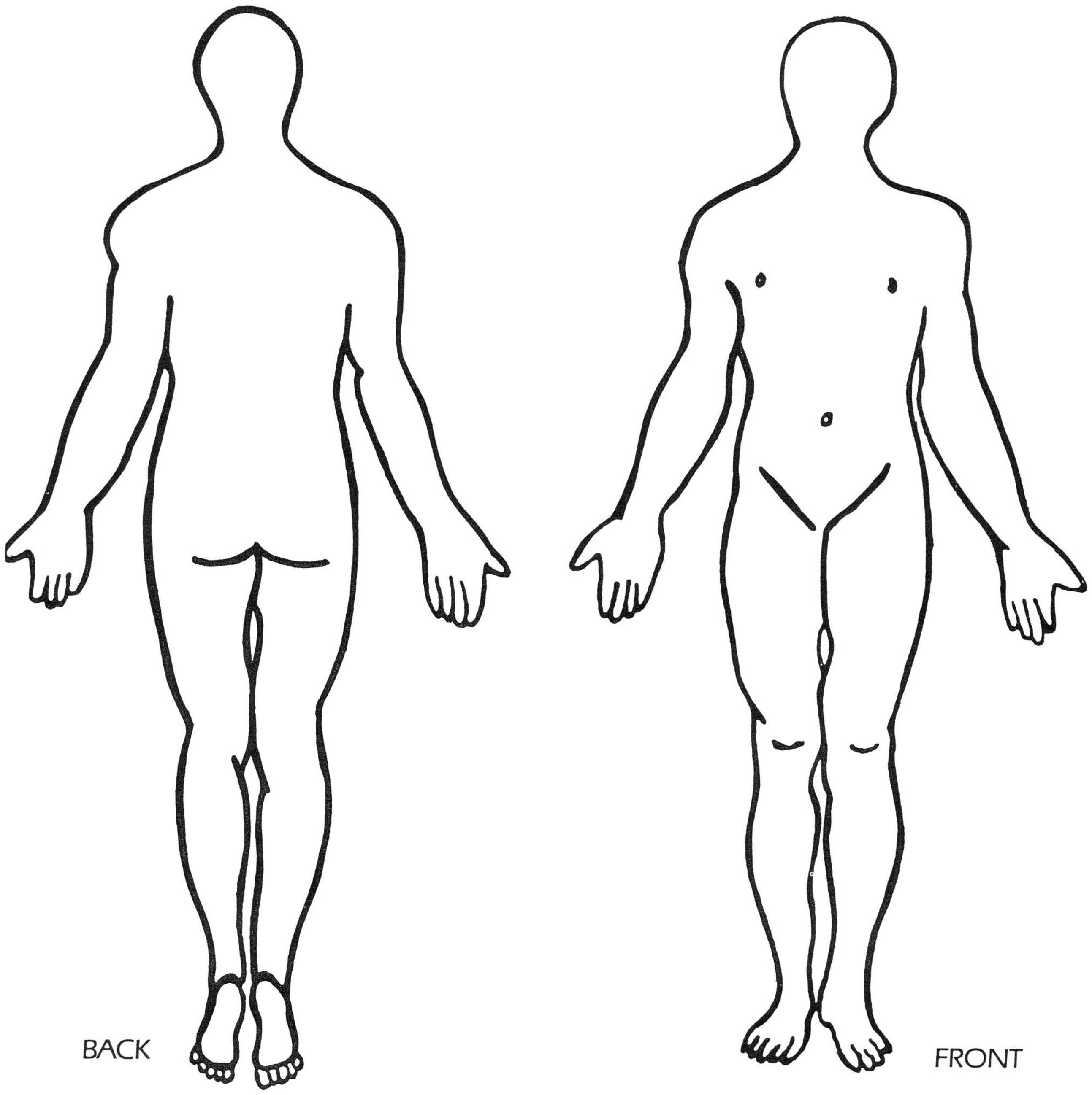

Exhibit 4–6 The Final Form of the History and Physical

Spec Exam and Report

November 9, 1984

Allergies- None
Other Illnesses- None
Medications-None

CHIEF COMPLAINT: Low back pain with radiation into the left leg.

HISTORY:
H.B. is a 31-year-old male with a chief complaint of pain in his low
back radiating into his left lower extremity. On 2/2/83 while working
as a racer he leaned over to pick up a tire to place on his racing
vehicle and felt a pull in his back with the gradual onset of pain in
his low back. He was seen by a chiropractor and rested, but always
had residual soreness in his back, though it was somewhat better. In
11/83 after a prolonged episode of sitting he experienced pain
radiating into the left lower extremity. On April of 1984 for no
known reason he had a severe exacerbation of the pain in his low back,
which was accompanied with severe numbness and tingling in the left
leg. He now finds that the numbness and tingling persist and he is
still having some aching in his back although this was helped by
chiropractic manipulation. He has had a variety of physical therapy
modalities which have not made any difference in the level of his
pain, and he has tried several blocks. These have not been effective
for him.   He now finds that he has stiffness and soreness in his low
back that radiates into the left leg, but is permanently bothered by
the numbness and tingling after prolonged walking. He states that he
is healthy other than his back problem. His pain and function remain
a two on a scale of 1-4 with his occupation a four.

RELATION TO ACTIVITY:
He finds that activities do not make any difference in the level of
his discomfort unless prolonged. Resting is somewhat helpful although
sleeping makes no difference. Sitting for any length of time makes no
change in the level of his pain. Standing is not uncomfortable.
Walking for extensive periods is somewhat aggravating and gives him a
numbness and tingling in his foot. Bending forward pulls in his left
leg. Lifting does not seem to alter the level of his discomfort. He
is a race car driver and stuntman, but has not been able to continue
with any of his work. He has used manipulation which is helpful in
relieving his pain, but not the numbness. He has used exercises which
have not been very effective.

Exhibit 4–6 continued

```
SAMPLE WORKUP
Page 2


NEUROLOGICAL EFFECT:
100% of his pain and discomfort now are in his left leg with
significant radiation of pain as well as numbness and tingling.
Coughing and sneezing do not increase the level of his pain.

CHRONIC INFLAMMATORY FACTORS:
He is not stiff upon getting out of bed in the morning, but somewhat
after sitting.  He has not found that the weather makes any difference
in the level of his pain and he is not using heat modalities.

PHYSICAL EXAMINATION:  (patient exam form results)

SUMMARY OF HISTORY & PHYSICAL:
In summary of the history and physical, Mr. B. has a herniated disc
with left S1 radiculopathy.

X-rays show some spotty changes in his S-I joints and some ill-defined
margins on the right S-I joint, but with no spondylitic defects and no
major destructive degenerative changes present.

DIAGNOSTIC IMPRESSION:  Herniated disc, lumbar spine, with left S1-
radiculopathy.

RECOMMENDATIONS:    1. Six weeks of intensive physical therapy with
                       Marie James
                    2. Indocin-SR.
                    3. He is totally disabled.
```

Exhibit 4–7 Physical Examination

HEENT	negative		**Leg Lengths**	*Right*	*Left*
Chest	negative		Leg lengths	negative	negative
Cardiovascular	negative		Thighs	negative	negative
Abdomen	negative		Calves	negative	negative
Rectal	negative		Muscle spasm	negative	negative
Fundi	negative		Convexity scoliosis	negative	negative
Prostate	negative				

Pulses	*Right*	*Left*	**Tests**	*Right*	*Left*
Femoral	2+	2+	Babinski	negative	negative
Popliteal	2+	2+	Clonus	negative	negative
Pedal	2+	2+	Lasegue	negative	negative
			Flip	negative	negative
Range of Motion			Bowstring	negative	negative
			Foot dorsiflexion	negative	negative
Flexion	90°		Kernig	negative	negative
Extension	20°		Fabere	negative	negative
Left lateral flexion	10°		Hip range of motion	negative	negative
Right lateral flexion	10°		Gaenslen	negative	negative
Tape flexion	8 cm		Nafsinger	negative	negative
Chest expansion	3 cm		Femoral stretch	negative	negative

Muscle Strength	*Right*	*Left*			
Hip abduction	5/5	5/5			
Hip adduction	5/5	5/5	**Point Tenderness**		
Hip flexion	5/5	5/5			
Hip extension	5/5	5/5	Thoracic spine	negative	
Knee flexion	5/5	5/5	L1	negative	
Knee extension	5/5	5/5	L2	negative	
Ankle dorsiflexion	5/5	5/5	L3	negative	
Ankle plantar flexion	5/5	5/5	L4	negative	
Toes dorsiflexion	5/5	5/5	L5	negative	
Toes plantar flexion	5/5	5/5	S1	negative	
			S2–5	negative	
Reflex Grades	*Right*	*Left*	Coccyx	negative	
			Anterior spine	negative	
Patella	2+	2+			
Achilles	2+	2+		*Right*	*Left*
Posterior tibia	2+	2+	Sacroiliac joint	negative	negative
			Sciatic notch	negative	negative
Pain Radiation	*Right*	*Left*	Greater trochanter	negative	negative
			Ischial tuberosity	negative	negative
Thighs	negative	negative	Paraspinous	negative	negative
Calves	negative	negative			
Feet	negative	negative			
Big toe	negative	negative			
Little toe	negative	negative			

Sensory Function	*Right*	*Left*	**Straight-Leg Raising**	*Right*	*Left*
Light touch	within normal limits bilaterally		Supine	negative	negative
Pin prick	within normal limits bilaterally		Sitting	negative	negative
Vibratory	within normal limits bilaterally		Contralateral	negative	negative

Exhibit 4–7 continued

Neck examination is as follows:

Muscle Strength	Right	Left
Trapezius	5/5	5/5
Cuff	5/5	5/5
Deltoid	5/5	5/5
Rhomboid	5/5	5/5
Serrant	5/5	5/5
Pectoralis	5/5	5/5
Biceps	5/5	5/5
Triceps	5/5	5/5
Triceps supination	5/5	5/5
Triceps pronation	5/5	5/5
Wrist extension	5/5	5/5
Wrist flexion	5/5	5/5
Thumb	5/5	5/5
Grip	5/5	5/5
Intrinsics	5/5	5/5

Sensory Function	Right	Left
Light touch	within normal limits bilaterally	
Pin prick	within normal limits bilaterally	
Vibratory	within normal limits bilaterally	

Review of Systems

PERRLA	negative
Gag	negative
Tongue	negative
Smile	negative
Hearing	negative
Sight	negative
Thyroid	negative
Neck mass	negative
Bruits:	negative
Carotids	negative
Subclavicular	negative
Axillary	negative

Range of Motion

Flexion	within normal limits
Extension	within normal limits
Left flexion	within normal limits
Right flexion	within normal limits
Left rotation	within normal limits
Right rotation	within normal limits

Tests	Right	Left
Spurling	negative	negative
Adson	negative	negative
Allen	negative	negative
Tinel elbow	negative	positive
Tinel wrist	negative	negative
Phalen	negative	negative
Referred biceps	negative	negative
Hoffman	negative	negative

Point Tenderness		
Occiput	negative	
C1	negative	
C2	negative	
C3	negative	
C4	negative	
C5	negative	
C6	negative	
C7	negative	
T1	negative	
T2	negative	

	Right	Left
Paraspinous	negative	negative
Sternocleidomastoid	negative	negative
Scapula	negative	negative
Bicipital groove	negative	negative
Rotator cuff	negative	negative
Trapezius	negative	positive
Anterior spine	negative	negative

Reflex Grades	Right	Left
Biceps	2+	2+
Brachioradialis	2+	2+
Triceps	2+	2+
Patella	2+	2+
Achilles	2+	2+

Tests	Right	Left
Babinski	negative	negative
Clonus	negative	negative
Chaddock	negative	negative
Oppenheimer	negative	negative

Foot	Right	Left
Vibratory	intact	intact
Pin Prick	intact	intact
Pulses	intact	intact

Exhibit 4–8 Morbidity Classifications

Pain
1. No pain to mild pain, minimal discomfort with activity
2. Moderate pain, may take non-narcotic medication
3. Constant low-grade or severe intermittent pain, intermittent narcotic use, may interfere with sleep
4. Constant severe pain, regular narcotic use, minimal to no relief of pain

Occupation
1. Full
2. Part-time
3. Changed jobs
4. Unemployed

Function
1. No impairment
2. Impairment of function (no sports)
3. Ineffective community ambulator
4. Ineffective household ambulator

Chapter 5

Plain X-Rays in Lumbar Disc Disease

James C. Thomas, Jr., M.D.

The value of plain roentgenograms in the management of a lumbar disc disease patient has always been controversial. Evidence shows that adult patients who present with sciatica or backache without a definite history of trauma should not have x-rays initially, as 80 percent of these patients will improve within a month with conservative treatment. Initial conservative treatment should be based on clinical impression and is seldom altered by findings on plain x-rays. An exception would be the possible case of lumbar discitis, where roentgenograms are necessary. Nachemson noted that, in a review of 68,000 roentgenographic examination reports over a ten-year period, very little was learned that was previously unsuspected. Clinically unsuspected positive findings in patients 20–50 years of age were obtained only once every 2,500 examinations.[11]

The clinician also faces the dilemma of interpreting x-ray results once plain films have been obtained. Information such as spondylolysis, facet trophism, Schmorl's nodes, and mild lumbar scoliosis may or may not be significant. Clearly, the clinician must interpret all findings on plain roentgenograms in association with the patient's subjective complaints and objective findings.

Plain x-rays do have a great value in management of patients with lumbar disc disease. They are not necessarily helpful in conservative management, but once it appears that a patient will require surgical intervention, their importance increases dramatically. First, x-rays allow the physician to establish whether or not lumbar spine instability is present. Second, they help to identify other conditions possibly responsible for the patient's discomfort. Finally, they enable identification of

segmentation anomalies, present in up to 30 percent of all patients, which could lead to surgery at the wrong level. Any one of these three conditions, if undetected, could lead to failure of posterior decompression for lumbar disc disease.

GONADAL DOSE

The relationship of the gonads to the lumbar spine makes plain roentgenograms of the lumbar spine genetically significant. There are three ways to reduce gonadal dose:

1. Using rare-earth screen/green sensitive film combinations reduces gonadal dose by requiring lesser amounts of radiation for equivalent image quality.[10]
2. For both men and women, various gonadal shields are available that substantially reduce gonadal dose.
3. The most effective way to limit gonadal dose is to reduce the number of films in the standard series from five to two; the standing anterior–posterior (AP) and a standing lateral lumbar film on a large 14 × 17 inch cassette. The other views should be reserved for appropriate clinical situations (to be discussed).

ROENTGENOGRAPHIC EXAMINATION

When the decision to take roentgenograms has been made, the specialist should choose the appropriate views from the list of views available (Table 5–1). Ordering every view for each patient should be avoided because this leads to unnecessary gonad and radiation exposure. Most common disorders can be observed with a limited number of radiologic views, specifically a standing AP and lateral of the lumbar spine. A clinician must judge, based on the patient's subjective symptoms and objective findings, when to order the more specialized views.

TECHNICAL CONSIDERATIONS

There are several technical points to consider in plain x-ray examination. The lateral projection views of the lumbar column are best performed with the patient in the standing or upright position. This requires a different technique and different equipment, but results in an anatomical view of the spine. The lumbar disc spaces appear more visible in the upright position. A deformity such as spondylolisthesis or scoliosis will be more apparent in the upright position.

Lateral Lumbar Views

In the standard lumbar series of five films, a standing lateral lumbar film and a spot lateral of the lumbosacral joint is generally ordered. The central ray should be positioned 1 cm above a metal marker on the most cephalad point of the iliac crest for the lateral lumbar standing film. This will result in a film centered over the L3–4 interspace or the L4 vertebral body, centering the x-ray close to the region of most importance. In a study performed with this technique, if the film was obtained on a 28 × 35.5 cm film, the area between T12 and mid-sacrum was clearly visualized on every lateral radiograph. Consequently, the standing spot lateral film can be reserved for specific cases when the lumbosacral joint must be visualized. This allows reduction of total gonadal dose and probably gives the same amount of information.[2]

When a spot lateral film is performed with the patient standing, it is not necessary to angle the central ray 5° caudal. However, when this film is performed with the patient in the lateral recumbent position, it is necessary to angle the central beam 5° caudal to obtain a good view of the lumbosacral joint.

The Anteroposterior View

A standing anteroposterior on a large 14 × 17 inch cassette will give the spine specialist much information. Lumbar scoliosis, diffuse idiopathic skeletal hyperostosis, leg length discrepancy, and often disease of the hip joint can be detected. To obtain all of this information, the film must be performed with a large cassette, and the patient must be standing completely upright with both knees totally straight.

The Ferguson View (30° Cephalic AP of the Lumbosacral Junction)

The Ferguson view, or the spot anteroposterior lumbosacral projection, is an important plain film. With the patient supine, the central x-ray beam is directed 25–30° cephalad through the midline at an imaginary line joining the anterosuperior iliac spines. Technicians estimate this angle from the patient's standing posture. The Ferguson view illustrates the presence of many conditions, including lumbosacral transitional vertebrae, sacroiliac joint sclerosis, and an occasional short segmental lumbar scoliosis, which may indicate the presence of a far-out syndrome. The Ferguson view may also demonstrate spondylolysis of the pars interarticularis of the L5 vertebra.[9] The central beam should be centered toward the midline parallel to the most cephalad point of the line joining the iliac crest.

Oblique Views of the Lumbar Spine

Forty-five degree oblique views of the lumbar spine are usually taken to detect unilateral or bilateral spondylolysis. These views are highly controversial. Studies have been performed which indicate that oblique radiographs were useful in only 2.4 percent of all cases, specifically in diagnosing unilateral spondylolysis.[14] Another report indicated that oblique views yielded additional information in only 12 percent of 500 cases. The "extra information" in over one-half of the patients (33 of 59) was degenerative apophyseal joint changes.[13] As these are often associated, on the lateral projection, with hypertrophic spurring or disc space narrowing, perhaps the pars views were not necessary.

Another study indicates that spondylolysis can best be detected with oblique views; a false-negative rate without oblique views was 20 percent.[8] This study of 1,743 soldiers noted that the incidence of spondylolysis in those aged 18–30 was 2.5 times that of patients 31–50 years of age. The conclusion was that oblique x-rays may be more important in the younger age group to demonstrate spondylolysis. To decrease the gonadal dose this report recommended restricting the oblique view from L3 to the sacrum since spondylolisthesis is rare above the L3 vertebra.

As oblique views do have a low yield of information, and as the gonadal dose from the oblique views is larger than those from either frontal or lateral views, it is recommended that these views be eliminated from the routine series and reserved for adolescents or young adults with symptomatic spondylolysis or possible acute fracture of the pars interarticularis. When a pars fracture is suspected, but not confirmed, on a 45° oblique view, a 30° and 60° oblique view may be beneficial.

Table 5–1 Plain x-rays of the lumbar spine

1. Lumbar AP standing (on 14 × 17 inch cassette)
2. Lumbar lateral standing (on 14 × 17 inch cassette)
3. Standing spot lateral
4. Left and right 45° oblique view of the pars
5. Ferguson view (30° cephalic AP of the lumbosacral junction)
6. AP pelvis
7. Knuttsen bending views
8. Lateral bending views

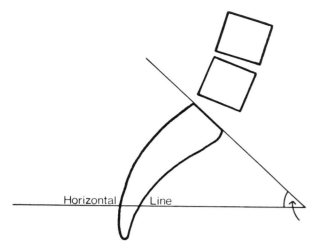

Figure 5–1 The sacrohorizontal angle is the angle between the superior border of S1 and the horizontal plane.

Source: Reprinted with permission from *Journal of Bone and Joint Surgery* (1983;65A:771), Copyright © 1983, Journal of Bone and Joint Surgery, Inc.

Oblique views will rarely be needed in patients older than 30. Recall that a computerized tomographic scan with serial sagittal reconstruction capability can also demonstrate spondylolysis, and a technetium-99 bone scan will determine if the patient has an acute pars fracture. Thus, other diagnostic tests are available to diagnose spondylolysis or acute fractures of the pars.

SPECIFIC CONDITIONS DETECTABLE ON PLAIN X-RAYS

Congenital Anomalies

In large population studies, increased or decreased lumbar lordosis has nothing to do with increased back pain.[6] However, similar studies have shown that a sacral horizontal angle of greater than 70 degrees is associated with increased back pain (Figure 5–1).[23] Asymmetrical lumbosacral facet joint orientation, *facet trophism*, can be detected on plain x-rays and has also been implicated in early degeneration of the lumbar disc at that level.

Lumbosacral Transitional Vertebra

The term *lumbosacral transitional vertebra* (LSTV) should probably replace previously used terms such as *lumbarization* or *sacralization*. The term *transitional* indicates changes simulating a characteristic of a preceding or succeeding vertebra. A lumbosacral transitional vertebra is one that does not meet all the criteria for either a lumbar vertebra or a sacral vertebra. Detection of an LSTV is important, for the disc below the LSTV is at least mildly rudimentary in every case and unlikely to cause problems. The Ferguson view is the best view for detection of such a vertebra.

What constitutes an LSTV has always been controversial. It was initially thought that vertical widening of a transverse

process greater than 19 mm indicated an anomaly [(Figure 5–2), type IA or IB].[16] This is the most frequent anomaly, but the anomaly is a forme fruste of a true LSTV. The incidence of disc herniation with this anomaly is not any different from the normal population.[2]

What appears to be clinically significant is the presence of a unilateral or bilateral articulation (diarthrodial joint present) or a unilateral or bilateral fusion of the transverse process to the sacrum [(Figure 5–2) type IIA-B, IIIA, IIIB, or IV]. Castellvi et al demonstrated that a herniated nucleus pulposus did not occur at the level of the lumbosacral transitional vertebra.[2] There was one exception: Of the 11 patients who had type IIA LSTV (Figure 5–2), one patient had a documented herniated nucleus pulposus.

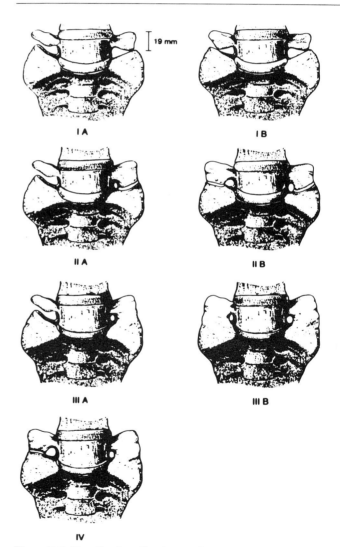

Figure 5–2 Classification of lumbosacral transitional vertebrae according to radiomorphological and clinical relevance with respect to lumbar disc herniation.

Source: Reprinted with permission from *Spine* (1984;9:493–495), Copyright © 1984, JB Lippincott Company.

The question of whether an LSTV is associated with an increased incidence of low back pain has always been debated. The paper of Tini et al shows that the 6.7 percent incidence of LSTV in 4,000 patients with low back pain did not differ significantly from the 5 percent incidence of LSTV in the control population of 1,873 patients.[17]

Consequently, the presence of a disc herniation at an LSTV should be irrefutable prior to surgical decompression. Surgical or posterior decompression at the wrong lumbar level is seen most often in association with a lumbosacral transitional vertebra present.[22]

Spine Phylogeny

Wigh's excellent work suggests that the spine specialist should also understand the variations of human phylogeny of the spine.[21] The spine may have 23, 24, or 25 presacral segments, with the variation usually an addition or subtraction in the thoracic or lumbar areas. The cervical spine is a constant count of seven, except in rare deformities such as Klippel-Feil syndrome. Besides variations from the standard count of 12 thoracic and 5 lumbar vertebrae, and the variations of the lumbosacral transitional vertebra, there is the thoracolumbar transitional vertebra. A short twelfth rib is usually present in this transitional anomaly and it should be identified by noting a complete facet at the root of the pedicle (Figure 5–3). When all anomalies are considered, Wigh notes that 33 percent of patients may have an anomalous spine.

With a high percentage of variants in spine anatomy in the normal population, failure to recognize variants with roentgenographic interpretation preoperatively may lead to surgical decompression at the wrong level. All clinicians should label transitional or suspected transitional vertebra and use this terminology when describing pathology on plain x-rays, computerized tomography, or myelography. For example, a herniated nucleus pulposus seen on computerized tomography in a patient with a transitional L5 should be described as a herniated nucleus pulposus at the L4–5 transitional level (Figure 5–3). This way all treating clinicians will understand that someone has recognized the presence of a transitional lumbar vertebra.

HERNIATED NUCLEUS PULPOSUS

Herniated nucleus pulposus is associated with normal spine roentgenograms in 55 percent of all cases.[4] Weitz's report shows that lateral bending radiographs may demonstrate the level of herniated nucleus pulposus. Weitz states that in patients who have a lumbar list, "the angle of deformity is localized to one disc space, and this angle deformity persists whether the patients bend to the left or to the right."[19] He reports that this deformity can be demonstrated at the level of disc space by performing adequate bending films to the right and to the left, and taking comparison anteroposterior plain roentgenograms.

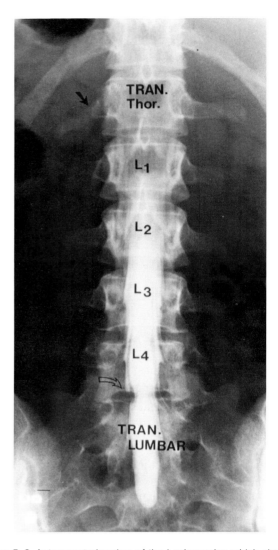

Figure 5–3 Anteroposterior view of the lumbar spine which shows a transitional thoracic vertebra. This is demonstrated by the dark arrow, pointing to the short thoracic rib. Note that the short rib is angled inferiorly and also the complete facet at the root of the pedicle. Then there is a transitional lumbar vertebra, type IIB. Note the herniated nucleus pulposus depicted by the light arrow at the L4 transitional lumbar vertebra.

The plain films are taken with the patient standing, and the anteroposterior x-ray beam is centered 1 inch above the iliac crest and angled cephalad 15 degrees. Three views, a neutral view with the patient upright and one each with maximal bending to the left and to the right are taken. Weitz insists that the back remain flush against the x-ray table, that the patients bend from the waist, and that the knees remain straight. Lines are drawn parallel to the vertebral body at each vertebra. At the level of disc herniation, impaired lateral bending is detected (Figure 5–4).

The lateral bending films are diagnostically helpful in difficult cases, specifically in lateral disc herniations, which are

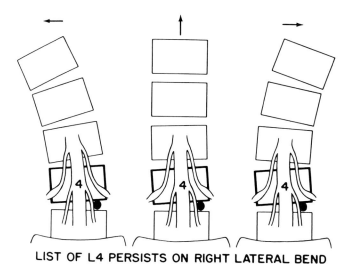

LIST OF L4 PERSISTS ON RIGHT LATERAL BEND

Figure 5–4 Figure demonstrates how herniated disc (dark spot) causes impaired lateral bending to right.

Source: Reprinted with permission from *Spine* (1981;6:384), Copyright © 1981, JB Lippincott Company.

often difficult to detect on myelography and where the CT scan can occasionally be equivocal.

THE NARROW LUMBAR DISC

Torgersen and Dotter demonstrated that roentgenographic evidence of disc degeneration is more likely to be present in a symptomatic group of patients than in an asymptomatic group.[18] However, a single narrow lumbar disc may be of no clinical significance.[11] Clinicians often ascribe low back pain to such a degenerative disc, but it should be noted that Anderssen et al showed that assessment of disc space height as interpreted from lateral roentgenograms can vary widely, because of differences in central roentgen ray orientation and differences among the interpreters of the roentgenograms.[1]

LUMBAR SPINE INSTABILITY

Clinical instability has been defined by White and Panjabi as "the loss of the ability of the spine under physiologic loads to maintain relationships between vertebrae in such a way that there is neither initial damage nor subsequent irritation to the spinal cord or nerve roots and, in addition, there is no development of incapacitating deformity or pain due to structural changes."[20]

Failure to demonstrate lumbar spine instability prior to surgical intervention is a source of failure of posterior decompression of the lumbar spine. The Knuttsen bending views, which are performed with the pelvis relatively fixed, demonstrate instability well. The Knuttsen bending views are performed in a flexed and extended position. The flexed posi-

tion is performed by having the patient sit on a stool and bend forward. The lateral projection is centered 1 inch above the iliac crest (Figure 5–5a). For the extension view, the patient is asked to stand upright with the right side of the buttocks against the table (Figure 5–5b). The patient then bends backward at the lumbosacral junction as much as possible. The extension view is then taken with again the beam centered 1 inch above the iliac crest.

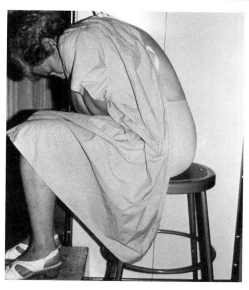

Figure 5–5a Knuttsen view—The patient sits on a stool with the feet placed on a small foot stool and flexes forward as far as possible. The lateral projection is centered 1 inch above the iliac crest.

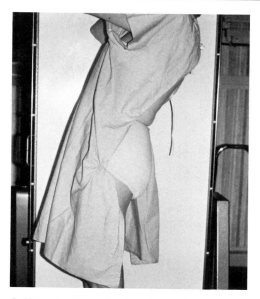

Figure 5–5b This is the extension view in the Knuttsen series. The patient stands upright with the right side of the buttocks against the x-ray table and extends backward at the lumbosacral junction as much as possible.

Posner et al have indicated that instability may occur in flexion with horizontal displacement of the superior vertebral body anteriorly (spondylolisthesis) or horizontal displacement posteriorly in extension (retrolisthesis). Their study also determined that the angulation of the lumbar and lumbosacral disc has maximal ranges in flexion and extension (Figure 5–6). Study results indicate that the lumbar spine (L1–5) and the lumbosacral joint behave differently (Table 5–2). Instead of using absolute numbers for displacement, it is suggested that *percentage* of horizontal displacement be used. All numbers provided by Posner et al were the displacements that could occur in a physiologically loaded, intact spine. The conclusion was that it may be illogical to assume that displacements of this magnitude indicate radiographic instability. It would appear from this report that spondylolisthesis must be 2.5 mm in flexion and retrolisthesis must be 3 mm in extension before radiographic instability is present (Figure 5–7,a-c).[12]

Knuttsen views are somewhat painful for patients, and these views should not be used to evaluate a lumbar fusion. Instead, lateral recumbent bending views are recommended. For this view of a previous lumbar fusion, the patient lies in the left or right lateral recumbent position and flexes forward and extends backward as far as possible. Films are taken at max-

Table 5–2 Clinical Guidelines to Define Displacements of the Intact FSU

	Flexion (mean ± 1 SD)		Extension (mean ± 1 SD)
	Lumbar	Lumbosacral	
Z^C (maximum)	1.7 mm ± 0.6 mm	1.0 mm ± 1.2 mm	2.1 mm ± 0.7 mm
$Z^C\%$ (maximum)	6% ± 2%	4% ± 4%	7% ± 2%
Θ^C (minimum)	−6° ± 4°	5° ± 7°	16° ± 10°

imal flexion and extension. Not only is this position easier for the patient, but also these films can be more easily superimposed than the Knuttsen films. A fused segment should superimpose on the flexion and extension view, with appropriate motion above the fused segment, if the fusion is considered solid. Although anteroposterior tomography is probably the precise method for detection for pseudarthrosis,[3] bending views are the best available method for detection of pseudarthrosis in an office setting. Posterior decompression, in the presence of instability or pseudarthrosis, will often be unsuccessful.

Kirkaldy-Willis uses lateral bending films (previously described) to demonstrate instability.[7] We note this particular demonstration of instability for the sake of completeness.

LEG LENGTH DISCREPANCY

Leg length discrepancy can be detected on the standing AP lumbar spine film performed with a large 14 × 17 inch cassette. The patient should be instructed to keep both knees perfectly straight during the film. A line is then drawn perpendicular to the vertical axis directly across the superior aspect of the femoral head and through the opposite hip joint. The presence of leg length discrepancy may then be detected by noting where the line intersects the contralateral femoral head. Studies have shown that congenital or gradually developing leg length discrepancy of up to 4 cm is not associated with an increased incidence of low back pain.[6] However, acquired acute shortening, such as that following a fracture, of as little as 1.3 cm is associated with an increased incidence of back pain.[23]

CONCLUSION

Plain roentgenograms of the lumbar spine are usually not necessary in the management of acute low back pain. When roentgenograms are taken, the full series is often not necessary, as adequate information can be obtained from the standing anteroposterior view and the standing lateral lumbar spine film. Specialized views, such as oblique views, the coned lateral view, the Ferguson view, and bending views should be ordered judiciously in appropriate clinical situations.

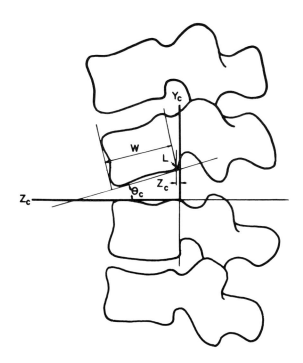

Figure 5–6 Z^C represents horizontal displacement of superior vertebra. $Z^C\%$ is percentage of horizontal displacement. $(\Theta)^C$ is the angulation at the lumbar disc.

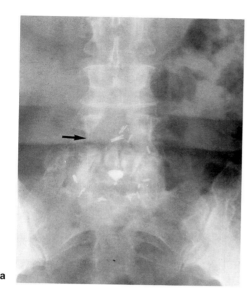

Figure 5–7a AP of lumbar spine showing previous lumbosacral fusion and resection of pars (denoted by dark arrow) of L4.

a

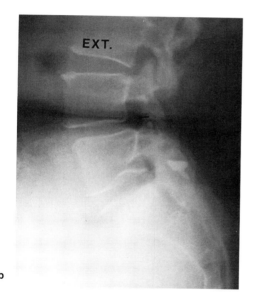

b

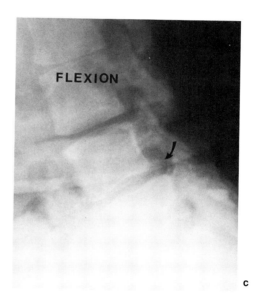

c

Figure 5–7b and **Figure 5–7c** Figures 7b and c demonstrate increased spondylolisthesis in flexion.

Plain films are most helpful when a patient is being considered for surgical decompression. They usually allow the clinician to decide in the office whether other conditions are present, such as lumbar spine instability, which may prevent the posterior decompression from being successful. Plain films also allow the clinician to adequately delineate segmentation anomalies, which can lead to surgical decompression at the wrong level.

REFERENCES

1. Anderssen G, Schultz A, Nathan A, Irstam L: Roentgenographic measurement of lumbar intervertebral disc height. *Spine* 1981;6.

2. Castellvi AE, Goldstein LA, Chan DK: Lumbosacral transitional vertebra and the relationship with lumbar extradural defects. *Spine* 1984;9:493–495.

3. Clater JIJ, Dawson EG, Bassett LW: The role of tomography in the evolution of the postoperative spinal fusion. *Spine* 1984;9:686–689.

4. Edeiken J, Pitt NJ: The radiologic diagnoses of disc disease. *Orthop Clin North Am* 1978;71:405–417.

5. Gehweiler JA Jr, Daffner RH: Low back pain, the controversy of radiologic evaluation. *AJR* 1983;140:109–112.

6. Hult L: The Munk Fors investigation. *Acta Orthop Scand* 1954; (suppl 16):74–114.

7. Kirkaldy-Willis WH: *Managing Low Back Pain*, New York, Churchill Livingstone, 1983, p 81.

8. Lipson E, Bloom RA, Denai G, Robin GC: Oblique Lumbar Spine Radiographs: Importance in Young Patients. *Radiology*, 1984;151:89–90.

9. Lipson E, William RA: Anteroposterior Angulated View. *Radiology* 1983;149:315, 316.

10. Moilanen A, Kokko-Marja-Liisa, Pitkanen M: Gonadal dose reduction in lumbar spine radiography. *Skeletal Radiol* 1983;9:153–156.

11. Nachemson A: The Lumbar Spine: An Orthopaedic Challenge. *Spine* 1976;1:59–71.

12. Posner I, White AA, Edwards WT, Hays WC: A Biomechanical Analysis of the Clinical Instability of the Lumbar and Lumbosacral Spine. *Spine* 1982;7:374–389.

13. Rhea J, Delua S, Llerwelyn H, Boyd R: The oblique view: An unnecessary component of the initial adult lumbar spine. *Radiology* 1980;134:45–57.

14. Roberts F, Keshore P, Cunningham N: Routine oblique radiography of the pediatric lumbar spine: Is it necessary?'' *AJR* 1978;131:297–298.

15. Scavome JB, Latshow RF, Weidner WA: Anterior, posterior and lateral radiographs: An adequate lumbar spine examination. *AJR* 1981; 136:715–717.

16. Southworth JD, Bersack SR: Anomalies of the lumbosacral vertebra in 550 individuals without symptoms referrable to the low back. *AJR* 1950; 6H:624–634.

17. Tini PG, Weiser C, Zinn WM: The transitional vertebra of the lumbosacral spine: its radiological classification, incidence, prevalence, and clinical significance. *Rheumatol Rehabil* 1977;16:180–185.

18. Torgersen WR, Dotter WE: Comparative roentgenographic study of the asymptomatic and symptomatic lumbar spine. *JBJS* 1976;58A:850–853.

19. Weitz E: The lateral bending sign. *Spine* 1981;6:383–397.

20. White AA, Panjabi MM: *Clinical Biomechanics of the Spine*, Philadelphia, JB Lippincott Co, 1978.

21. Wigh R: The thoracolumbar-lumbosacral transitional junctions. *Spine* 1980;5.

22. Wiltse LL: Personal Communication, November 1984.

23. Wiltse LL: Lumbosacral spine: Reconstruction. *Orthopaedic Knowledge Update-I*, 1984;245–258.

24. Wiltse LL: The effect of the common anomalies of the lumbar spine upon disc degeneration and low back pain. *Orthop Clin North Am* 1971; 2:569–581.

Chapter 6

CT of Lateral Spinal Stenosis

Kenneth Heithoff, M.D.
Charles D. Ray, M.D.

Lumbar lateral spinal stenosis is an entity given relatively little credence prior to the use of computed tomography (CT) for the study of the lumbar spine. A few pioneers, such as Kirkaldy-Willis, recognized the entity, but without a radiographic imaging modality to demonstrate lateral bony nerve root entrapment, they found it difficult to convince others of its importance.

As the only satisfactory radiographic modality capable of showing lateral entrapment of the spinal nerve roots by bone and soft tissue, CT has led to an increased awareness of lateral spinal stenosis as a cause of lumbar sciatica and also as a significant factor in failed back surgery syndrome. Burton and Kirkaldy-Willis found lateral spinal stenosis as the etiology in 60 percent of 450 patients with failed back surgery syndrome. This combined study illustrates the extreme importance of recognizing and conceptually understanding spinal stenosis so that accurate decompression of the stenosis may be performed.

TECHNIQUE

Axial images are not easily translated to surgical topographical anatomy. Thus, the information is often not clearly communicated from the diagnostic radiologist to the surgeon. Sagittal reformatted images (soon 3-D) obtained from stacked, adjacent, nonangled axial images provide a more understandable depiction of the extent and severity of the lateral spinal stenosis for both radiologist and surgeon.

Reformatted images are performed as a routine part of all lumbar spine examinations (Figure 6–1, a-c). These images are essential to understanding the bony pathology and are particularly valuable in evaluating the presence and severity of cephalo-caudad narrowing of the intervertebral nerve root canals. Cephalo-caudad stenosis cannot be accurately evaluated and quantified by axial images alone (Figure 6–2, a-e). Since most lateral spinal stenosis occurs at the L5–S1 level, a routine examination includes 3 mm table incrementations at L5–S1 and 5 mm incrementations from L5 to L3. This provides improved resolution of the L5–S1 intervertebral nerve root canals on the sagittal reformatted images. Phantom studies indicate that the resolution of the sagittal reformatted images is equal to that of table incrementation.

In addition these studies were used to select an optimum window width, that would neither artificially enlarge nor diminish the apparent size of the intervertebral nerve root canals. A window setting of 350 to 400 and a level of 50 on the GE 9800 Scanner was determined to be optimum. Widths wider than this tend to artificially enlarge the canals and narrower settings constrict the canals. Some lateral nerve root entrapment is, in part, secondary to disc protrusion, and relatively narrow window settings are useful in depicting both soft-tissue and bony nerve root entrapment. These settings allow visualization of the nerve roots as they emerge from the canal and also of nerve root compression.

Routine, equally spaced sagittal reformatted images must be obtained throughout the entire intervertebral nerve root canal since lateral stenosis and entrapment of the nerve root within the canal may be a focal phenomenon. A routine examination should provide five to six sagittal reformatted images of each intervertebral nerve root canal spaced at 10-pixel (2.3 mm) increments. If necessary, for evaluation of central

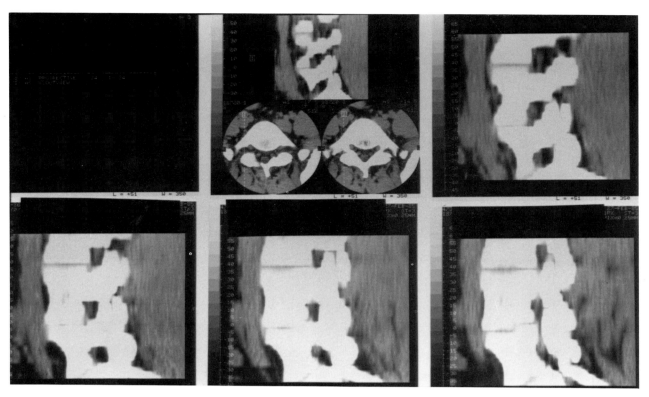

Figure 6–1a Technique of routine sagittal reformatting. Note that sagittal reformatted images are performed at regular intervals of 2.3 mm through each of the intervertebral nerve root canals and a midsagittal reformatted image is obtained. This requires five to six images of each intervertebral nerve root canal in most patients. Images are displayed from lateral to medial. Note the trapezoid appearance of the far lateral aspect of the L5–S1 intervertebral nerve root canal with a more narrow cephalo-caudad dimension. This is the normal configuration of the far lateral aspect of the intervertebral nerve root canal. Note that the scan of the very medial aspect of the intervertebral nerve root canal is elongate in its cephalo-caudad dimension indicating that one is imaging at the margin of the lateral recess. When observing these various configurations, one can be sure that the entire intervertebral nerve root canal has been studied.

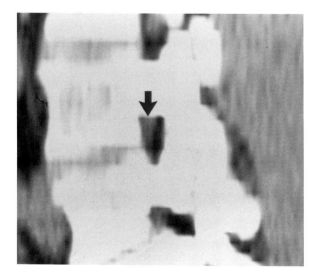

Figure 6–1b Normal sagittal reformatted images of the lower lumbar spine. Note the visualization of the nerve roots within the ventral aspects of the intervertebral nerve root canals (arrow) and the epidural fat dorsal to the nerve roots.

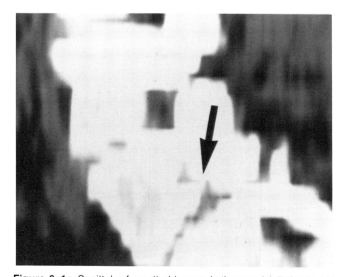

Figure 6–1c Sagittal reformatted image. Lytic spondylolisthesis with severe lateral spinal stenosis at L5–S1 on the right due to severe loss of disc height and overgrowth of the pars superior resulting in marked constriction of the intervertebral nerve root canal (large arrow). Note the normal appearance of the L3–4 and L4–5 foramina.

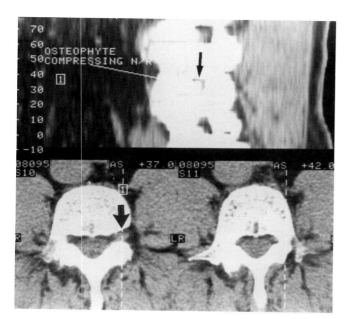

Figure 6–2a Severe bony lateral spinal stenosis at L4–5 with a normal appearing axial image of the cephalad aspect of the intervertebral nerve root canal. The anteroposterior dimension of the intervertebral nerve root canal is normal and there is epidural fat ventral to the L4 nerve root ganglia (large arrow). The ganglia was slightly larger than its companion on the right. This was caused by the cephalo-caudad compression of the nerve root ganglia by the large osteophyte shown on the sagittal reformatted image (small arrow). The thin slice sections obtained in high resolution axial CT imaging allow one to entirely miss a significant cephalo-caudad stenosis, if the images are not reformatted.

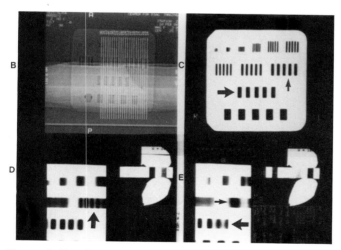

Figures 6–2b-e Phantom study demonstrating the resolution of sagittal reformatted images is equal to the table incrementation.

(b) Lateral computed radiograph of the phantom with localization of the axial images. (c) Axial image of the phantom demonstrating the position of the 3 mm (small arrow) and 5 mm (large arrow) spacing. (d) Sagittal reformatted images of the stacked axial images with 3 mm table incrementation shows resolution of the 3 mm bars (arrow). (e) Sagittal reformatted image obtained from 5 mm slice spacing shows resolution of the 5 mm spacing (large arrow) but failure to resolve the 3 mm spacing (small arrow).

disc protrusion and listhesis, a single midsagittal reformatted image can be obtained. Additional oblique images paralleling the pedicle of L5 may be required in patients with far lateral (far-out or extraforaminal) stenosis. Scanning techniques that utilize angled, noncontiguous scanning are less than desirable, since they greatly prolong reformatting times, effectively precluding this part of the exam.

LUMBAR SPONDYLOSIS AND STENOSIS

The pathogenesis of degenerative lumbar spondylosis and stenosis leads to a conglomerate of degenerative changes including (1) loss of disc height, (2) ligamentous laxity with rotational instability, (3) spondylolisthesis and retrolisthesis, (4) degenerative hypertrophy of the facets, (5) degenerative osteophyte formation, (6) thickening of the ligamentum flavum, and (7) fibrocartilagenous overgrowth at the margin of a degenerated, unstable disc. Therefore, a variety of configurations may be present that lead to nerve root entrapment.

In contrast with central spinal stenosis, which is usually seen at one or more lumbar spinal levels (typically L4–5 and above), bony lateral spinal stenosis most often occurs at the lumbosacral level. For purposes of this presentation, these L5–S1 stenoses will be discussed since they are frequently more complex than those at any other spinal segment. Several entities occur commonly at this level that do not occur more proximally because of the configuration of the sacrum and the presence of unique anatomic degenerative (uncinate) spurs arising from L5. Once the principles are understood, they may be extrapolated to the higher lumbar vertebral spaces.

The margins of the L5–S1 intervertebral nerve root canals are composed of the pedicles of L5 and S1 superiorly and inferiorly, the superior articular processes of L1 dorsally, the L5 vertebral body and L5–S1 intervertebral disc ventrally, and laterally by the iliolumbar and corpro-transverse ligaments. Any one of these structures may interface with nerve roots and produce nerve root impingement. Morphologically, this may result in narrowing of the intervertebral nerve root canal in the cephalo-caudad and anterior posterior dimensions as well as in a circumferential narrowing because of a combination of these stenoses. The major classification of lateral spinal stenosis should be divided according to the anatomic narrowing, i.e., front-back stenosis and up-down stenosis, since these correspond to specific anatomic pathologic entities.

UNCINATE SPURS

Usually, lateral stenoses are due to a multiplicity of degenerative and proliferative processes that cause the intervertebral nerve root canal to narrow in one or more of its several dimensions. Recently, it has become apparent that cephalo-caudad stenosis at L5–S1 resulting from spurs (uncinate) arising from the dorsolateral aspect of L5 is the most common

Figure 6–3 Uncinate spurs at L5–S1.

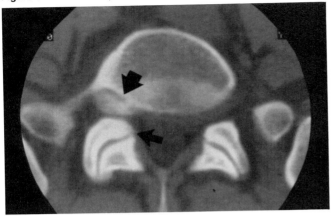

Figure 6–3a Axial CT showing a large focal uncinate spur projecting dorsally into the right L5–S1 intervertebral nerve root canal completely occludes the anteroposterior dimension of the canal at the level of the spur (large arrowhead). Note the smooth, oval appearance of this osteophyte. At surgery, these osteophytes are covered by smooth, fibrous tissue and annular attachments. Note also the enlargement of the superior articular process of S1, which contributes to the antero-posterior narrowing (small arrow).

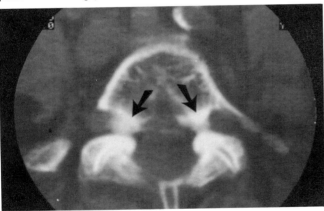

Figure 6–3b Axial CT shows bilateral, focal, large, uncinate spurs pro-ducing severe impingement on the intervertebral nerve root canals at L5–S1 bilaterally (arrows).

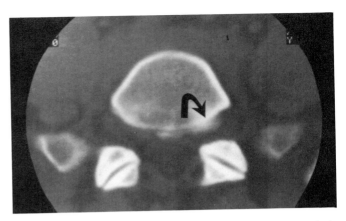

Figure 6–3c Unilateral, moderate-sized, uncinate spur that projects into the ventral aspect of the intervertebral nerve root canal. Although there is epidural fat within the dorsal aspect of the intervertebral nerve root canal, the L5 nerve root is found to lie entirely within the ventral aspect of the intervertebral nerve root canal and becomes compressed between the uncinate spur, which arises from the dorsal aspect of the L5 vertebral body and the pedicle of L5 cranially.

cause of lateral spinal stenosis at this level. In most cases, there is a degenerative narrowing or collapse of the L5–S1 disc space in association with the development of these postero-lateral osteophytes.

Uncinate spurs are anatomic correlates of the uncinate spur-ring found in the cervical spine. Cross-sectional anatomic specimens of human embryos have shown that these uncinate processes exist as separate ossification centers, distinct from the vertebral body of L5.[1] The exact etiology of uncinate spurs in the adult is believed to be the result of disruption or tearing of the annular and/or Sharpey's fibers from the vertebral end plates and the uncinate process. These osteophytes are visu-alized on standard CT axial images as dense rounded bony structures that project dorsally and laterally into the inter-

vertebral nerve root canal from the vertebral body of L5. The posterolateral location of these spurs correlates anatomically with the uncinate spurs found in the degenerating cervical spine. As they enlarge, they project into the intervertebral nerve root canal and impinge upon the caudal surface of the L5 nerve root or nerve root ganglion, causing compression of the ganglia against the pedicle of L5 (Figure 6–3, a-f). A surgeon will find these bony processes covered by tough, smooth tissue; ligaments; or portions of the annulus.

UP-DOWN STENOSIS

As the spinal nerve root emerges from the thecal sac, small dural ligaments attach the nerve ventrally to the posterior longitudinal ligament, annulus, and fascia covering the pos-terior and lateral aspect of the vertebral body and intervertebral disc. Anatomical and surgical dissections have proven their presence (Figure 6–4, a-b).[2] The emerging neural structure (root, ganglia, and spinal nerve) remains relatively fixed in the ventral portion of the canal because (1) of the close proximity of the root to the inferior aspect of the pedicle as it courses through the canal to exit beyond, (2) of the filamentous fibrous extradural ligaments that anchor the nerve root sleeve as it traverses the canal, and (3) of a normally slight outward trac-tion of the spinal nerve.

The nerve lies against the vertebral body caudal to the pedicle, almost like a rope passing around a pulley. These natural structures may slide a bit in and out of their foramina, but they have little or no ventral-dorsal mobility. Postero-lateral osteophytic (uncinate) spurs that arise from the ver-tebral body therefore narrow that ventral portion of the canal where the nerve root structures are found, namely the con-

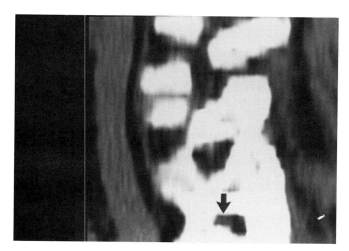

Figure 6–3d Sagittal CT reformatted image of the patient in 6–3c cephalo-caudad stenosis secondary to the uncinate spurring. On this image, note the mild narrowing of the ventral aspect of the intervertebral nerve root canal and the clear delineation of the L5 nerve root ganglia within the ventral aspect of the nerve root canal (arrow) and the absence of neural structures in the dorsal one-half of the intervertebral nerve root canal, which is filled with epidural fat.

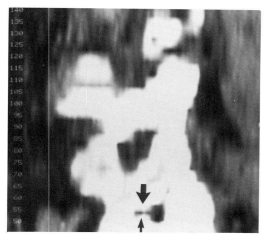

Figure 6–3e Sagittal reformatted image of the same patient as 6–3c taken just lateral to the sagittal plane of 6–3c showing severe cephalo-caudad narrowing of the ventral aspect of the intervertebral nerve root canal. The nerve root ganglia is markedly compressed between the uncinate spur caudally (small arrow) and the pedicle of L5 cranially (large arrow). Note again that the dorsal aspect of the intervertebral nerve root canal contains no neural tissue but rather epidural fat. This portion of the canal is easily probed by instruments during surgery with the false impression that no stenosis exists despite the severe stenosis existing ventrally within this same canal.

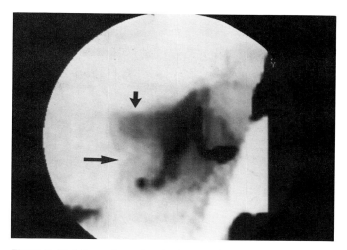

Figure 6–3f A three-dimensional reformatted image showing the presence of a moderately large, uncinate spur (large arrow) and the position of the L5 nerve root ganglia between the pedicle of L5 and the uncinate spur (small arrow). Again, note the large expanse of the dorsal aspect of the canal which does not contain neural elements.

surgery that results from unrecognized lateral stenosis because myelography is negative in these cases. The reason that myelography is negative is that the compression of the nerve occurs at or beyond the ganglia distal to the termination of the nerve root sheath.

The anteroposterior dimension of that portion of the intervertebral nerve root canal that lies cephalad to this spur may be normal. A thin-section axial image obtained through this portion of the canal will not detect the osteophyte. The bony canal will appear normal with epidural fat lying both anterior and posterior to the nerve root ganglia that lies within this cephalad aspect of the canal. In many cases, the only clue to cephalo-caudad compression of the L5 nerve root ganglia is an asymmetric enlargement on the affected side resulting from cephalo-caudad compression of the ganglia. This compression produces an expansion of the ganglia in the axial plane. Sagittal reformatted images, however, clearly define the severity of the cephalo-caudad narrowing and the position and degree of compression of the L5 nerve root ganglia (Figure 6–5a). Similar cephalo-caudad stenosis may be caused by osteophytes arising from the margin of the L5–S1 disc, or focal irregular more lateral osteophytes (Figure 6–5b).

LYTIC SPONDYLOLISTHESIS

Lytic spondylolisthesis is another entity commonly associated with up-down stenosis. Associated disc space narrowing on plain films is an accurate indicator of the presence of lateral stenosis or far-out stenosis in patients with greater than 20 percent lytic spondylolisthesis. Lateral spinal stenosis is rarely detected in the absence of disc space narrowing. Conversely, lateral spinal stenosis is commonly present in patients with both lytic spondylolisthesis and degenerative disc space nar-

stricted space between the spur caudally and the pedicle cranially. Conversely, the dorsal portion of the nerve root canal may be widely potent in these cases, and may easily accept a surgical probe. Therefore, surgical probing of a canal does not exclude significant lateral stenosis at L5–S1 because of uncinate spurring. This makes preoperative CT diagnosis and evaluation essential in the prevention of failed lumbar spine

Figure 6–4 Ligamentous nerve root attachments fixing the position of the lumbosacral nerve roots.

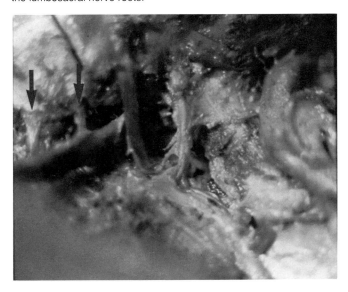

Figure 6–4a Cadaveric dissection showing small ligamentous attachments to the lumbar nerve root (arrows).

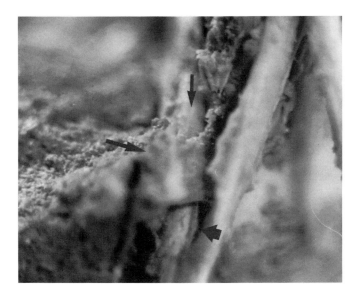

Figure 6–4b Cadaver specimen showing the broad, thick, "sickle" ligament defining the far lateral aspect of the L5–S1 intervertebral nerve root canal (large arrows) and containing the exiting L5 nerve root (small arrow).

Figure 6–5 Cephalo-caudad stenosis with compression of nerve root ganglia.

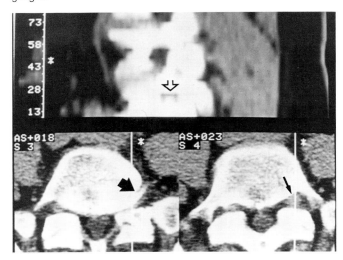

Figure 6–5a Adjacent axial images and sagittal reformatted image of cephalo-caudad lateral spinal stenosis at L5–S1 on the left produced by large osteophytes arising from the margin of the L5–S1 disc (large arrow). The axial image through the nerve root canal shows a normal AP diameter and a "too large" left L5 nerve root ganglia (small arrow). The sagittal reformatted image shows the marked narrowing of the cephalo-caudad dimension of the intervertebral nerve root canal caused by the osteophytes (arrowhead).

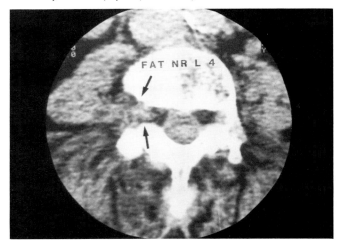

Figure 6–5b Marked enlargement of the exiting right L4 nerve root ganglia due to marked cephalo-caudad compression. Note that the anteroposterior dimension of the axial image through the plane of the ganglia is normal and the cephalo-caudad compression is not detected on the axial image.

rowing (Figure 6–6, a-d). In most patients, the forward slip of the vertebral body, pedicle, and pars of L5 is associated with a caudal settling of that vertebra as the disc space narrows, with entrapment and compression of the L5 nerve root between the pedicle and proximal stump of the pars cranially and the L5–S1 disc and body of S1 caudally. As described by Wiltse et al, entrapment of the L5 nerve root may occur far laterally,

between the transverse process of L5 and the sacrum (the far-out syndrome) (Figure 6–7, a-e).

Axial images of lytic spondylolisthesis show distortion of the intervertebral nerve root canal with elongation of the anteroposterior dimension of the canals because of the ventral slip of L5. Preimpingement swelling of the L5 nerve root often occurs. Sagittal reformatted images are the most useful in

Figure 6–6 Spondylolisthesis with lateral spinal stenosis.

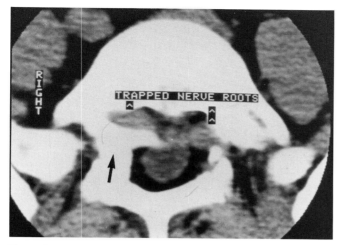

Figure 6–6a Axial CT image at L5–S1 in a patient with spondylolysis of L5, grade I spondylolisthesis, and severe disc space narrowing. Note the marked enlargement of the L5 nerve roots as they lie medial to the pedicle of L5. Also note the marked medial projection of the superior pars on the right (arrow). The marked enlargement of the nerve roots is due to preimpingement swelling as well as cephalo-caudad compression.

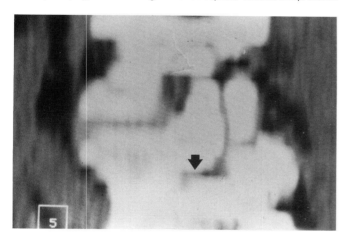

Figure 6–6b Sagittal reformatted image of the patient in 6–6a showing the slitlike configuration of the cephalo-caudad dimension of the right L5–S1 intervertebral nerve root canal (arrow).

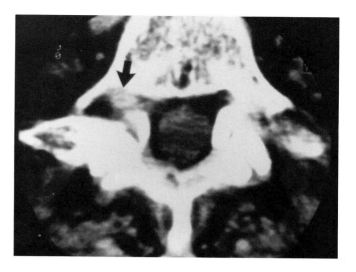

Figure 6–6c Axial CT of a patient with lytic spondylolisthesis at L5–S1 demonstrating an enlarged right L5 nerve root ganglia in a canal which appears to have an adequate anteroposterior dimension (arrow).

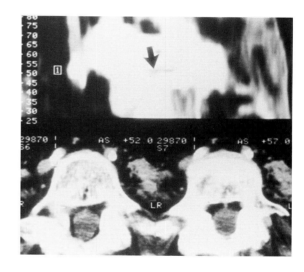

Figure 6–6d Sagittal reformatted image of the patient in 6–6c again showing a slitlike cephalo-caudad dimension of the right L5–S1 intervertebral nerve root canal (arrow).

delineating nerve root compression both within the intervertebral nerve root canal and also laterally between the transverse process of L5 and the sacrum (Figure 6–8). Coronal and oblique reformatted images are occasionally useful.

Posterolateral bulging of the L5–S1 disc annulus and/or lateral disc herniations at L5–S1 may contribute to the L5 nerve root impingement. Marked narrowing of the cephalo-caudad dimension of the intervertebral nerve root canal results in compression and flattening of the L5 nerve root ganglia, which can completely replace the epidural fat within the canal. Distinguishing between the density of the compressed nerve root ganglia and that of a degenerative bulging or laterally

herniated L5–S1 disc is often difficult or impossible. Again, parasagittal reformatted images may be helpful (Figure 6–9).

With advancing age, the vertebral bodies frequently reduce in height but widen at the end plate margins. The pedicle, however, increases in diameter and may alter its normally oval configuration into a larger, more rounded shape. The changes are observed best on plain films of the lumbar spine. In effect, this represents an apparent relative descent of the pedicle in the vertebral body.

The pedicles approach each other downward, further restricting the cephalo-caudad (up-down) diameter of the foramen. Disc margins, along which the annulus attaches,

Figure 6–7 Far-out stenosis.

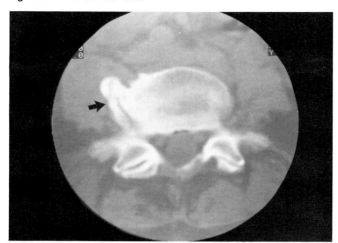

Figure 6–7a Axial CT at L5–S1 showing very large, cauliflower osteophyte arising at the margin of the L5–S1 disc (arrow).

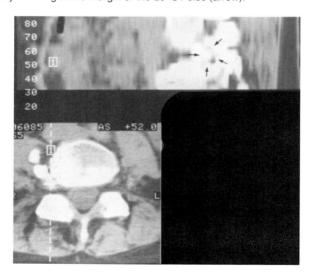

Figure 6–7b Sagittal reformatted image showing the marked impingement of this osteophyte on the intervertebral nerve root canal and compression of the exiting right L5 nerve root ganglia (arrows).

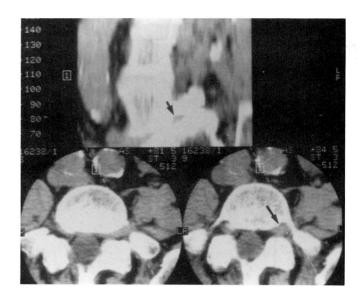

Figure 6–7c Preoperative adjacent axial images and oblique reformatted image obtained through the long axis of the pedicle of (dashed line) L5 demonstrating a very far lateral, lateral spinal stenosis occurring at the very lateral and inferior aspect of the L5 pedicle. Note the enlargement of the left L5 nerve root ganglia due to preimpingement swelling (large arrow), and the severe narrowing of the far lateral aspect of the left L5–S1 intervertebral nerve root canal on the sagittal reformatted image (small arrow).

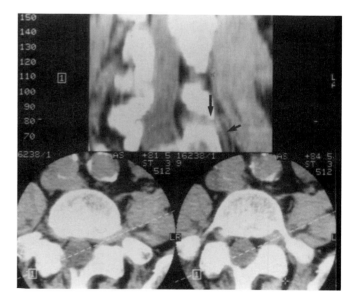

Figure 6–7d Oblique reformatted image in the long axis of the intervertebral nerve root canal (dashed line) showing the focal narrowing of the very lateral aspect of the intervertebral nerve root canal. The normal pedicle of an L5 vertebra has an arcuate configuration with the very caudal margin of the pedicle also being most lateral (arrow). Because of this anatomic configuration of the pedicle of L5, far lateral stenosis at the very lateral margin of the nerve root canal is not uncommon. Note the exiting L5 nerve (small arrow).

become more prominent and often calcified. These bars of the disc margin, especially the uncinate spur, further contribute to up-down narrowing as discussed earlier (Figure 6–10, a-e).

FRONT-BACK STENOSIS

For a considerable period of time hypertrophy of the superior articular facet was considered the major cause of lumbar lateral spinal stenosis. As the disc space collapsed, it seemed plausible that the superior articular facet would rise up in the foramen and compress the nerve cephalad against the pedicle. However, although facet hypertrophy is commonly associated with lateral stenosis, the hypertrophied superior articular proc-

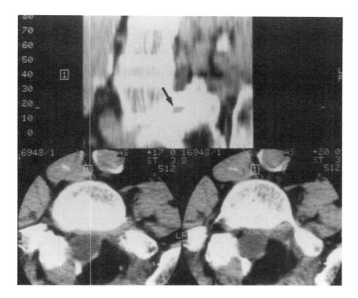

Figure 6–7e Postoperative adjacent axial and oblique reformatted image (dashed line) of the same patient as 6–7a and 6–7b. Note that despite a very generous hemilaminectomy and medial facetectomy, the far lateral and inferior margin of the pedicle is retained and the oblique sagittal reformatted image through the long axis of the pedicle shows that the far lateral stenosis is uncorrected (arrow). The width of the stenosis is only millimeters wide; however, persistent severe nerve root impingement resulted in no improvement postoperatively in this patient. Subsequent surgery with removal of the pedicle resulted in complete relief of the left-sided sciatica.

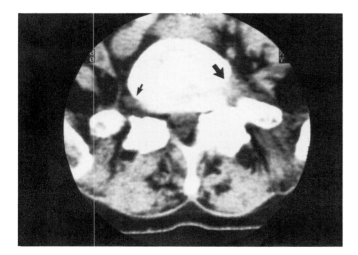

Figure 6–8 Postimpingement swelling of the left L5 nerve root ganglia due to severe left-sided L5–S1 bony stenosis. Note the triangular configuration of the soft-tissue density of the nerve root due to containment of the inflammation by the iliolumbar ligament (arrow). The swollen left L5 nerve root ganglia fills the entire triangular space contained by the ligament. Note the normal right L5 nerve root ganglia (small arrow).

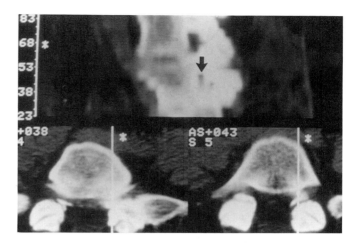

Figure 6–9 Pinhole stenosis. Note the marked concentric narrowing of the left L5–S1 intervertebral nerve root canal due to large osteophytes arising from the margin of the L5–S1 disc and hypertrophic overgrowth of the superior articular process (arrow).

Figure 6–10 Degenerative spondylisthesis and stenosis.

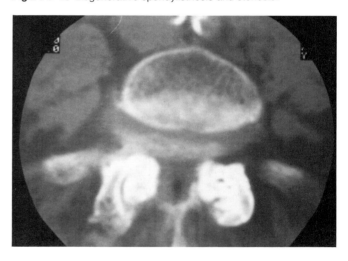

Figure 6–10a Note the marked hypertrophic overgrowth of the L4–5 facets in this patient with degenerative spondylolisthesis. Despite the demonstration of marked spondylosis of the facets on the plain films, the CT clearly shows that no hypertrophic overgrowth into the intervertebral nerve root canals is occurring and that the spondylosis is directed dorsally. Therefore, lateral spinal stenosis is easily excluded by CT examination.

ess almost always lies dorsal to the nerve with resultant anteroposterior compression of the nerve ganglia against the dorsal aspect of the vertebral body by the enlarged facet (Figure 6–11, a-d). A combination of facet hypertrophy and osteophytic spurring may produce severe anteroposterior stenosis.

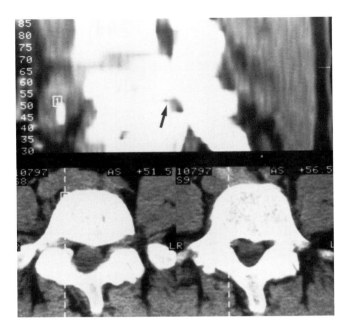

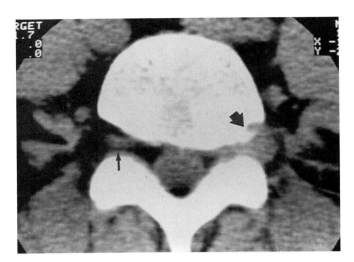

Figure 6–10d Axial CT image at L4–5 showing marked swelling of the exiting left L4 nerve root ganglia due to osteophytic impingement (arrow). Note the normal right L4 nerve root ganglia (small arrow).

Figure 6–10b Small focal uncinate spur at L5–S1 on the right producing mild to moderate impingement of the exiting L5 nerve root. Although small, this osteophyte was shown at surgery to be producing specific and focal impingement on the exiting nerve root (arrow).

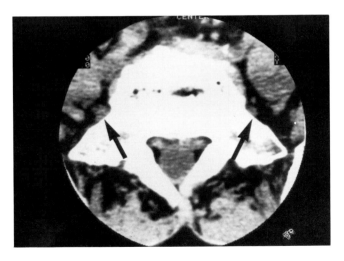

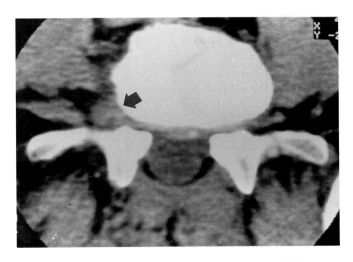

Figure 6–10e Postoperative axial CT image at the L5–S1 level in a patient with a wide central decompressive laminectomy. Note failure to remove the superior articular processes of S1 and persistent marked swelling of the exiting right L5 nerve root ganglia (arrow). The patient was unrelieved of his right-sided sciatica following this surgical procedure. A second procedure consisting of a complete right-sided L5–S1 facetectomy relieved the patient's symptoms.

Figure 6–10c Note the discrepancy of the size of the L5 nerve roots as they lie on the sacral ala (arrows). The left L5 nerve root is smaller than normal and consistent with atrophy. This patient had marked bony stenosis of the left L5–S1 intervertebral nerve root canal. The patient had no current symptomatology but had a past history of chronic right-sided sciatica that gradually remitted.

disc) are present and lead to severe multidimensional concentric bony stenosis. Sagittal reformatted images show a ''pinhole'' intervertebral nerve root canal in these cases (Figure 6–12, a-d).

(BURNED-OUT) STENOTIC CASE

Computed tomography with sagittal reformatted images accurately depicts the degenerative anatomic processes that lead to lateral spinal stenosis. With CT, one can clearly define

This combination is the most common cause of front-back stenosis.

In the most severe cases, all elements of bony hypertrophy (consisting of the dorsolateral osteophyte arising from the vertebral bodies, thickening of the pedicle, overgrowth of the superior articular process, and degenerative narrowing of the

Figure 6–11 Subarticular recess stenosis.

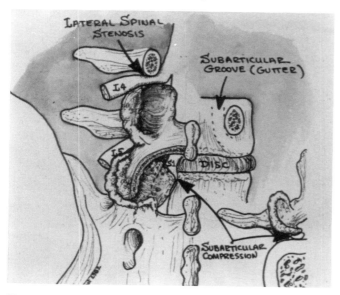

Figure 6–11a Line drawing demonstrating the position of the subarticular recess in the face and axial planes. The subarticular recess is a pathologic recess that is due to medial hypertrophy of the degenerated superior articular process. Nerve root impingement may be due either to osteophyte formation, bulging of the disc annulus within a trefoil spine or a combination of both.

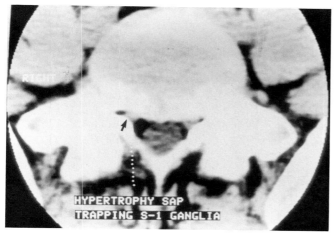

Figure 6–11b Right-sided bony subarticular recess compression of the right S1 nerve root due to inward projection of the base of the superior articular process of S1 as it joins the lamina (arrow). Note the flattening of the right S1 nerve root ganglia in a young woman with right-sided sciatica. This subarticular recess stenosis was surgically confirmed. The importance of this degree of subarticular recess impingement was not appreciated on the preoperative CT examination and surgery was performed on the basis of clinical symptomatology.

those degenerative processes that merely involve the facet joints without encroachment on the canal (Figure 6–13, a-f). In most cases, CT visualization of bony nerve root compression correlates closely with the clinical symptomatology, particularly if swelling of the affected nerve root is observed.

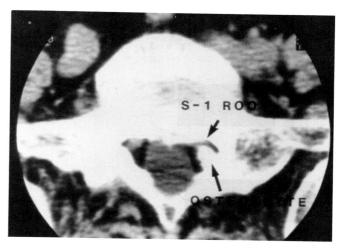

Figure 6–11c Focal osteophyte arising from the medial and caudal aspect of the left L5–S1 facet joint with marked compression of the left S1 nerve root (arrows).

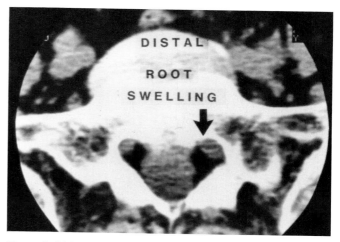

Figure 6–11d Axial CT image of the same patient shown in 6–11c. Note the postimpingement swelling of the left S1 nerve root (arrow).

However, there are patients who have definite, and sometimes severe, bony stenosis without the associated clinical symptomatology. Degenerative bony overgrowths and lateral stenosis result from chronic processes occurring over a span of years. Many of these patients, if questioned carefully, reveal a history of sciatica in the distribution of the affected nerve root. This may be followed slowly by symptomatic regression, with or without conservative management. In other words, the painful sciatica may disappear, although some weakness or other loss of nerve function may remain. In some of these longstanding cases, the CT findings are both a severe bony stenosis and a nerve root smaller than its companion on the opposite side. This suggests atrophy of the affected nerve root as a cause of the cessation of clinical symptomatology (Figure 6–13, a-f). This is one form of a ''burned-out'' sciatica syndrome.

Figure 6–12 Myelography and enhanced CT imaging of subarticular stenosis.

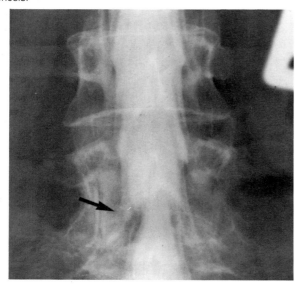

Figure 6–12a Myelogram showing bilateral impingement of the L5 nerve root sheaths and narrowing of the metrizamide column at the level of the L4–5 disc. The larger defect on the left (arrow) was misinterpreted as a disc herniation.

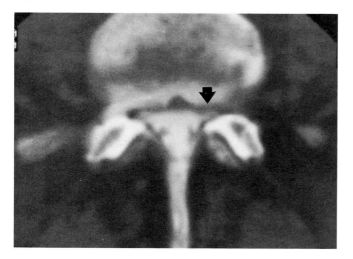

Figure 6–12b Metrizamide-enhanced axial CT scan following the myelogram of 6–12a showing moderate subarticular compression of the left L5 nerve root by the hypertrophied superior articular process and compression between the margin of the disc ventrally and the superior articular process dorsally (arrow). There is no disc herniation present. It is common for subarticular recess stenosis to be misinterpreted as disc herniation on the basis of myelography alone.

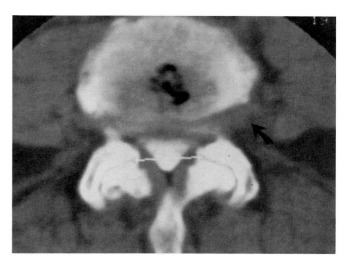

Figure 6–12c Moderate central stenosis and bilateral subarticular recess stenosis in a patient with degenerative spondylolisthesis and constriction of the thecal sac as well as impingement of the L5 nerve roots. Lateral stenosis with swelling of the left L4 nerve root ganglia was also present (arrow).

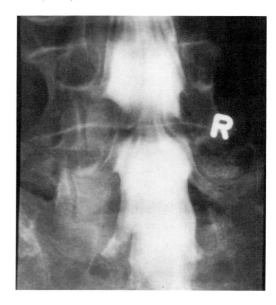

Figure 6–12d Myelogram of the patient shown in 6–12c. Note the displacement of the L5 nerve roots and the widening of the left L5 nerve root secondary to the subarticular compression.

SUBARTICULAR STENOSIS

The subarticular recess is that space within the anterolateral portion of the central spinal canal lying ventral to the base of the superior articular process at its junction with the lamina and dorsal to the intervertebral disc. The subarticular recess is a lateral extension of the central canal and occurs when the canal has a trefoil configuration in conjunction with bulging of the disc or when there is medial hypertrophy of the base of the superior articular process or lamina. Not to be confused with the lateral recess of the intraosseous portion of a trefoil spine, the subarticular recess is a pathologic entity not present in the normal spine.

Focal osteophyte overgrowth arising from the medial margin of the superior articular facet may produce subarticular

Figure 6–13 Degenerative spondylolisthesis with central subarticular and lateral stenosis.

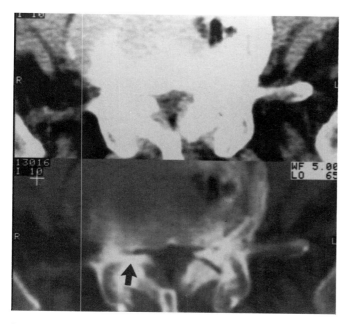

Figure 6–13a Severe central spinal stenosis in a patient with degenerative spondylolisthesis at the L4–5 level. Note the marked erosion and remolding of the superior articular processes that project medially into the central spinal canal to form a very narrowed subarticular recess (arrow). Note the marked constriction of the thecal sac, primarily by bony hypertrophy but also by thickening of the ligamentum flavum and minimal central bulging of the disc annulus.

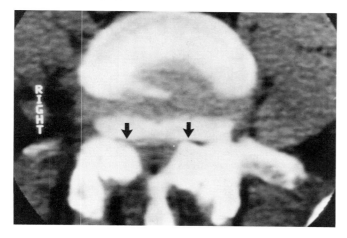

Figure 6–13b Severe central spinal stenosis primarily due to moderate central bulging of the disc annulus and considerable thickening of the ligamentum flavum. The thecal sac measures approximately 3 mm and is triangular in configuration (arrows). CT clearly delineates between central stenosis due to soft-tissue encroachment and bony stenosis.

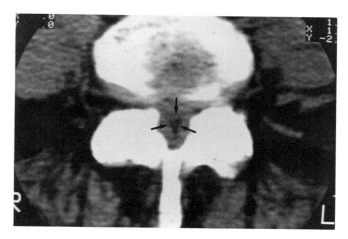

Figure 6–13c Marked central stenosis and bilateral subarticular recess stenosis due to anterior subluxation of the intact neural arch of L4 in a patient with L4–5 degenerative spondylolisthesis. The inferior articular processes of L4 lie in a plane ventral to the superior articular processes of L5 secondary to marked erosion of the medial aspect of the superior articular processes and overriding of the inferior facets (arrows).

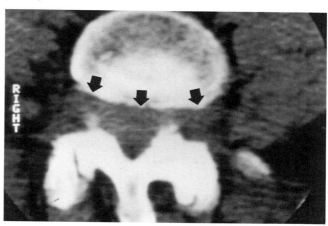

Figure 6–13d Axial image just cephalad to image 6–13c showing the marked fibrotic reaction at the margin of the L4–5 disc due to instability. This fibrotic reaction often incorporates the exiting L4 nerve roots in patients with severe spondylolisthesis making distinction of the nerve roots difficult (arrows). Note the marked overriding of the neural arch of L4 and the erosion of the medial aspect of the superior articular processes of L5.

recess impingement with entrapment of the nerve root as it traverses the intervertebral disc at that level. In the more common form of subarticular recess stenosis or entrapment, the nerve is pressed dorsally by a disc bar against the superior ventral edge of the lamina or base of the superior articular process of the segment below. Either form of subarticular recess does not affect the nerve root exiting at that level, but only the one exiting at the next lower level.

As previously described, the extradural nerve root is tethered ventrally by ligamentous attachments to the posterior longitudinal ligament and disc margin. Therefore, although degenerative processes producing subarticular recess impingement are slowly progressive and chronic, the nerve root becomes entrapped within the subarticular recess because of

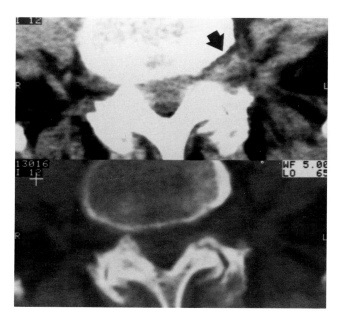

Figure 6–13e Lateral spinal stenosis at L4–5 on the left in the patient shown in 6–13a. Again, note the marked erosion and remolding of the articular facets and the rotatory instability of the spine with rotation of the spinous process toward the patient's left. Note the irregularity and enlargement of the left L4 nerve root within the intervertebral nerve root canal (arrow).

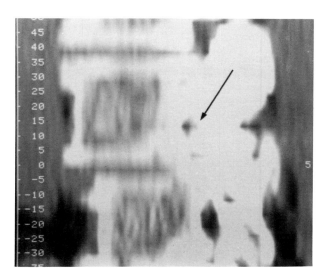

Figure 6–13f Lateral computed radiograph of the patient shown in 6–13a and 6–13e demonstrating the severe bony lateral spinal stenosis at L4–5 on the left (arrow). Note the normal appearance of the L3–4 and L5–S1 intervertebral nerve root canals.

its immobility. When subarticular recess narrowing becomes severe, the affected nerve root often is not well visualized. Metrizamide-enhanced scans confirm the constant position of the affected nerve roots within the far anterolateral aspect of the central canal and clearly delineate the compression of the nerve roots. Swelling of the affected nerve roots within the nerve root sheath may be visualized and is strong confirmative evidence of the pathologic significance of the subarticular narrowing and nerve root compression. Myelograms performed in the absence of CT show displacement and broadening of the affected nerve roots and often are misinterpreted as showing disc herniation.

DEGENERATIVE SPONDYLOLISTHESIS

Degenerative spondylolisthesis occurs most commonly at the L4–5 level. Hallmarks of this entity on axial images are (1) marked degenerative changes of the zygapophyseal joints, (2) severe hypertrophic overgrowth and fragmentation of the superior and inferior articular facets, and (3) erosion of the medial aspect of the superior articular processes with consequent anterior subluxation of the intact neural arch of the vertebral body above. This commonly produces severe central and subarticular recess stenosis.

In addition to the bony constriction, a thickening of the ligamentum flavum and degenerative bulging of the disc annulus occurs. Also, the disc annulus becomes prominent

because of the anterior subluxation of the vertebra above. Although the exiting nerve roots are usually indistinct as a result of fibrotic reaction at the margin of the affected disc extending laterally into the intervertebral nerve root canals, bony lateral spinal stenosis is unlikely.

It appears that lateral spinal stenosis is associated with degenerative spondylolisthesis only when there is an associated posterolateral osteophyte projecting into the intervertebral nerve root canal and/or rotational instability with more prominent anterior subluxation of the lamina and inferior facet on one side.

SUMMARY

The vast majority of lateral stenosis cases may be diagnosed and pathologic changes carefully mapped using axial CT scanning plus sagittal and off-axis image reformatting. The recommended general terminology for bony stenosis of the lumbar spine is central, subarticular, lateral, and extraforaminal or far-out. Lateral stenosis refers only to stenoses occurring within the confines of the intervertebral nerve root canal.

A suggestion for classifying lateral stenosis is given based on simple descriptions of the planes of narrowing of the lumbar neural foramina. By far, the most common is up-down stenosis, where the ganglia is pressed upward (cephalad) into the pedicle of that segment by a disc bar or spur immediately inferior (caudad). This is an important concept since at the L5–S1 level, the L5 nerve root is held within the ventral aspect of the L5–S1 intervertebral nerve root canal by surgically and anatomically definable ligamentous attachments. Thus, the L5 nerve root may be severely compressed in the cephalo-caudad dimension within the ventral half of the intervertebral nerve root canal while the dorsal half of the canal remains devoid of neural tissue and filled with epidural fat. The operating surgeon unaware of this situation may conclude incorrectly that no stenosis is present when he or she probes the patent uninvolved dorsal portion of the intervertebral nerve root canal and finds it to be "patent." Therefore, lateral spinal stenosis cannot be excluded at surgery unless the nerve root is directly visualized and followed throughout the entire intervertebral nerve root canal. Since far lateral visualization requires extensive bony decompression, it is imperative that any patient submitted to laminectomy for nerve root decompression have a preoperative CT scan of the lumbar spine to exclude and/or clearly define the etiology and location of the lateral spinal stenosis. Degenerative bony lateral nerve entrapment has been seen in patients in their teens and twenties. There is no patient group in which lateral spinal stenosis secondary to traumatic and/or degenerative spondylosis does not occur.

Surgery in the face of unsuspected lateral spinal stenosis has led to innumerable second and third operative procedures and is possibly the most common cause of failed back surgery syndrome seen. CT of the lumbar spine is incomplete with axial images alone. Reformatted images are necessary to detect and adequately quantify cephalo-caudal stenosis throughout the intervertebral nerve root canal.

Lateral stenosis is a commonly found entity and a natural concomitant of degenerative disc disease. Therefore, routine reformatting is essential, and intermittent or case-by-case image reformatting (in those cases in which the axial images suggest stenosis) cannot be justified since axial images of pure cephalo-caudal stenosis may appear normal. Neither can reserving reformatting be justified "for those patients in whom lateral stenosis or complex anatomy is suspected." Although evidence of the lesions responsible for cephalo-caudal stenosis (i.e., loss of disc height, uncinate spurring, etc.) is present on the axial images, on the basis of review of numerous reports and outside studies composed of only axial images, it must be concluded that lateral stenosis is often missed with this technique. Once the cephalo-caudal dimension of stenosis is clearly appreciated by sagittal reformatted images, accurate interpretation of axial findings is much facilitated.

Screening with plain films may suggest lateral stenosis in patients with severe spondylosis and concomitant disc space narrowing; however, both plain films and myelography are nonspecific and inadequate for the clearer depiction and diagnosis of lateral spinal stenosis.

BIBLIOGRAPHY

Burton CV, Heithoff KB, Kirkaldy-Willis WH, et al: Computed tomographic scanning and the lumbar spine: Part II: Clinical considerations. *Spine* 1979;4:354.

Burton CV, Kirkaldy-Willis WH, Yong-Hing K, et al: Causes of failure of surgery on the lumbar spine. *Clin Orthop* 1981;157:191.

Burton CV: How to avoid the "failed back surgery syndrome." in *Lumbar Spine Surgery: Indications, Techniques, Failures and Alternatives*, Cauthen JC (ed). Baltimore, Williams & Wilkins Co, 1983.

Burton CV: High resolution CT scanning: The present and future. *Orthop Clin North Am* 1983;14:539.

Burton CV: Diagnosis and treatment of lateral spinal stenosis: Implications regarding the "failed back surgery syndrome." In *Spine Update 1984*, Genant HK, Chavetz N, Helms CA (eds): San Francisco: Department of Radiology, University of California, San Francisco, 1984.

Carrera GF, Haughton VM, Syversten A, et al: Computed tomography of the lumbar facet joints. *Radiology* 1980;134:145.

Cauthen JC (ed): *Lumbar Spine Surgery: Indications, Techniques, Failures and Alternatives*. Baltimore, Williams & Wilkins Co, 1983.

Ciric I, Mikhael MA, Tarkington JA, et al: The lateral recess syndrome: A variant of spinal stenosis. *J Neurosurg* 1980;53:433.

Colley DP, Dunsker SB: Traumatic narrowing of the dorsolumbar spinal canal demonstrated by computed tomography. *Radiology* 1978;120:95.

Crock HV: Isolated lumbar disc resorption as a cause of nerve root canal stenosis. *Clin Orthop* 1976;115:109.

Epstein JA, Epstein BS, Lavine LS, et al: Lumbar nerve root compression at the intervertebral foramina caused by arthritis of the posterior facets. *J Neurosurg* 1973;39:362.

Epstein JA, Epstein BS, Lavine LS, et al: Degenerative lumbar spondylolisthesis with an intact neural arch (pseudospondylolisthesis). *J Neurosurg* 1976;44:139.

Glenn WV: Further investigation and initial clinical use of advanced CT display capability. *Invest Radiol* 1975;10:479.

Glenn WV: Image generation and display techniques for CT scan data: Thin transverse and reconstructed coronal and sagittal planes. *Invest Radiol* 1975;10:497.

Glenn WV, Rhodes ML, Altschuler EM, et al: Multiplanar display computed body tomography applications in the lumbar spine. *Spine* 1979;4:282.

Heithoff KB: High resolution computed tomography of the lumbar spine. *Postgrad Med* 1981;70:193.

Heithoff KB: High-resolution computed tomography in the differential diagnosis of soft tissue pathology of the lumbar spine, in Genant HK, Chafetz N, Helms CA (eds): *Computed Tomography of the Lumbar Spine*, San Francisco: Department of Radiology, University of California, San Francisco, 1982.

Heithoff KB: Pathogenesis and high-resolution computed tomographic scanning of direct bony impingement syndromes of the lumbar spine, in Genant HK, Chafetz N, Helms CA (eds): *Computed Tomography of the Lumbar Spine*, San Francisco: Department of Radiology, University of California, San Francisco, 1982.

Heithoff KB: Computed tomographic assessment of the postoperative spine, in Genant HK, Chafetz N, Helms CA (eds): *Spine Update 1984*, San Francisco: Department of Radiology, University of California, San Francisco, 1984.

Heithoff KB, Ray CD: Principles of the computed tomographic assessment of lateral spinal stenosis, in Genant HK, Chafetz N, Helms CA (eds): *Spine Update 1984*, San Francisco: Department of Radiology, University of California, San Francisco, 1984.

Kirkaldy-Willis W, McIvor GWD: Spinal stenosis. *Clin Orthop* 1976;115:2.

Kirkaldy-Willis W, Wedge JH, Yong-Hing K, et al: Pathology and pathogenesis of lumbar spondylosis and stenosis. *Spine* 1978;3:319.

Kirkaldy-Willis W, Heithoff KB, Bowen CVA, et al: Pathological anatomy of lumbar spondylosis and stenosis, correlated with the CT scan, in Post MJD (ed): "Radiographic Evaluation of the Spine: Current Advances with

Emphasis on Computed Tomography,'' New York, Masson, 1980, pp. 34–35.

Lancourt JE, Glenn WV, Wiltse LL: Multiplanar computerized tomography in the normal spine and in the diagnosis of spinal stenosis: A gross anatomic-computerized tomographic correlation. *Spine* 1979;4:379.

Moon KL, Genant HK, Helms CA, et al: Musculoskeletal applications of nuclear magnetic resonance. *Radiology* 1983;147:161.

Naidich TP, King DG, Moran CJ, et al: Computed tomography of the lumbar thecal sac. *J Comput Assist Tomogr* 1980;4:37.

Quencer RM, Murtagh FR, Post MJD, et al: Postoperative bony stenosis of the lumbar spinal canal: Evaluation of 164 symptomatic patients with axial radiography. *AJR* 1978;131:1059.

Ray CD, Heithoff KB: Techniques for decompression of lumbar spinal stenosis ''guided'' by high-resolution CT scans. *Mod Neurosurg* 1982; 1:31–36.

Verbiest H: A radicular syndrome from developmental narrowing of the lumbar vertebral canal. *J Bone Joint Surg* [Br] 1954;36:230.

Wiltse LL, Kirkaldy-Willis W, McIvor GWD: The treatment of spinal stenosis. *Clin Orthop* 1976;115:83.

Chapter 7

Multiplanar CT in the Diagnosis of Disc Herniation

Stephen L.G. Rothman, M.D.
William V. Glenn, Jr., M.D.

To date, computed tomography (CT) is the method of choice for the diagnosis of disc bulge, protrusion, or extrusion. Just like any other radiographic procedure, however, the reliability of results is directly related to the method of examination. Many different scanning techniques have been developed over the past few years.

Proper CT examination of the spine should include closely spaced axial scans that are reformatted into a complete series of sagittal and coronal images (Figure 7–1, a–d).[1] When possible, the coronal images should be curved to conform to the curvature of the lumbar spine.[2] All of the images must be photographed twice, once for bone detail and once for soft-tissue detail. This type of examination produces a complete series of anatomical images so that no areas of potential pathology are accidentally left unstudied.

Commonly, CT examinations include one or two sagittal reformations at random or through the middle of the spinal canal. This is adequate only if the particular views chosen happen to show the abnormality. Quite often the symptom-producing lesion will not be on the one or two selected views, and the diagnosis may be missed entirely. Virtually all functioning scanners are now capable of full series accurate sagittal and coronal reformations. The responsibility rests with the clinician to insist on an adequate examination.

Some facilities scan patients only through the disc spaces with the gantry tilted perpendicular to the long axis of the spinal canal.[3] This method is inadequate for several reasons: (1) sequestered disc fragments may wander from the disc space and could be overlooked; (2) small lesions of the vertebral body will be missed; and (3) reformation is impossible.

One study has shown the inadequacy of this tilted gantry scanning method.[4] Although the authors state that CT is not as accurate as myelography, the appropriate conclusion to be drawn from their study is that tilted gantry CT is less reliable than myelography. This is not necessarily the case with the complete multiplanar reformatted study.

THE DIAGNOSIS OF DISC DISEASE

One must be as precise as possible within the limitations of the methodology to define the type of disc pathology. The degenerated intervertebral disc space is frequently narrowed, often contains gas, and is only rarely associated with symptom-producing nuclear herniation. More commonly, the patient complains of mechanical back pain rather than radiculopathy. When the degenerative process is severe and the zygapophyseal joints become degenerated and osteoarthritic ridges form, symptoms of recess or foraminal stenosis may dominate. In patients with narrowed spinal canals, the pseudoclaudication syndrome may be present.

The diffusely bulging disc poses the greatest dilemma, both radiologically and clinically. It is extremely difficult to define precisely the amount of bulge of the annulus from axial scans alone. This is because the posterior bony border of the adjacent vertebrae is not on the same slices as the bulging disc. Measuring the extent of the disc bulge or protrusion on sagittal views is much more precise. It is important to realize that the margins of the disc may insert several millimeters above the vertebral end plate posteriorly. This sometimes appears abnormal on axial CT views (Figure 7–2, a–c).

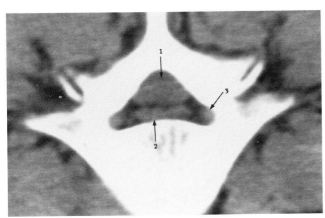

Figure 7–1a Axial CT at the L5–S1 level demonstrates: (1) thecal sac, (2) epidural veins, and (3) exiting L5 root.

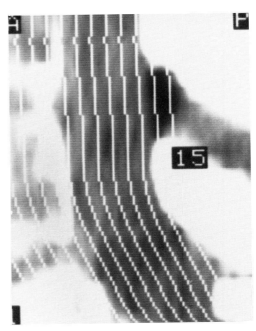

Figure 7–1c Sagittal reformation with computer-generated curves for the production of curved coronal reformation.

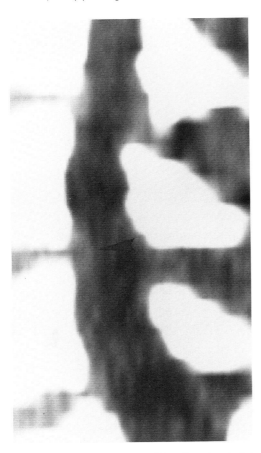

Figure 7–1b Sagittal reformatted view. Note the minor bulging of the annulus fibrosis at L4–5.

In patients with an adequately sized spinal canal, 3 mm of posterior convexity of the annulus may be a manifestation of the normal aging process, and in most cases, should be considered borderline-normal. Marked diffuse symmetrical bulging may produce clinical signs, especially when the spinal cord is

trefoil in shape or congenitally narrowed (Figure 7–3, a–b). It is important to realize that CT provides accurate detail of anatomy. The significance of the particular finding must be related to the patient's complaints. Minor asymptomatic diffuse disc bulge is common in middle-aged and older adults.

An objective grading scheme can be used whereby the amount of soft-tissue extradural disc or annulus can be quantitated on sagittal reformatted scans. Grade I is a normal scan with no obvious measurable convexity on the sagittal images. Grade II scans reveal 2 mm of measurable convexity but should always be considered within normal limits. Grade III scans have 3 mm of extradural soft tissue within the canal, and while usually normal must be considered as borderline. Three millimeters of disc protrusion in a 9 mm spinal canal is much more likely to be significant than when found in a 20-mm-wide spinal canal. A Grade IV disc protrudes 5 mm into the spinal canal and is likely to be a significant lesion, especially if it lies laterally within the spinal canal. Grade V is defined as an extradural soft-tissue mass greater than 6 mm; these masses are most likely severe neurocompressive lesions.

DISC PROTRUSION OR HERNIATION

When the posterior margin of the disc extends symmetrically across, beyond the bony margins, there may or may not be true nuclear protrusion. Williams et al.[5] demonstrated that fissuring and protrusions are grossly underestimated by the axial CT. When the posterior border of the annulus is locally bulging, protrusion of nuclear material is likely. Distinguish-

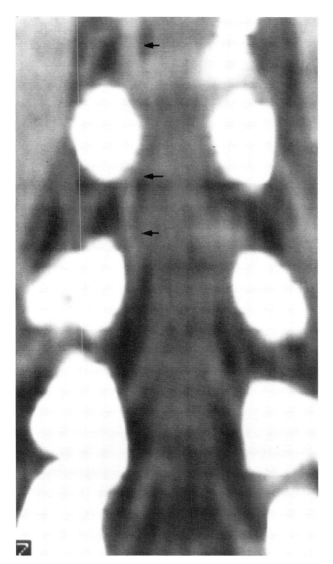

Figure 7–1d The curved coronal view is an image produced along the plane of one of the curves. Note the symmetry of the exiting nerve roots and the descending epidural venous chain (arrow).

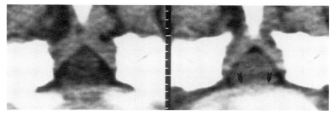

Figure 7–2a Axial CT scan, which appears to demonstrate diffuse bulging of the annulus.

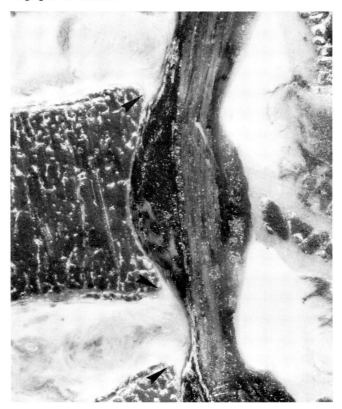

Figure 7–2b Anatomical cross-section through the lumbar spine. Note the insertion of the disc several millimeters above and below the vertebral end plates at both visualized levels. This is a normal anatomical variant.

Source: Courtesy of Dr. Wolfgang Rauschning, Uppsala, Sweden.

ing between localized protrusion of nuclear material and true extrusion of the entire nucleus is not usually possible as long as migration of the disc fragment has not occurred. On axial scans, the localization of the protrusion is evaluated. Nuclear material appears lighter on the CT image than does the cerebrospinal fluid (CSF) within the thecal sac. This nuclear material is nearly the same radiographic density of the ligamentum flavum. Therefore, it will be a lighter shade of gray than any of the surrounding soft-tissue structures (Figure 7–4, a–b).

The amount of extradural soft-tissue mass is also best measured on the sagittal views. Standard flat coronal or curved

coronal reformations reveal well-defined localized high attenuation defects with clear margins. The protruding fragment may actually appear to lie against one of the descending nerve roots. Root displacement, as seen on the axial or curved coronal reformations, is a subtle but useful correlative sign in determining the significance of borderline lesions (Figure 7–5).

In difficult cases, one must rely on secondary signs to aid in the diagnosis. One of the most important signs is asymmetry of the epidural fat. Fat appears very dark black on the CT image and acts as a natural contrast agent, allowing the neural and vascular structures to be seen easily. In most individuals, the

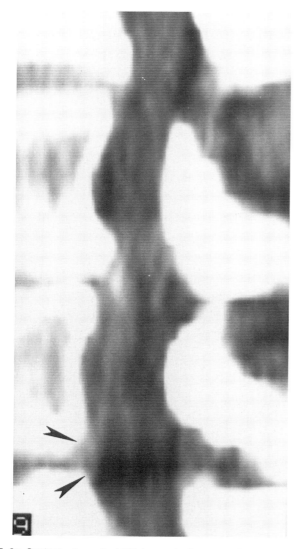

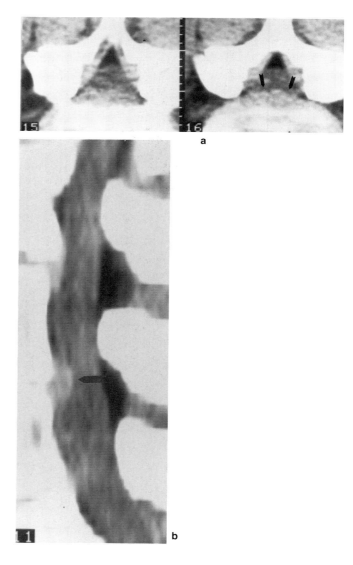

Figure 7–2c Sagittal reformatted CT demonstrating normal convexity of the annulus fibrosis at L5–S1 appears a lighter gray. Note that on the sagittal view one gets an accurate representation of the amount of extradural soft-tissue indentation on the spinal canal. A moderate bulge of the disc is seen at L4–5.

Figure 7–3 Axial (a) and sagittal (b) views on a patient with 5 mm of diffuse symmetrical bulge of the annulus. This patient has a relatively narrow spinal canal, which is considerably compressed by this diffuse annular bulge.

epidural fat surrounding the roots is very symmetrical. Even subtle asymmetry may be important (Figure 7–6). Occasionally, the displaced nerve root appears larger than its contralateral mate. This finding commonly correlates precisely with the patient's radiculopathy.

Gas is commonly seen within the lumbar disc spaces on routine lateral radiographs in both symptomatic and asymptomatic patients. This gas can also be seen on CT scans. Occasionally, bubbles of gas are noted beyond the confines of the normal disc space. For this to occur, there must be either displacement of the annulus posterior to the gas shadow or entrapment of gas in an extruded disc fragment. Sometimes a

sizable soft-tissue mass can be identified and associated with the gas, but quite often this is not the case. In surgery, the gas-filled bulging annulus can be punctured, which results in the audible sound of escaping gas. Gas protruding from the disc into the spinal canal may be an important sign of symptom-producing disc herniation (Figure 7–7, a–b).

Not all gas bubbles in the spinal canal come from the disc space. Nitrogen gas may remain in the epidural soft-tissue spaces for several days following epidural steroid injection, lumbar puncture, or any other invasive manipulation. These gas bubbles are frequently far from the disc space and are of no consequence (Figure 7–8).

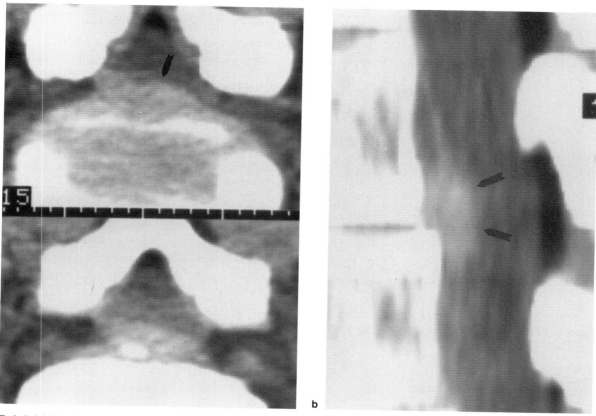

Figure 7–4 Axial (a) and sagittal (b) views demonstrate a large soft-tissue disc herniation. The extruded disc is higher in attenuation, and therefore, a lighter gray than the thecal sac.

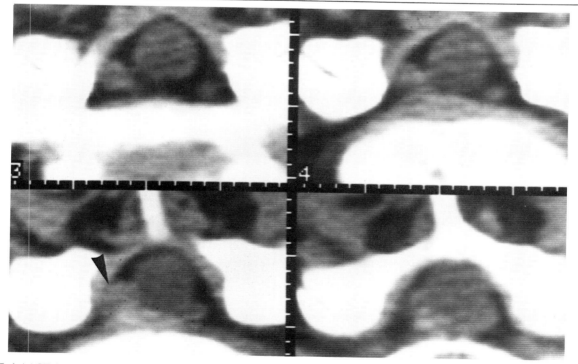

Figure 7–5 Axial CT demonstrating localized left-sided disc herniation. The S1 root is displaced posteriorly and is larger than its contralateral mate (arrow).

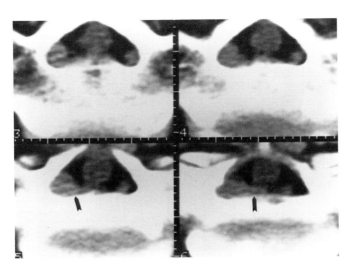

Figure 7–6 There is subtle asymmetry of the epidural fat adjacent to the S1 nerve root and an apparent difference in size of the descending roots.

DISC EXTRUSION OR SEQUESTRATION

Extruded disc fragments pose several unique diagnostic problems because the fragments may wander far from the site of annulus rupture. Often the fragment may lie tight within the lateral recess or may be tucked up underneath the pedicle. On axial-only CT, it may be difficult to determine from which disc space the extruded fragment originated because upward and downward migration occurs with almost equal frequency. The sagittal reformatted image will almost always show contiguity of the fragment with the involved disc space or separation of the posterior longitudinal ligament or annulus. On coronal views, thecal displacement and root asymmetry are easily seen (Figure 7–9, a–b).

The diagnosis of a migrating fragment is most easily missed when disc space-only axial CT is performed. Even the proponents of this limited examination acknowledge this limitation.[6] But this is yet another reason that a complete examination must be performed on all patients.

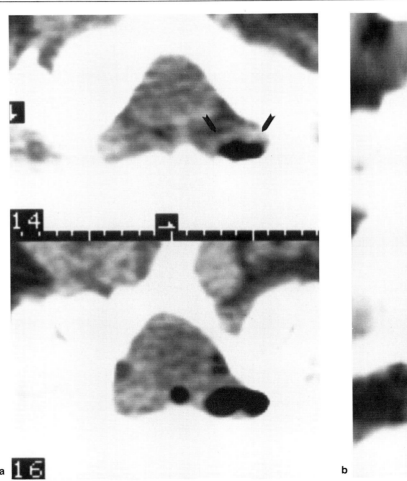
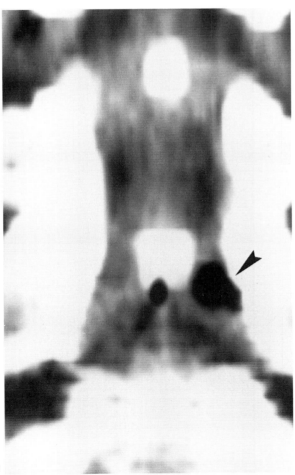

Figure 7–7 Axial (a) and coronal (b) views of a patient with a large bubble of gas extruded into the spinal canal (arrows). The disc herniation must extend posterior to the bubble of gas.

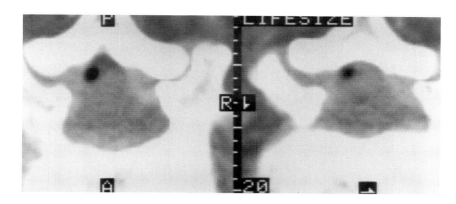

Figure 7–8 Gas bubbles posteriorly within the spinal canal. Remnant from an epidural steroid injection.

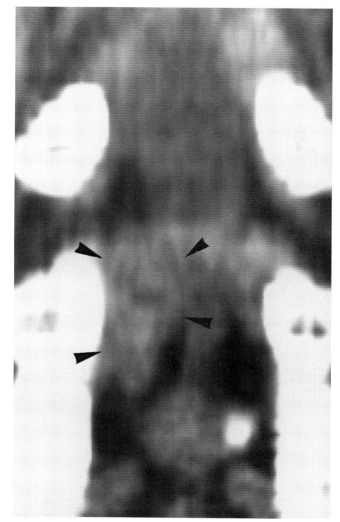

Figure 7–9a Curved coronal reformation of a patient with a large extruded disc fragment. Note displacement of the thecal sac away from a clearly demarcated, high-density disc fragment.

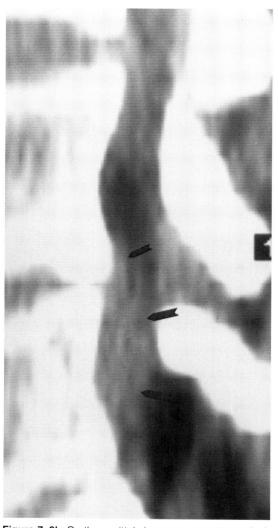

Figure 7–9b On the sagittal view, one can note continuity of the disc fragment with the L4–5 interspace (arrow).

Even nonmigratory fragments may be difficult to diagnose when they become very large. This seeming contradiction is evident in instances where the entire thecal shadow is oblit-erated by a huge disc fragment. It may be extremely difficult to decide whether the central canal shadow is a normal thecal sac or whether it is a disc fragment. In many instances these cases have been read on axial images as normal but subsequent myelography has shown a total extradural block. The problem is obviated by sagittal reformation on which the upper and lower extension of the fragment is always clearly visualized, as a distinct high-density shadow, very different from the normal thecal sac above and below the block (Figure 7–10, a–b).

LATERAL AND FAR LATERAL DISC HERNIATION

True disc herniation may occur laterally to the spinal canal, either within the neural foramen or lateral to the foramen. These two conditions pose unique diagnostic and therapeutic problems. In neither case will myelography show any hint of the abnormality because the afflicting mass is far lateral to even the most prominent dural root sheaths. The therapeutic problem occurs because the symptoms will relate to the nerve root exiting from the neural foramen rather than the disc space above.

An example of far lateral disc herniation is shown in Figure 7–11, a–d. The patient complained of pain in the anterior aspect of the right thigh and drew the illustrated pain pattern as part of his clinical history. The drawing and history conform to a radiculopathy of the L3 nerve root. Classical surgical doctrine would place the offending lesion at the L2–3 interspace rather than near the origin of the nerve root. The CT, however, clearly shows that the abnormality is within the neural foramen, one level below the expected site of abnormality.

Although they are quite uncommon, true extraforaminal disc herniations are significant because they cannot be diagnosed myelographically and produce symptoms one level higher than expected. It is important that the diagnosis be made accurately because a routine laminectomy stands no chance of allowing surgical exposure of the disc (Figure 7–12, a–b). Some other type of lateral approach would be necessary for removal of the offending fragment.

THE DIFFERENTIAL DIAGNOSIS OF DISC HERNIATION

Several normal structures and anatomical variants may, on occasion, be confused with herniated discs. In all patients, at least a portion of the epidural venous plexus can be identified. Vascular structures being of high attenuation may, on occasion, masquerade as sequestered fragments. Prominence of the epidural plexus tends to occur near the vascular pedicle of the vertebral body, and therefore, the interosseous venous channel immediately adjacent to the vessels makes the diagnosis obvious.

Conjoined nerve roots and other anomalies of the root sheaths and dura may also produce confusing shadows on the axial CT scans. Figure 7–13, a–b, shows a patient with asymmetry of the intraspinal structures. The nerve root on the left

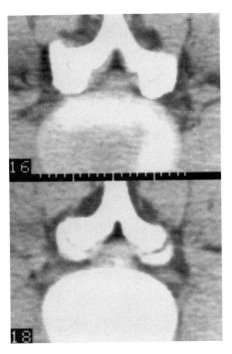

Figure 7–10a Axial CT demonstrates subtle high density within the spinal canal. The disc fragment nearly fills the canal but is difficult to identify.

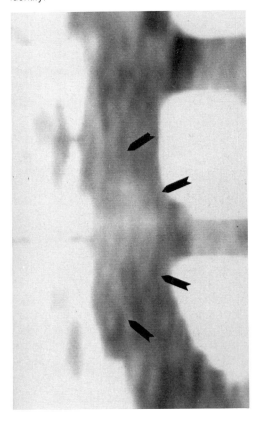

Figure 7–10b On the sagittal view note that the upper and lower extent of the huge disc herniation is clearly visualized.

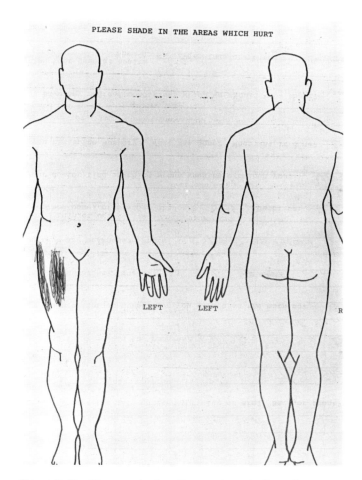

Figure 7–11a Diagram of pain pattern as drawn by the patient.

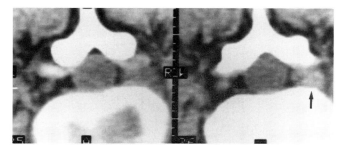

Figure 7–11b Axial CT demonstrating disc fragment within the right neural foramen.

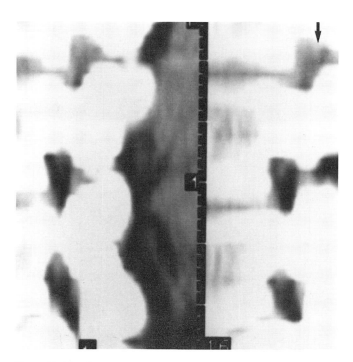

Figure 7–11c Sagittal reformation shows a large disc herniation in the foramen. Note the absence of fat at L3 compared to L4 and L5.

Source: Reprinted from *Multiplanar CT of the Spine* (p 126) by SLG Rothman and WV Glenn Jr, Aspen Publishers Inc, © 1985.

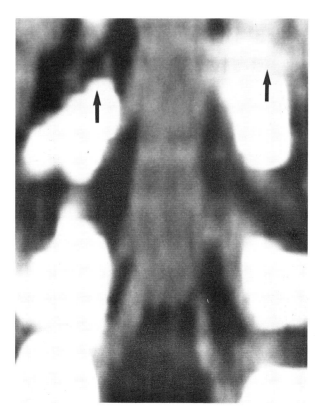

Figure 7–11d Coronal view. Note foraminal asymmetry.

side is surrounded by fat. On the right, there is a conical-shaped structure that appears to be contiguous with the theca. The epidural fat is asymmetrical. Does this patient have a disc fragment obliterating the epidural fat or nerve root sheath abnormality? While it is possible, with experience, to state that this particular axial picture represents a conjoined root, the differentiation from disc herniation is confirmed by the curved coronal reformation.

Note that in the conjoined root anomaly, the aberrant root pouch arises at a level between the two contralateral roots. On

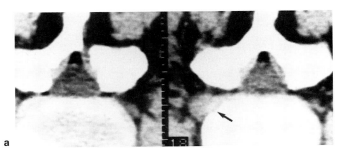

coronal scans, each of the exiting roots is clearly seen surrounded by fat. There is definitely no disc filling the spinal canal. It would be inappropriate to make the diagnosis of root abnormality on only a lateral myelographic film. Similarly, it is inappropriate to make the CT diagnosis of root anomaly on the axial view alone. Regardless of the modality, the diagnosis of conjoined root is made with certainty in the frontal plane.

Although extradural compression of neural structures in the lumbar spine is most often due to disease of the disc, one must

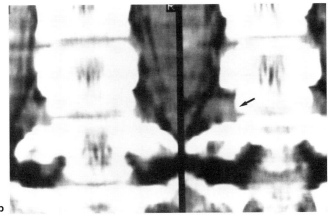

Figure 7–12 Axial (a) and curved coronal reformation (b) on a patient with an extraforaminal disc herniation (arrows).

Source: Reprinted from *Multiplanar CT of the Spine* (p 127) by SLG Rothman and WV Glenn Jr, Aspen Publishers Inc, © 1985.

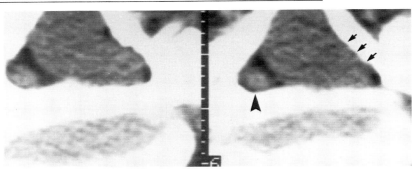

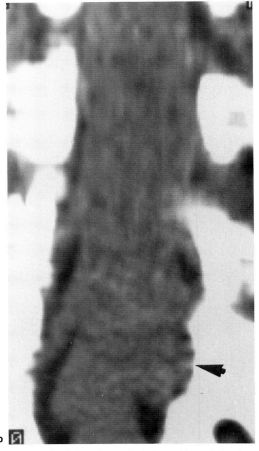

Figure 7–13 Conjoined nerve root. Axial CT (a) demonstrates a normal nerve root surrounded by fat on the left and a conical-shaped lucent structure on the right. Curved coronal reformation (b) demonstrates this to be a dural anomaly. Note its origin between the contralateral two nerve roots.

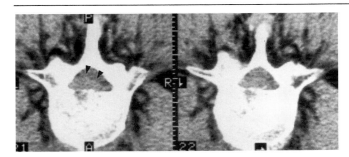

Figure 7–14a Axial views showing soft-tissue extradural lesion (arrow-

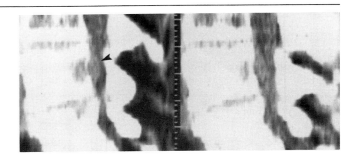

Figure 7–14b Sagittal reformatted image showing soft-tissue lesion in

always exclude other more ominous lesions. Figure 7–14, a–c, is a scan of a patient with radiculopathy. Note a soft-tissue extradural lesion that is nearly indistinguishable on the axial scans from a typical disc herniation. The sagittal view defines the position of the mass to be far from the disc space and to be associated with a pathological fracture of the vertebral end plate.

The differentiation of recurrent disc herniation from postoperative scar is considered to be very difficult. Various authors have suggested that in order to make this differentiation, intravenous or intrathecal iodinated contrast media have to be injected.[7] However, in the great majority of cases, this differentiation can be made on standard noncontrast CT when appropriate sagittal and coronal views are performed.

Key to this differentiation is the realization that a herniated disc is a localized foreign body that projects into the spinal canal. Its radiographic density is higher than the exiting nerve roots. When viewed in the frontal or lateral planes, herniated discs will have definable borders.

Postoperative fibrosis, on the other hand, is a diffuse interstitial process that insidiously replaces the epidural fat surrounding the theca and exiting roots. Its radiographic density is the same as the exiting nerve root and scar will not have clearly defined borders (Figure 7–15, a–b).

While it is true that in the axial plane the differentiation between a disc and a scar may be very difficult, diagnosis is usually obvious on the sagittal and coronal views. On the coronal images, a scar frequently extends over several vertebral segments. A scar also tends to engulf the exiting nerve roots and may extend out through the neural foramen. The thecal sac can be pulled toward the side of the fibrosis rather than pushed away from the side of a sequestered disc fragment.

On the sagittal view, one can almost always identify the normal annulus fibrosis because it is higher in attenuation than the thecal sac. The presence of a homogeneous intraspinal process and a normal-appearing annulus fibrosus excludes the possibility of a recurrent disc herniation.

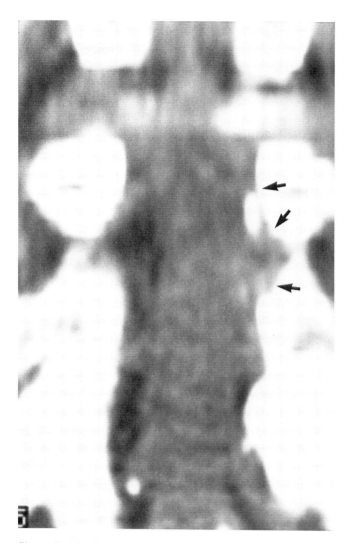

Figure 7–15a Curved coronal reformation on a patient with postoperative fibrosis. Note that the thecal sac is pulled toward the side of the low attenuation. Epidural fat is absent over a long segment (arrows).

Source: Reprinted from *Multiplanar CT of the Spine* (p 266) by SLG Rothman and WV Glenn Jr, Aspen Publishers Inc, © 1985.

THE DIFFERENTIAL DIAGNOSIS OF RADICULOPATHIC SYNDROMES

Nuclear herniation accounts for many, but not all, cases of lumbar radiculopathy. Recognizing those other anatomical abnormalities that may mimic disc syndromes or that may coexist with disc herniation is important.

Lateral Recess Stenosis

The lateral recess is a conical structure bounded laterally by the pedicle, anteriorly by the vertebral body, and posteriorly by the lamina and articular processes. Within the lateral recess the nerve roots exit from the thecal sac and begin their down-

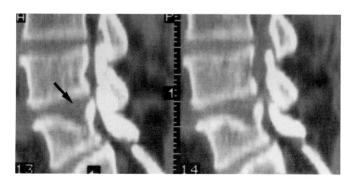

Figure 7–14c Both window sagittal images showing pathologic end plate fracture (arrow).

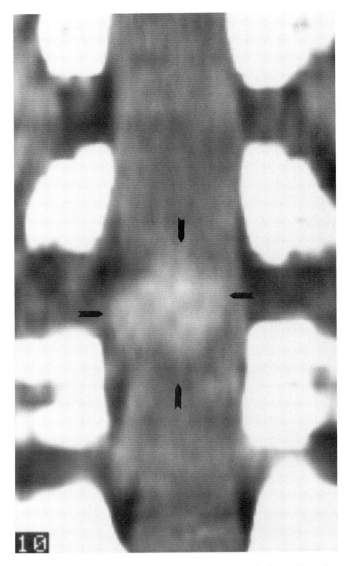

Figure 7–15b Patient with disc herniation, coronal plane. Note the high-density soft-tissue mass with clearly defined borders—the hallmark of disc herniation.

ward sloping extradural course toward the neural foramina. Compression of the nerve in the lateral recess is most often due to bony overgrowth of the articular processes in patients with congenital trefoil-shaped spinal canals.

The recess is divided into upper and lower portions. Neural compression in the upper third of the recess is due to overgrowth of the inferior articular process and deformity of the lamina at the higher disc space level, while neural compression in the lower one-third of the recess is due to bony overgrowth of the superior articular process at the lower disc space level (Figure 7–16, a–b).

This seemingly minor anatomical detail has major surgical implications. Radiculopathic pain resulting from compression of the L5 root in the lateral recess may, in fact, be due to

compression at either the L4–5 disc space level or at the L5–S1 level. A discectomy and facetectomy at L4–5 will therefore *not* relieve the recess stenosis in the lower one-third. An L5–S1 laminectomy will do nothing for nerve entrapment in the upper one-third of the recess. The anatomical deformity, which is best evaluated in the axial projection, must be described carefully in order to guide the appropriate surgical approach.

Neural Foraminal Stenosis

Compression of one of the exiting roots within the neural foramen may be due to bony ridges from the vertebral end plates, overgrowth and spurs of the articular processes, subluxation of the articular processes, periarticular soft-tissue swelling, or intraforaminal disc herniation (Figure 7–17, a–d). Symptoms of all of the above will relate to the nerve within the foramen. Surgery is, however, indicated one level

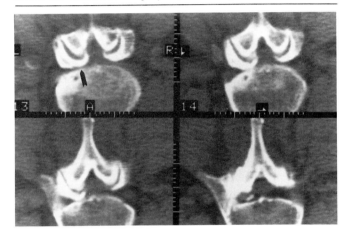

Figure 7–16a Axial CT scan demonstrating prominence of the superior articular process and compression of the lateral recess.

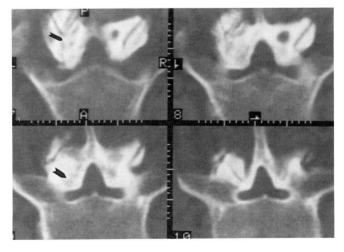

Figure 7–16b Compression of lateral recess resulting primarily from bony overgrowth of the lamina and prominence of the inferior articular process.

lower than one would expect if the radiculopathy were due to disc herniation. Because the exact cause of pain is now deter-

minable, surgical approaches have been described that are tailored to the individual abnormality.[8]

Extraforaminal Root Compression

Wiltse describes two special instances where the L5 nerve root is compressed between the transverse process of L5 and the ala of the sacrum. This occurs at the concavity of a degenerated scoliosis and in patients with severe spondylolisthesis. Wiltse terms this entity the far-out syndrome.[9] The surgical approach to relieve this radiculopathy is obviously different from all of the previously mentioned entities (Figure 7–18).

SUMMARY AND CONCLUSION

When properly performed, computed tomography provides the surgeon with the equivalent of a complete set of plain films, tomograms, and a myelogram for all but the intrathecal structures. Careful analysis of CT images in frontal, lateral, and axial planes permits the exact assessment of anatomical disc herniation and its consequences and all those anatomical abnormalities that may tend to cause poor surgical results. Careful preoperative analysis of the CT data will allow the surgical approach to be tailored to the cause of the patient's back pain or radiculopathy. Such an approach will greatly improve the treatment of radiculopathic syndromes.

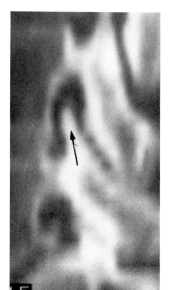

Figure 7–17a Neural foraminal stenosis resulting from subluxation of the facets with the inferior articular process of L5 herniated into the neural foramen.

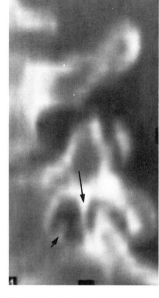

Figure 7–17b Foraminal stenosis resulting from bony overgrowth and ossification of the joint capsule and superior fibers of the ligamentum flavum, as well as bone spurs from the inferior end plate of L5.

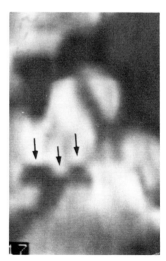

Figure 7–17c Neural foraminal compression resulting from horizontal orientation and callus from a spondylolisthesis.

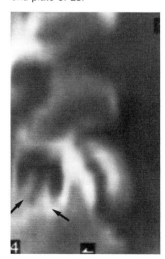

Figure 7–17d Bilateral railroad track bony spurs arising from the inferior end plate of L5 and the superior end plate of the sacrum.

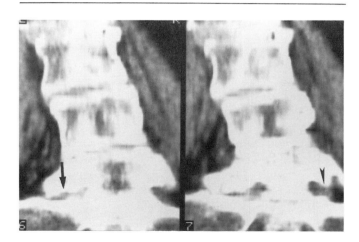

Figure 7–18 Curved coronal reformation demonstrating far-out syndrome. Note the compressed L5 nerve on the left (arrow) and the normal L5 nerve on the right (arrowhead).

REFERENCES

1. Rothman SLG, Glenn WVG Jr: *Multiplanar CT of the Spine*. Baltimore, University Park Press, 1985, pp 1–18.

2. Rothman SLG, Dobben GD, Rhodes ML, Glenn WVG, Azzawi YM: Computed tomography of the spine. *Radiology* 1984;150:185–190.

3. Haughton VM: *Intervertebral Disc Degeneration in Computed Tomography of the Spine*. New York, Churchill Livingstone, 1983, pp 23–38.

4. Bell GR, Rothman RH, Booth RE, Cuckler JM, Garfin S, Herkowitz H, Simeone JA, Dolinskas C, Hann SJ: A study of computer assisted tomography. *Spine* 1984;9:549–536.

5. Williams AL, Haughton VM, Meyer GA, Ho KC: Computed tomographic appearance of bulging annulus. *Radiology* 1982;142:403–408.

6. Teplich JG, Haskins ME: CT and lumbar disc herniation. *Radiol Clin North Am* 1983;21:259–288.

7. Teplich JG, Haskins ME: Intravenous contrast enhanced CT of the postoperative lumbar spine: Improved identification of recurrent disc herniation, scar, arachnoiditis, and discitis. *AJNR* 1984, 5:373–383.

8. Camp P, Kerber CW: Planning and performing spine surgery with CT/MPR: a primer for radiologists, in Rothman SLG and Glenn WVG Jr (ed): *Multiplanar CT of the Spine*. Baltimore, University Park Press, 1985, pp 293–307.

9. Wiltse LL, Guyer RD, Spencer CW, Glenn WVG Jr, Porter IJ: Far-out syndrome. *Spine* 1984;9:31–41.

Chapter 8

Contrast-Enhanced Computed Tomographic Scanning

Scott Kingston, M.D.

Computed tomography (CT) of the spine has become a mainstay in the evaluation of patients with diseases and related disorders of the spine. It has supplemented and largely replaced many of the older conventional diagnostic procedures. Its excellent contrast and spatial resolution allows the observer to examine the bony structures including all adjacent soft tissues that were difficult, if not impossible, to demonstrate on other radiographic examinations. With the information obtained on serial axial CT scan images, computer manipulation can display the data in a multidirectional format for viewing in the coronal, sagittal, or oblique planes (Figure 8–1).

TECHNIQUE

High resolution CT scanning can be performed with relative ease and comfort for the patient. A lateral digital scout view of the spine is obtained for means of localization and positioning. Either contiguous or overlapping 5 mm thick axial scans are obtained at 5 or 4 mm increments, respectively, when studying the lumbar spine. Thinner sections can be obtained for improved spatial resolution in certain instances but this prolongs the examination and adds an extra burden of heat build-up within the x-ray tube.

Since 95 to 98 percent of lumbar disc herniations occur at the L4–L5 and L5–S1 levels, the three lowermost lumbar disc levels are routinely examined. Of course, any site of concern can be examined by means of localization on the scout view. Other investigators have advocated scanning only through the disc spaces but incur the risk of not detecting an extruded or se-

questered disc fragment that might have migrated away from the disc space.

It is important to scan as parallel to the intervertebral disc space as possible. This sometimes necessitates tilting the scanning gantry in areas of excessive lordosis, particularly common at the L5–S1 interspace (Figure 8–2).

Once the information is acquired on the axial images, reformations can then be obtained in the sagittal, coronal, or oblique planes if needed. These reformations may offer valuable information to the surgeon but should not be relied upon solely since the spatial resolution is decreased in contrast to the data obtained on the original axial scans. These reformatted images may be helpful in evaluating compromise of the spinal canal in trauma cases where it is necessary to evaluate alignment of bony fragments (Figure 8–3) and soft-tissue masses (e.g., herniated nucleus pulposus, ligamenta flava hypertrophy, tumors) or in the postoperative patient. Oblique reformations through the neural foramina may also be helpful in evaluating for significant stenoses.

INTRATHECAL CONTRAST ENHANCEMENT

Although diagnostic information can be obtained from a noncontrast CT scan, it is sometimes advantageous to introduce a water-soluble contrast medium (e.g., metrizamide) into the subarachnoid space. This can be performed in one of several ways. A low dose (usually 4–5 cc) of isotonic metrizamide (170–180 mg/ml iodine) can be injected into the subarachnoid space via the lumbar or cervical route. With the

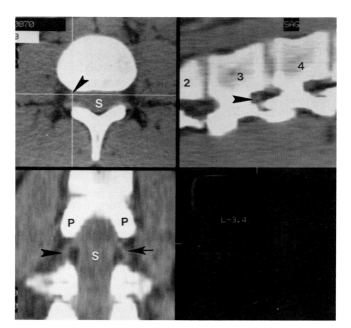

Figure 8–1 Computed multiplanar reformations. Axial (upper left), sagittal (upper right), and coronal (lower left) reformations are produced from the information obtained on the axial CT images. The white cursor lines allow any point in any plane to be imaged on the computer. The exiting right L3 nerve (arrowhead) is seen coursing below the pedicle of L3 through the neural foramen. Note the surrounding fat, which appears black on the CT image. The opposite L3 nerve (arrow) is noted on the coronal view.

patient in a Trendelenburg or reverse Trendelenburg position, the contrast can be pooled into the area to be studied. Prior to scanning, the patient is then rolled over several times to allow for adequate mixing of contrast with the cerebrospinal fluid

(CSF). Because of the low dose and concentration of metrizamide, the procedure can be performed on an outpatient basis. For those inpatients who are studied with metrizamide myelography, the same protocol can be used for mixing the metrizamide with the CSF; however, it is wiser to postpone scanning for at least several hours to allow further absorption of metrizamide and to ensure a more satisfactory concentration of contrast for CT scanning. The intrathecal metrizamide will result in an improved contrast resolution and ability to distinguish soft tissues of subtle density differences which may not be as apparent on routine noncontrast CT scans.

NORMAL ANATOMY

On the noncontrast CT scan, the dural sac appears round or oval and is of uniform density lower than that of the intervertebral disc. Following the intrathecal administration of metrizamide, the dural sac, spinal cord, and nerve roots are demonstrated with clarity (Figure 8–4) because of the difference in density between the metrizamide and adjacent soft tissues. The outline of the thecal sac is easily highlighted against the abundant anterior epidural fat and posterolateral ligamenta flava and facet capsules. The anterior internal vertebral venous channels and posterior longitudinal ligament are easily distinguished from the thecal sac following the instillation of contrast medium.

Typically, the intervertebral disc-thecal sac interface produces a smooth midline concavity or linear posterior margin (Figure 8–4). Variations at the L5–S1 disc level may include a flat or slightly convex margin. Alterations in the configuration of the disc's appearance on CT and secondary deformity of the dural sac should be carefully scrutinized in evaluating ·the abnormal disc.

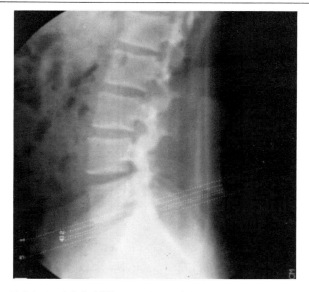

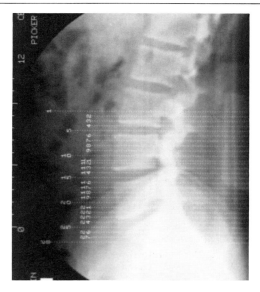

Figure 8–2 Lateral digital CT scout views of the lumbosacral spine. In addition to multiple overlapping scans from L3 to the sacrum, angled scans parallel to the L5–S1 disc space are obtained.

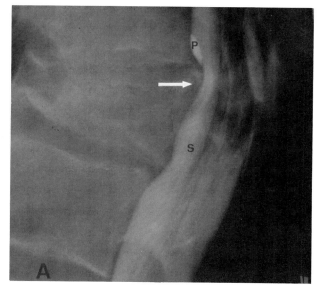

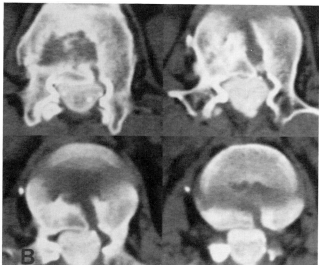

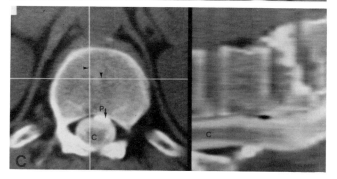

Figure 8–3 Thoracic compression fracture. (a) Conventional metriza-mide thoracic myelogram shows posterior displacement of the vertebral body compression fracture (white arrow). S is the thecal sac and P is the pantopaque droplet. (b) Precise relationship between the dural sac and the fractured vertebral body is well demonstrated on serial transaxial CT scans following myelography. (c) Intersecting cursor lines (arrow-heads) demonstrate how sagittal reformations could be obtained in any plane for a more thorough evaluation. C is the spinal cord.

THE BULGING OR HERNIATED DISC

In general, the different density of the intervertebral disc from the dural sac and other soft tissues results in different CT attenuation values. The scanner records this information and consequently constructs an image assigning various shades of gray according to these CT attenuation values.

Unfortunately, only the peripheral margin of the interverte-bral disc can be analyzed with respect to the disc-thecal sac interface, nerve roots, and epidural fat. This does not prevent the making of a correct diagnosis in the majority of cases. For instance, a bulging annulus fibrosus can be detected when there is a symmetrical concentric extension of disc material beyond the periphery of the adjoining vertebral body end plates (Figure 8–5). This often results in flattening of the ventral aspect of the dural sac or obliteration of some of the anterior epidural fat in the anterolateral recesses of the spinal canal.

A more focal asymmetric soft-tissue mass having disc den-sity would be more diagnostic of a herniated nucleus pulposus. In cases where there are subtle density differences between the disc and thecal sac, the intrathecal administration of contrast can be used for enhancement of the disc-thecal sac interface (Figures 8–6 through 8–8). This is often desirable in obese pa-tients since the CT-generated images are often "noisy" as a result of artifacts and result in grainy images with poor density discrimination of the soft tissues.

Following routine metrizamide myelography and CT my-elography, the acquired multiple transaxial scans can then be used in reformatting the images in the sagittal, coronal, or oblique planes (Figures 8–9 and 8–10). This allows the sur-geon to conceptualize the pathology in different perspectives.

In addition to the obvious deformity of the thecal sac result-ing from a herniated nucleus following metrizamide enhance-ment, the lumbar root sleeves should be carefully inspected for any signs of displacement or nonfilling, which may signify a subtle herniation not demonstrated on myelography (Fig-ure 8–11).

THE POSTOPERATIVE PATIENT

Following lumbar surgery, the degree of postoperative epi-dural fibrosis is quite variable. Some patients may demonstrate minimal scarring in the anterolateral epidural space from pre-vious discectomy while others may reveal exuberant fibrosis in the entire spinal canal encompassing the dural sac and com-pletely obliterating the normal epidural fat. The poor soft-tissue discrimination may completely conceal the location and outline of the thecal sac. In such patients, it is essential to perform CT myelography either following a conventional myelogram or a low-dose injection. Either case will suffice in highlighting the thecal sac. In certain instances, there is evi-dence of retraction of the thecal sac or nerve root adjacent to the soft tissue within the canal in the postoperative patient.

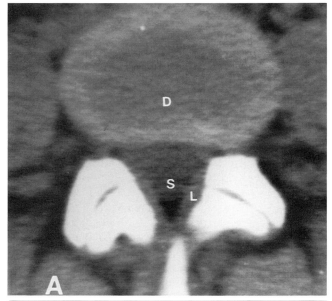

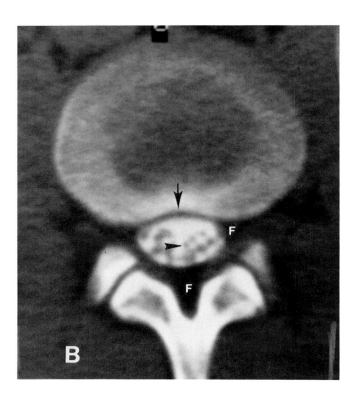

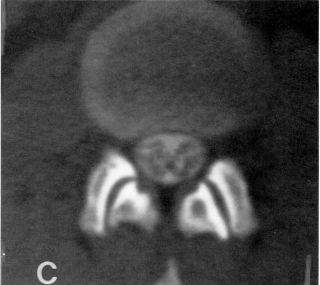

Figure 8–4 Anatomy of a normal lumbar intervertebral disc space. (a) Plain CT scan compares the higher density of the disc (D) with the lower density of the thecal sac (S). L is the ligamentum flavum. (b) Following myelography, a contrast enhanced CT image depicts the individual nerve roots (arrowhead) within the enhanced subarachnoid space of the thecal sac. Note the central concavity (arrow) at the posterior margin of the vertebral body. F is the epidural fat within the neural foramen and spinal canal. (c) Metrizamide enhanced CT scan showing the "spider" appearance of the tip of the conus medullaris with the adjacent nerve roots.

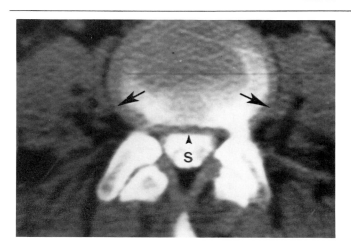

Figure 8–5 Typical appearance of a bulging annulus fibrosus with flattening (arrowhead) of the ventral aspect of the dural sac (S). There is symmetric extension of disc material beyond the margins of the vertebral end plates.

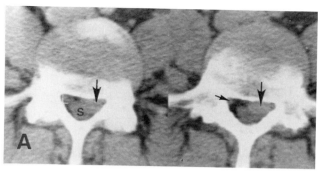

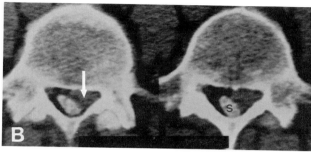

Figure 8–6 Plain and contrast enhanced CT scans demonstrating a large disc herniation. (a) Axial CT scans reveal a large soft-tissue mass (large black arrow) projecting posterolaterally within the spinal canal and extending inferiorly into the left lateral recess replacing the epidural fat. The mass is contiguous to the dural sac (S). Note the lumbar nerve root (small black arrow) on the opposite side surrounded by epidural fat. (b) After the intrathecal administration of metrizamide, the compression of the dural sac (S) is highlighted and is easily distinguished from the herniated nucleus pulposus (white arrow).

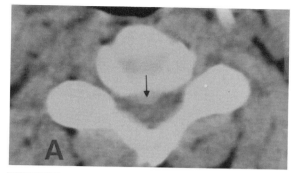

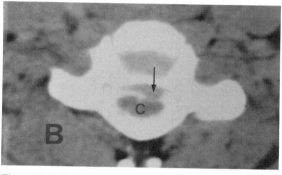

Figure 8–7 Two different cervical disc herniations. (a) Focal midline disc herniation. Note the higher density of the disc (arrow) compared with that of the thecal sac. Also note the paucity of epidural fat in the cervical area in contrast with the lumbar spine. (b) Metrizamide CT scan of a different patient reveals compression of the anterior subarachnoid space with minimal deformity of the left hemicord resulting from a herniated nucleus pulposus (arrow). The herniation is clearly highlighted with contrast in the subarachnoid space. (c) is the spinal cord.

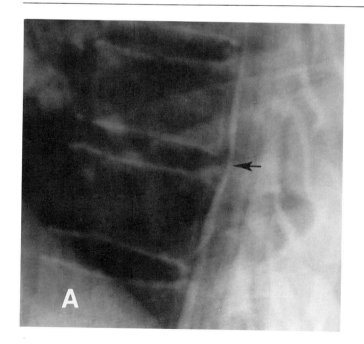

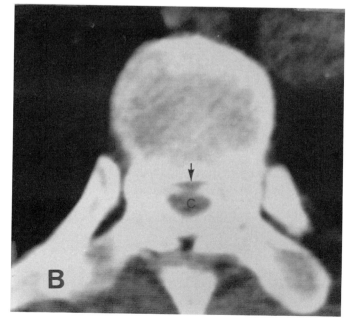

Figure 8–8 Thoracic disc herniation. (a) Metrizamide myelogram reveals a small ventral extradural defect (arrow). (b) A small disc herniation (arrow) is seen on the CT scan. There is compression of the anterior subarachnoid space but no deformity of the spinal cord (C).

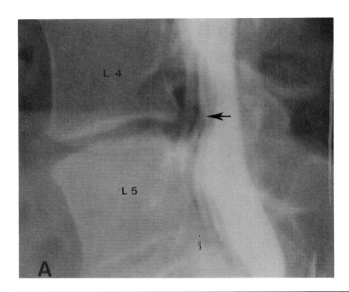

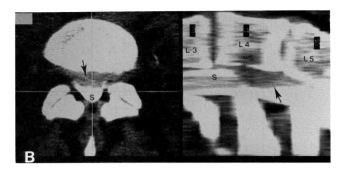

Figure 8–9 Metrizamide myelogram and contrast enhanced CT scan demonstrating a large herniated nucleus pulposus. (a) Myelogram shows a large L4–L5 disc herniation (arrow) that has migrated cephalad from the disc space. (b) Transaxial CT scan and sagittal reformation depicts the true extent of the herniation (arrow) above and below the L4–L5 disc space. S is the dural sac.

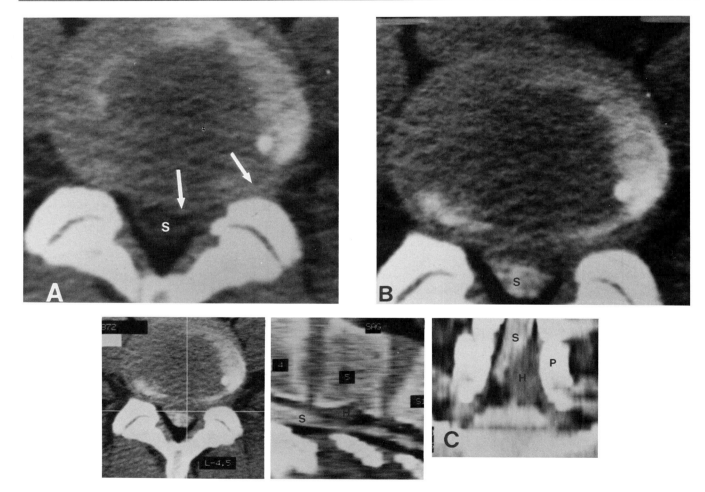

Figure 8–10 Large disc herniation with coronal and sagittal reformations. (a) Noncontrast CT scan shows a left lateral herniation (white arrow) with obvious deformity of the thecal sac (S) and extending into the neural. (b) Metrizamide enhanced CT scan demonstrates compression of the thecal sac to better advantage. (c) Transaxial (left), sagittal (middle), and coronal (right) reformations. Note the disc material extending caudal to the L4–L5 disc space and to the left of the thecal sac (S). H is herniation and P is the L5 pedicle.

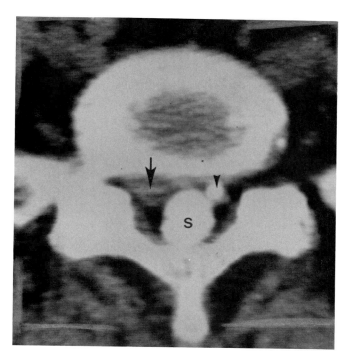

Figure 8–11 Nonfilling of the right nerve root sheath resulting from a posterolateral herniation (arrow). Note the opposite nerve root sheath (arrowhead) and thecal sac (S), which enhance normally with metrizamide.

This would indicate that epidural fibrosis is more likely a consideration rather than a recurrent disc herniation, which would be expected to produce more of a mass effect with displacement of the thecal sac or nerve root (Figure 8–12).

Certain CT scanners are equipped with a "blink" mode device for highlighting soft tissues with different densities (Figure 8–12). This method may be constructive in identifying other soft tissues within the spinal canal that may mimic disc herniations (e.g., prominent epidural veins, epidural fibrosis, neurogenic tumors, and cystic dilatation or diverticula of the lumbar nerve root sleeves).

NERVE ROOT ANOMALIES

The CT characteristics of the lumbar nerve roots are soft round tissues of homogeneous density with CT attenuation values similar to that of the thecal sac. In the "blink" mode, both nerve roots and thecal sac will normally blink simultaneously. For patients with a radiculopathy and unilateral enlargement of a nerve root, further evaluation can be obtained with CT myelography.

Conjoined nerve roots appear as soft-tissue masses larger than the expected size of a single nerve root (Figure 8–13). Because of potential confusion with a disc herniation, careful analysis with regard to the origin of the mass from the thecal sac and its course within the spinal canal and foramen will

disclose its true etiology. The absence of an adjacent normal nerve root on the same side as the mass, in conjunction with the mass splitting up into two smaller masses, should alert the interpreter to the possibility of conjoined nerve roots. Tracing the typical course of the exiting nerve root in its more lateral direction through the foramen with the caudal nerve root already within the subarticular recess would lend more support to the presumptive diagnosis.

In certain cases, it is necessary to perform a postmetrizamide CT scan for confirmation that the soft-tissue mass indeed represents a conjoined nerve root (Figure 8–14). Because the length of the conjoined nerve root sheath is shorter than the contralateral normal sheath, one may not expect enhancement of the entire soft-tissue mass especially distal to the takeoff of the more caudal nerve root. With interpretive expertise, this common anomaly should be readily diagnosed on CT and should not be confused with more serious problems.

Another consideration regarding an enlarged nerve root in the absence of any postimpingement edema is that of distinguishing between a neurogenic tumor or perineural cyst (diverticulum of a nerve root sheath). The latter entity is a normal variation and is of no clinical significance, but may appear more disturbing on plain CT. If the cysts become large enough, bony erosive changes of the subarticular recess or sacral foramina may occur and therefore simulate a neurogenic tumor. Intrathecal metrizamide definitively distinguishes these two entities since the benign perineural cyst accumulates the contrast and enhances on CT (Figure 8–15). Similar applications with metrizamide could be used for evaluating fluid density sacs adjacent to the thecal sac. Such examples include congenital meningoceles or pseudomeningoceles, if there has been violation of the dura in the postoperative patient.

MISCELLANEOUS

Computed tomography is undoubtedly more sensitive in its contrast and spatial resolution than conventional radiography. Its ability to reconstruct images in a variety of planes makes it highly desirable in situations where the etiology of the patient's symptoms is not apparent on routine radiographs.

Since CT requires only subtle differences in density to distinguish between various soft tissues, only a small amount of dilute metrizamide within the subarachnoid space is needed for demonstrating the thecal sac, which might not be otherwise visually apparent. Hence, in the case of a subarachnoid block on myelography, the extent of the obstructing lesion (e.g., fracture fragment, herniated nucleus pulposus, epidural hematoma, tumor, or bony stenosis) can be better delineated on the contrast CT scan (Figures 8–16 through 8–19).

In the rare patient with either a congenital or post-traumatic syrinx, the intrathecal introduction of metrizamide will not only enhance the subarachnoid space, but may reveal the syrinx within the spinal cord on delayed images (sometimes

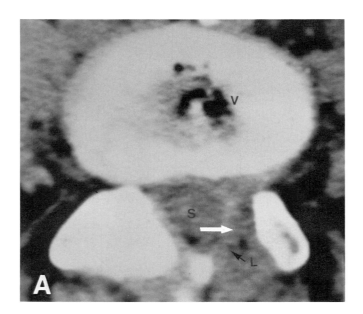

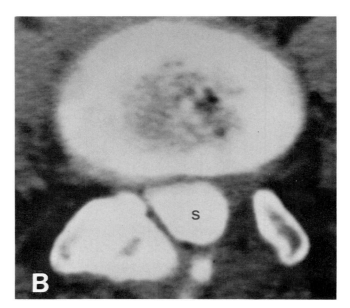

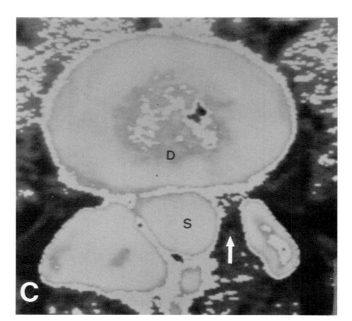

Figure 8–12 Postlaminectomy patient with postoperative scarring. (a) The left half of the spinal canal is filled with soft tissue (white arrow) encasing the left half of the dural sac (S). V is the vacuum disc and L is laminectomy defect. (b) Enhancement of the dural sac with metrizamide fails to show compression but rather retraction to the left because of epidural fibrosus. (c) "Blink" mode helps distinguish the intervertebral disc (D) from scar tissue (white arrow).

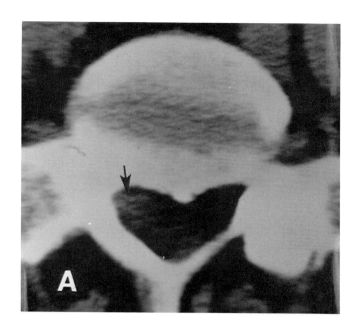

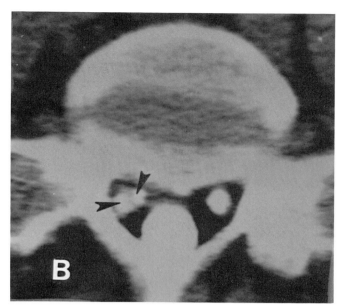

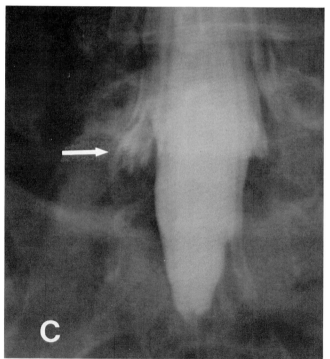

Figure 8–13 Conjoined nerve roots at the lumbosacral disc level. (a) A large right nerve root (arrow) is demonstrated on plain CT. (b) Following metrizamide myelography, a repeat CT scan shows both nerve root sheaths (arrowheads) to enhance. (c) Myelogram shows the conjoined L5 and S1 roots (white arrow) just below the L5 pedicle. Note the absence of an S1 nerve root in its normal location more inferiorly.

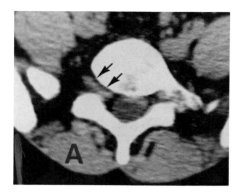 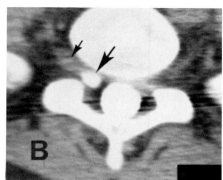

Figure 8–14 Conjoined nerve roots simulating a herniated disc. (a) High density soft-tissue mass (arrow) is seen within the right neural foramen. (b) There is enhancement of the medial soft-tissue mass (large arrow) with metrizamide. This represents a conjoined root of the right L5 and S1 nerve roots on myelography. The L5 nerve (small arrow) lateral to the foramen is not enhancing.

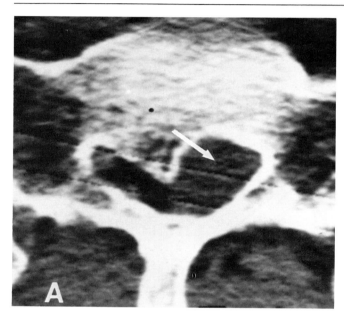

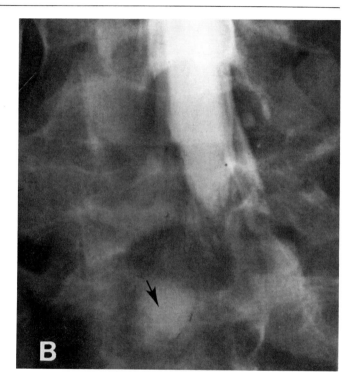

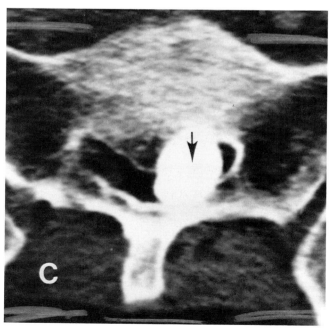

Figure 8–15 Perineural cyst simulating a neurogenic tumor. (a) There is a large soft-tissue mass (white arrow) causing bony erosion within the enlarged left sacral neural foramen. A neurogenic tumor was highly suspected. (b) There is faint pooling of contrast in the sacral area on the myelogram. (c) A repeat CT scan following the myelogram represents cystic dilatation of the nerve root sheath. The ability of the CT scan to perceive slight differences in density offers a definite advantage over conventional radiography.

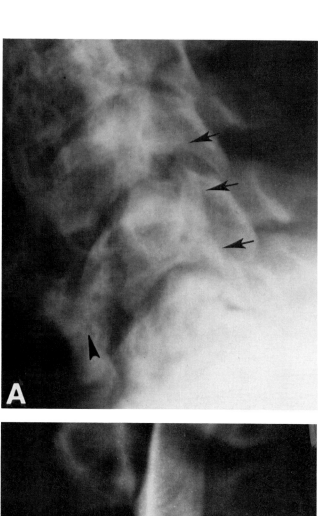

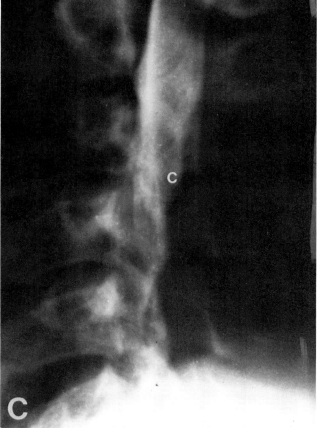

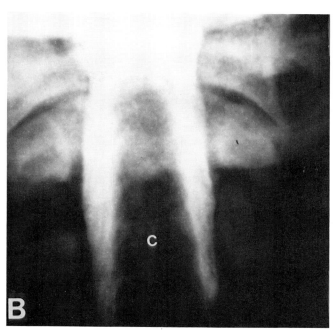

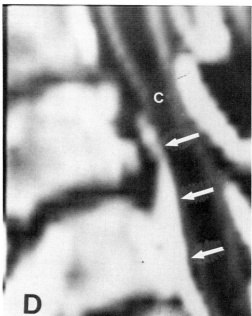

Figure 8–16 Calcified posterior longitudinal ligament (PLL) producing a high grade subarachnoid block. (a) Lateral view of the cervical spine revealing marked anterior bony proliferation (black arrowhead) characteristic of diffuse idiopathic skeletal hyperostosis (DISH). Heavily calcified posterior longitudinal ligament (black arrows) was noted in retrospect. (b) and (c) Apparent block on cervical metrizamide myelography. There is questionable widening of the spinal cord (C). (d) The true nature and extent of the obstructing lesion is displayed on these sagittal reformations of the cervical spine. Note that the spinal stenosis and apparent block is due to the calcified PLL (white arrows). Contrast is seen caudal to the site of obstruction on the enhanced CT image. Spurious widening of the cord (C) is due to compression in the anteroposterior dimension.

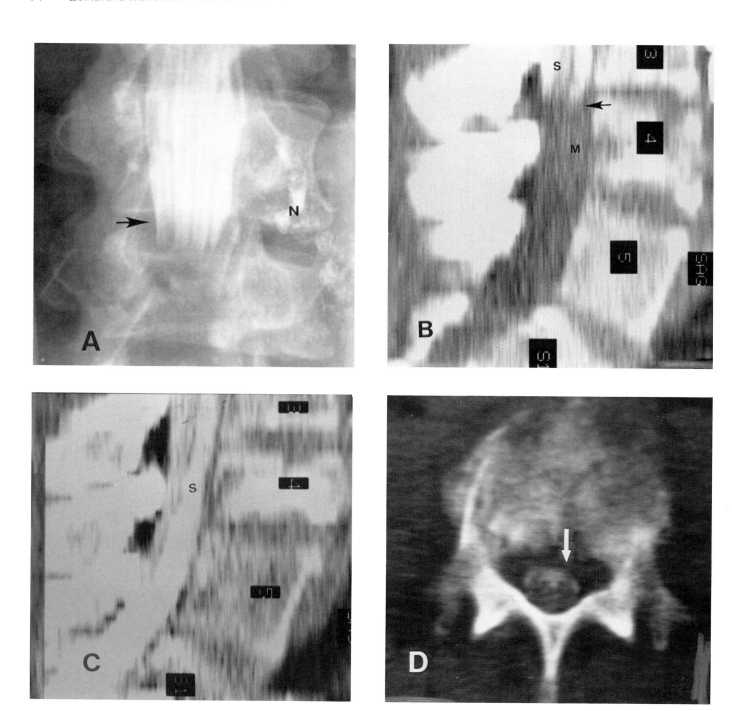

Figure 8–17 Metastatic tumor with complete subarachnoid block. (a) There is a complete block (large arrow) at the L3–L4 disc level. N is the opacified lymph nodes from lymphography. (b) CT sagittal reformation following lumbar myelography demonstrates destruction of L4 with a soft-tissue mass (M) within the spinal canal, which produces an extradural impression (arrow) on the thecal sac (S) causing the obstruction. (c) Although there is further loss of height of the L4 vertebral body, there has been resolution of the subarachnoid block on this follow-up CT myelogram following local radiation. (d) Transaxial CT scan on the follow-up study shows a more normal-appearing thecal sac and nerve roots despite residual tumor (white arrow) in the epidural space.

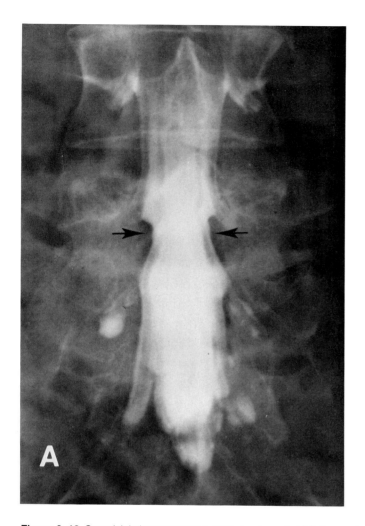

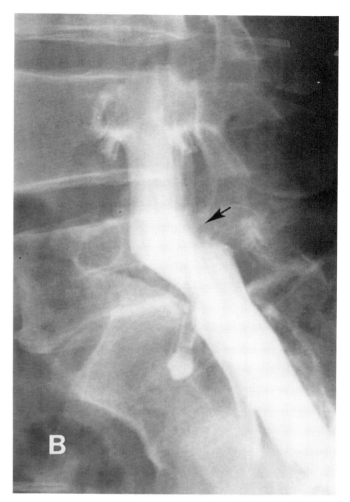

Figure 8–18 Spondylolytic compression of the dural sac. (a-b) Anteroposterior and oblique views of the myelogram demonstrate gross distortion with posterolateral compression (black arrows) of the dural sac. (c) Axial contrast-enhanced CT scan displays the relationship between the fibrocartilagenous soft tissues and ossific fragments of the pars defects (black arrowheads) to the dural sac (S).

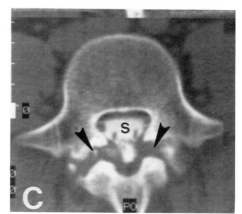

necessitating scanning 24 hours following the intrathecal metrizamide administration) (Figure 8–20). Sagittal reformations could then be utilized to demonstrate the cephalic and caudal extent of the cavity.

SUMMARY

The role of CT has grown considerably since its introduction in the mid-1970s and now plays a major part in the evaluation of patients with back pain and other disorders of the spine. Although the plain noncontrast CT examination can often be diagnostic, the intrathecal administration of a water-soluble contrast medium improves the diagnostic accuracy of dramatically highlighting the dural sac and adjacent nerve root sheaths. Of course, not every patient will require intrathecal contrast; however, if contrast enhancement is needed, a more efficient and comprehensive evaluation could be obtained with unparalleled diagnostic accuracy.

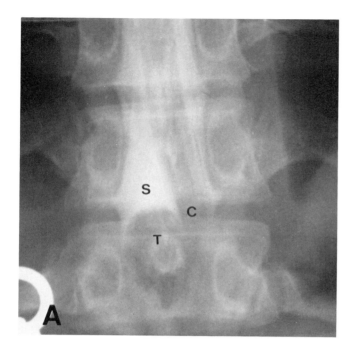
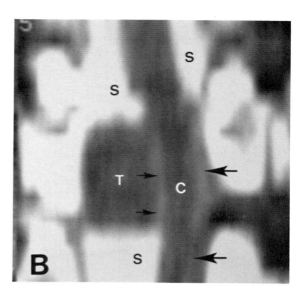

Figure 8–19 Delineation of an intradural, extramedullary tumor on contrast-enhanced CT. (a) Metrizamide myelogram demonstrates deviation of the lower spinal cord (C) to the left due to an intradural tumor mass (T). Note that contrast is within the upper portion of the dural sac (S) only and is not seen caudal to the lesion. (b) Delayed CT coronal reformation portrays the entire extent of the neuroma (T) surrounded by metrizamide within the dural sac (S). The deviated spinal cord (C) is surrounded by a thin rim of contrast (arrows).

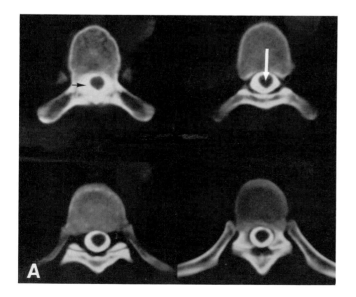
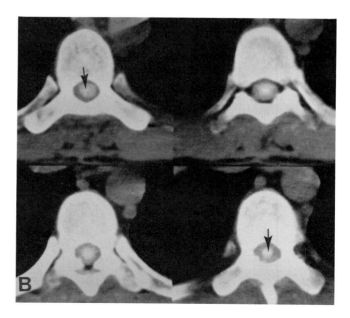

Figure 8–20 Demonstration of post-traumatic syringomyelia on CT. (a) Initial axial CT scans following myelography show abnormal enlargement and configuration of the lower thoracic spinal cord (white arrow) within the enhanced subarachnoid space (black arrow). (b) A large syrinx (arrow) is opacified on the delayed 24-hour CT scans as the cavity accumulates the contrast. The patient relates a past history of trauma that presumably resulted in spinal cord contusion and hematoma with subsequent cavitation and slow progression of weakness in the lower extremities.

BIBLIOGRAPHY

Aubin ML, Vignaud J, Jardin C: Computed tomography in 75 clinical cases of syringomyelia. *AJNR* 1981;2:199–204.

Ball MJ, Dayan AD: Pathogenesis of syringomyelia. *Lancet* 1972; 2:794–801.

Brant-Zawadzki M, Jeffrey, Jr RB, Minagi H: High resolution CT of thoracolumbar fractures. *AJNR* 1982;3:69–74.

Brant-Zawadzki M, Miller EM, Federle MP: CT in the evaluation of spine trauma. *AJR* 1981;136:369–375.

Brown BM, Brant-Zawadzki M, Cann CE: Dynamic CT scanning of spinal column trauma. *AJR* 1982;139:1177–1181.

Carrera GF, Williams AE, Haughton VM: Computed tomography in sciatica. *Radiology* 1980;137:433–437.

Dorwart RH, DeGroot J, Sauerland EK: Computed tomography of the lumbosacral spine: Normal anatomy, anatomic variants and pathologic anatomy. *Radiographics* 1982;2:459–499.

Dorwart RH, Genant HK: Anatomy of the lumbosacral spine. *Rad Clinics of NA* 1983;21:201–220.

Genant HK ed (1983) Spine Update 1984. Radiology research and education foundation, San Francisco.

Glenn WV, Jr, Rhodes ML, Altschuler EM, Wiltse LL, Kostanek C, Kuo YM: Multiplanar display computerized body tomography applications in the lumbar spine. *Spine* 1979;4:282–352.

Gulati AN, Weinstein R, Studdard E: CT scan of the spine for herniated discs. *Neuroradiology* 1981;22:57–60.

Harbin WP: Metastatic disease and the nonspecific bone scan: Value of spinal computed tomography. *Radiology* 1982;145:105–107.

Haughton VM, Syvertsen A, Williams AL: Soft tissue anatomy within the spinal canal as seen on computed tomography. *Radiology* 1980;134:649–655.

Haughton VM, Williams AL: *Computed Tomography of the Spine.* St. Louis, CV Mosby Co, 1982.

Helms CA, Dorwart RH, Gray M: The CT appearance of conjoined nerve roots and differentiation from a herniated nucleus pulposus. *Radiology* 1982;144:803–807.

Hirschy JC, Leve WM, Berninger WH, Hamilton RH, Abbot GF: CT of the lumbosacral spine: importance of tomographic planes parallel to vertebral end plate. *AJR* 1981;136:47–52.

Lee BCP, Kazam E, Newman AD: Computed tomography of the spine and spinal cord. *Radiology* 1978;128:95–102.

Naidich TP, McLone DG, Mutluer S: A new understanding of dorsal dysraphysm with lipoma (Lipomyeloschisis): radiologic evaluation and surgical correction. *AJR* 1983;140:1065–1078.

Post MJD, Green BA: The use of computed tomography in spinal trauma. *Rad Clinics of NA* 1983;21:327–376.

Shapiro R: *Myelography,* ed 3. Chicago, Year Book Medical Publishers, 1976.

Stratemeier PH: Evaluation of the lumbar spine: A comparison between computed tomography and myelography. *Rad Clinics of NA* 1983;21: 221–258.

Teplick JG, Haskin ME: Computed tomography of the postoperative lumbar spine. *AJR* 1983;141:865–884.

Teplick JG, Peyster RG, Teplick SK, Goodman LR, Haskin ME: CT identification of postlaminectomy pseudomeningocele. *AJR* 1983;140: 1203–1206.

Williams AL, Haughton VM, Meyer GA, Ho KC: Computed tomographic appearance of the bulging annulus. *Radiology* 1982;142:403–408.

Williams AL, Haughton VM, Syvertsen A: Computed tomography in the diagnosis of herniated nucleus pulposus. *Radiology* 1980;135:95–99.

Williams JP, Joslyn JN, Butler TW: Differentiation of herniated lumbar disc from bulging annulus fibrosus use of reformatted images. *J Comput Assist Tomogr* 1982;6:89–93.

Chapter 9

Magnetic Resonance Imaging of the Lumbar Spine

Bonnie Flannigan, M.D.

INTRODUCTION

Magnetic resonance imaging (MRI), a new diagnostic imaging technique, offers many advantages over other spine imaging modalities without sharing some of their disadvantages or hazards. Because it is a computer-based technology and produces similar cross-sectional images through the body, MRI has been compared with x-ray computed tomography (CT). However, it uses *no* ionizing radiation, is noninvasive, and imaging can be performed *directly* in any plane including nonorthogonal planes. Initially, MRI was felt to display the soft-tissue structures of the spine with increased contrast and resolution, but CT most elegantly displayed bone detail. However, MRI is being used increasingly for bone evaluation.

MRI involves interplay between radio waves and the hydrogen nuclei of the body in the presence of a magnetic field.[1] The patient is placed in a large magnet and following the pulsing of a specified imaging volume with a radio wave, a radio signal is emitted by the hydrogen nuclei within that imaging volume. This signal is detected by a receiver coil. With the aid of computer analysis, highly detailed images are formed. The intensity of the emitted signal reflects the density of hydrogen nuclei within the imaged volume and also two chemical parameters, which are called relaxation times T1 and T2. Both T1- and T2-weighted images can be obtained by varying imaging parameters (time between pulses, sampling time). The images are displayed in varying intensities of a gray scale. For example, fat is displayed as bright (high signal intensity) as compared with dense cortical bone, which is void of hydrogen nuclei and displayed as dark (low signal intensity or signal void). Muscle has an intermediate signal intensity and appears as a shade of gray. Cerebrospinal fluid (CSF) can be black or white depending on the imaging parameters. This is due to the intrinsic relaxation times (T1 and T2) of cerebrospinal fluid.

The patients are usually imaged in a supine position on a bed similar to that of a CT scanner. The bed is placed in a large body coil within the magnet. The body coil acts both as the transmitter and receiver of the radio wave signals. A surface coil can be substituted as a receiver coil, giving increased signal-to-noise ratio and increased spatial resolution. The surface coil is particularly valuable for fine detail of the lumbar spine. The patient must lie relatively still for approximately one hour. With newer technologies evolving, scanning times are constantly being reduced.

Early experience with MRI of the lumbar spine suggests it may obviate the need for myelography, x-ray CT, and/or discography. The ability to image the spine directly in multiple planes is superior to obtaining reformatted images with x-ray CT. Sagittal plane imaging of the lumbar spine allows evaluation of the intervertebral discs and MRI appears to be more sensitive to many disease processes including early disc degeneration. The avoidance of ionizing radiation and the noninvasive nature of the study are appealing to patients. Myelography involves hospitalization of the patient, and many untoward side effects have been described with the use of metrizamide. MRI combined with x-ray CT can often be substituted for myelography, thus saving the cost of hospitalization, as well as the adverse reactions.

There are certain limitations with MRI. Bone, calcifications, and cortical bone overgrowth (osteophytes) are not as well appreciated on MRI as they are with x-ray CT, with bone algorithms. Because of the paucity of hydrogen ions within bone, bony structures appear dark or as areas of signal void and can be difficult to define, particularly if they are adjacent to other dark structures such as cerebrospinal fluid. This problem can be eliminated by choosing the correct pulsing sequences. If the CSF is made white it will provide contrast between the CSF and adjacent bone spurs or degenerated disc material. Occasionally, large bony spurs will contain cancellous bone marrow (fat) and thus have a higher signal intensity.

MRI is contraindicated for patients who have cardiac pacemakers, intercranial clips, or metallic foreign bodies in vital structures including the eye. Patients have been safely imaged with Harrington rods and metallic hip protheses. Local artifact is present but is much less than with x-ray CT.

TECHNIQUE

Routine spine imaging is generally performed with a multi-slice spin echo (SE) pulse sequence in sagittal and axial planes. It is possible to obtain oblique axial images angled parallel to the disc spaces, similar to x-ray CT, with an angled gantry (Figure 9–1). Using this technique, simultaneous multiple angle slices can be obtained in one single sequence, thus being a time-efficient maneuver. By choosing different imaging parameters (repetition time and echo delay time) both T1- and T2-weighted images are obtained. T1-weighted images best outline anatomical detail and are identified by the CSF as being dark, whereas in T2-weighted images the CSF appears much brighter because of a higher signal intensity of the CSF,

producing a myelographic effect. T2-weighted images tend to enhance or accentuate pathology, particularly disc disease. T2-weighted images, however, require longer imaging times because of the longer repetition times (time between pulses) used.

Sagittal and parasagittal T1-weighted images of the lumbar spine demonstrate normal anatomy in Figures 9–2a and 9–2b with correlative cryomicrotome sections. Using T1-weighting, the cancellous bone marrow of the vertebral bodies containing fat is of relatively high signal intensity. The vertebral bodies are outlined by a thin, dark line representing compact cortical bone. The intervertebral discs are homogeneous in appearance and are of intermediate intensity. It is not possible to separate the nucleus pulposus from the annulus fibrosis with this pulsing sequence. The CSF is dark (signal void) and the conus and cauda equina are of intermediate intensity and thus outlined by the surrounding dark CSF. Parasagittal images (Figures 9–2c and 9–2d) demonstrate lower intensity nerve roots exiting under respective pedicles and surrounded by high intensity fat.

With T2-weighting, the discs separate into two components, the brighter nucleus pulposus and the surrounding dark annulus fibrosus. There is often a linear cleft identified within the nucleus itself.[2] Early disc degeneration is characterized by loss of disc height and a loss of the bright signal intensity within the nucleus pulposus. It is best appreciated on a T2-weighted image (Figure 9–3). Axial images (Figure 9–4) demonstrate normal structures with correlative cryomicrotomy. The dorsal root ganglia are identified bilaterally as fusiform swellings of intermediate signal intensity, exiting just under the pedicles and surrounded by the high intensity fat. The fat surrounds the thecal sac in a symmetrical manner as seen also in x-ray CT. Asymmetry of the fat is associated with pathology (i.e., disc disease, facet hypertrophy).

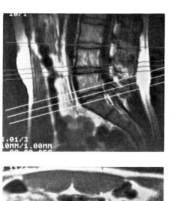
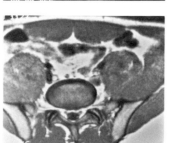
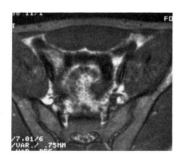
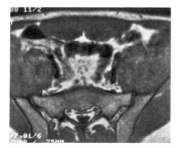

Figure 9–1 Sagittal scout view (upper left) with line cursors placed for acquisition of simultaneous multiple-angled, multiple-level axial plane images comparable to x-ray CT technology. Consecutive oblique axial images of the L5–S1 level are displayed. (SE 600/28)

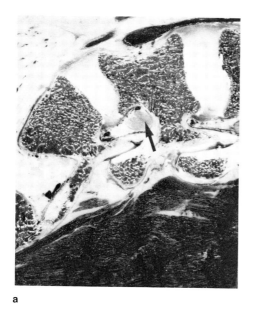
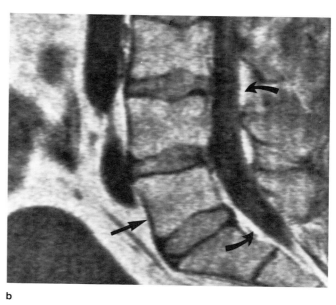

a

b

Figure 9–2a and 9–2b Midline sagittal crymicrotome section (a) and corresponding MR image (b) demonstrate the high signal intensity as a result of the epidural fat (curved arrows). The cancellous bone marrow containing fat (and hemastopoietic elements) within the vertebral bodies shows a relatively high signal intensity as compared with the dense cortical bone outlining the vertebral bodies (short arrow). The thecal sac filled with cerebrospinal fluid is depicted behind the vertebral bodies as an area of signal void. (SE/500/28)

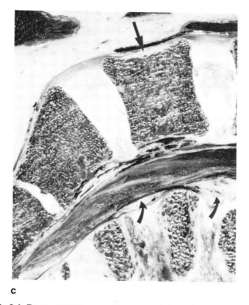
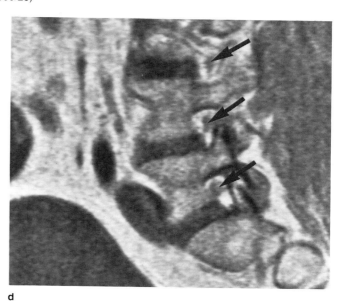

c

d

Figure 9–2c and 9–2d Parasagittal cryomicrotome (c) and corresponding MR image (d) demonstrate the lower-intensity nerve roots (arrows) exiting under the pedicles and surrounded by high-intensity fat. (SE 500/28)

The nerve roots can be seen at lower levels exiting laterally, again surrounded by the high intensity fat. The thecal sac is located centrally within the spinal canal and contains the dark CSF. The cauda equina are identified as layering posteriorly. Facet joints are demonstrated as is the articulating cartilage between the dense cortical bone of the superior- and inferior-articulating facets. The articulating cartilage has an intermediate signal intensity, as contrasted with the low signal intensity

of cortical bone. The ligamentum flavum is identified posteriorly and has an intermediate signal intensity.

MRI is advantageous in the imaging of pediatric patients and can be used as a screening technique to avoid radiation exposure. Excessive radiation from plain films, nuclear medicine scans, and other radiographic tests can also be avoided in young athletes who have repeated injuries requiring assessment.

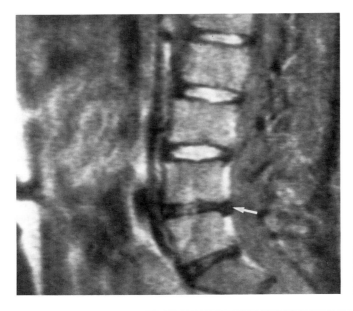

Figure 9-3 With T2 weighting (SE 2000/56) the nucleus becomes brighter than the surrounding annulus (upper three levels). Abnormal discs are demonstrated at L4–5 with a disc protrusion at L4–5 (arrow). CSF in the thecal sac has increased in intensity.

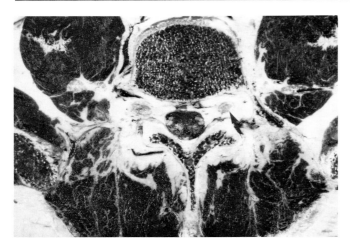

a

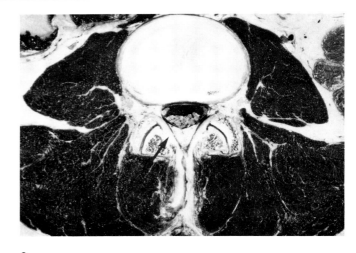

c

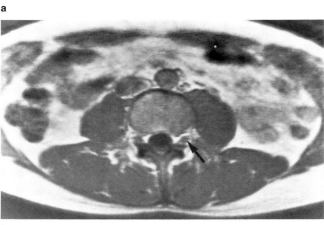

b

Figure 9-4a and 9-4b Axial cryosection with corresponding MR image (b) demonstrates the left dorsal root ganglia (arrow) surrounded by high intensity fat. (SE 500/28)

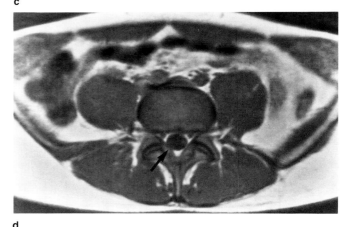

d

Figure 9-4c and 9-4d Axial cryosection and MR through the level of the facets demonstrates facet joints, ligamentum flavum (arrow) in the posterior spinal canal. Note the high intensity fat surrounding the thecal sac and nerve roots.

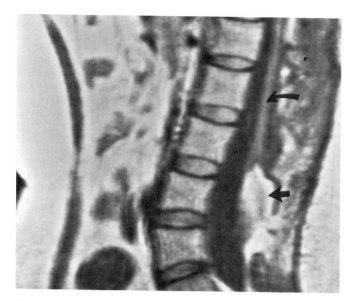

Figure 9–5 A tethered cord (curved arrow) is associated with a lipoma (arrow). (SE 500/28)

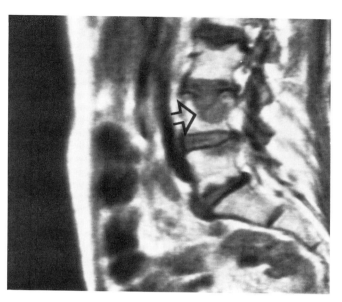

Figure 9–6 A focal area of decreased signal intensity is identified within the L4 vertebral body (arrow) in a patient with metastatic lung carcinoma. (SE 500/28)

Congenital malformations are well delineated, particularly in those patients with spinal dysraphism syndromes (tethered cords, lipomas, meningoceles, and diastematomyelia). These images can be invaluable for the surgeon planning for dissection of lipomas or closure of meningoceles. Myelography was performed reluctantly in the past for these patients because of the potential danger of anesthesia in the child. In addition, CT has not provided the necessary spatial resolution for defining the particular anomaly. MRI beautifully displays the pathoanatomy (Figure 9–5).

Primary and metastatic tumors are detected using MRI imaging. It is particularly well suited for the radiation therapist in detecting metastatic tumor blocks because of its direct sagittal plane imaging and because myelography can be obviated. Early experience suggests that MRI may be more sensitive to metastatic disease than nuclear medicine bone scanning techniques.

Several cases have been reported of patients who have had negative bone scans and abnormal MRI scans. If normal cancellous bone marrow is infiltrated with tumor tissue, the vertebral body demonstrates a decrease in signal intensity on T1-weighted images. This can be a focal, well-defined area of decreased intensity, an irregular area of decreased signal intensity, or it can involve the entire vertebral body as a homogeneous decrease in signal intensity often associated with a compression fracture. With T2 weighting, the area involved with tumor demonstrates increased signal intensity. MRI is particularly useful in patients with myeloma[3] where the bone scan may often be negative.

Figure 9–6 demonstrates the typical appearance of metastatic disease. It is often difficult to differentiate a metastatic compression fracture from an osteopenic compression fracture

in patients who have a malignancy and are osteopenic. The high signal intensity resulting from fatty bone marrow within the vertebral body is relatively well maintained in patients with osteopenia. However, in contrast, patients with metastatic compression fractures tend to demonstrate a relative decrease in signal within the compressed vertebral body because of infiltration of the tumor tissue into the bone marrow (Figure 9–7).

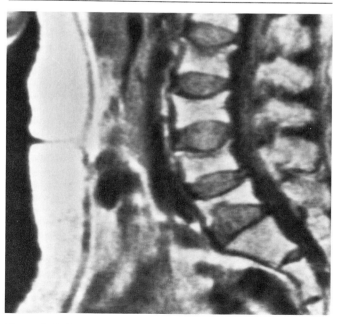

Figure 9–7 Compression of multiple vertebral bodies is present with preservation of the high intensity marrow in a patient with osteopenic compression fractures. (SE 500/28)

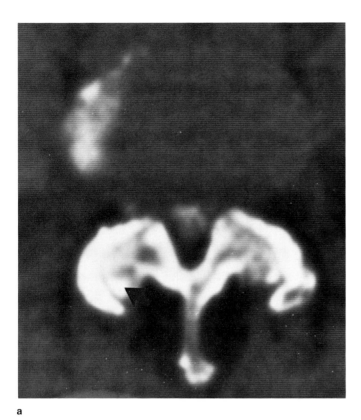

a

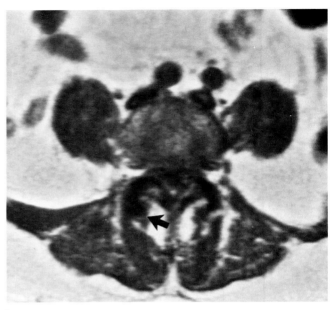

b

Figure 9–8a and 9–8b Hypertrophied facets are demonstrated on MRI (a) (SE 500/28) as areas of signal void (arrow) due to dense compact bone as contrasted with CT (b) where bone is white.

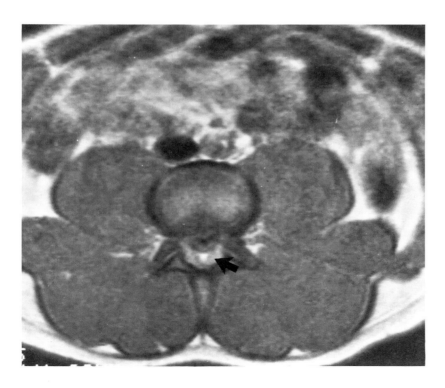

Figure 9–9 The ligamentum flavum is hypertrophied (arrow) in a young weightlifter with spinal stenosis. (SE 500/28)

MRI has been shown to be sensitive in the evaluation of vertebral osteomyelitis and discitis.[2,4] In osteomyelitis and discitis, the disc and the vertebral bodies above and below demonstrate a marked increase in signal intensity with T2 weighting. The normal internuclear cleft is often obliterated.[2,4]

MRI can be a useful diagnostic tool in the patient with "discogenic pain." Very early disc degeneration is recognized by a decrease in signal intensity on sagittal T2-weighted images as compared with adjacent normal disc levels. Often, the decreased disc height and decreased signal intensity of the disc itself is associated with either a focal or diffuse posterior disc protrusion.[5,7] Nerve root impingement can be diagnosed on parasagittal or axial images. Although bony changes are often better appreciated with x-ray CT, similar findings are identified with MR imaging as demonstrated in Figure 9–8.

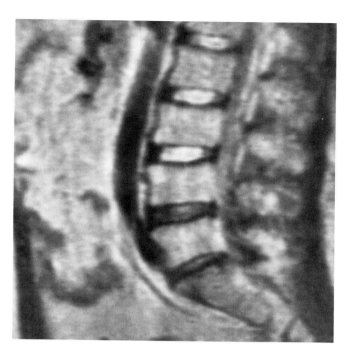

Figure 9–10b Similar findings are demonstrated with MRI where L4–5 and L5–S1 have a diminished signal intensity with disc protrusion. (SE 2000/56)

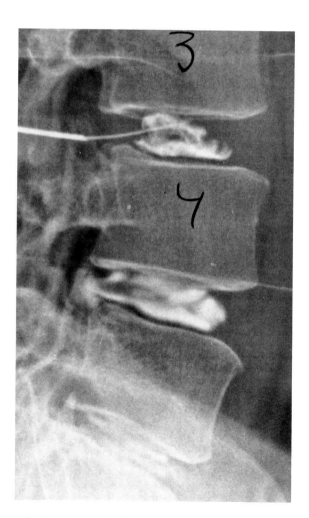

Figure 9–10a A three-level discogram demonstrates a normal disc at the L3–4 level and abnormal discs at L4–5 and L5–S1.

By recognizing the bony structures as being black or relatively dark and the fat as higher in signal intensity one can appreciate encroachment on the spinal canal and the neural foramina. Ligamentum flavum hypertrophy is demonstrated in Figure 9–9 in a patient with spinal stenosis.

MRI is helpful in preoperative planning, specifically in patients undergoing spinal fusion. With the use of sagittal T2-weighted MR imaging, the discs above and below the level of planned fusion can be evaluated for early degeneration and thus help direct a surgical plan of approach. If the discs above and below demonstrate a normal MRI intensity, discography can be avoided. Early experience[6] indicates that a normal disc on MR imaging correlates highly with a normal radiographic discogram study.[8] If the adjacent discs are of abnormal signal intensity, one can assume early degeneration and predict an abnormal radiographic discogram appearance (Figure 9–10).

In conclusion, with further advances in technology including shorter scanning times, thinner sections, and increased spatial resolution, MRI will become the clinical tool of choice for many patients with lumbar spine symptomatology. Its non-invasive nature, multiplanar capabilities, and the lack of ionizing radiation are particularly desirable for both the patient and physician.

REFERENCES

1. Bradley WG, Crooks LE, Newton TH: Physical principles of nuclear magnetic resonance, *Modern neuroradiology advanced imaging techniques.* in Newton TH and Potts DG: II. San Francisco, Clavadel Press, 1983, chap 3.

2. Modic MT, Pavlicek W, Weinstein MA, et al: Magnetic resonance imaging of intervertebral disk disease: Clinical and pulse sequence considerations. *Radiology* 1984;152:103–111.

3. Daffner RH, Lupetin AR, Dash N, et al: MRI in the detection of malignant infiltrations of bone marrow. *AJR* 1986;146:353–358.

4. Modic MT, Weinstein MA, Pavlicek W, et al: Nuclear magnetic resonance imaging of the spine. *Radiology* 1983;148:757–762.

5. Chafetz NI, Genant HK, Moon KL, Helms CA, Morris JM: Recognition of lumbar disk herniation with NMR. *AJNR* 1984;5:23–26; *AJR* 1983; 141:1153–1156.

6. Han JS, Kaufman B, El Yousef SJ, et al: NMR imaging of the spine. *AJNR* 1983;141:1137–1145.

7. Edelman RR, Shoukimas GM, Stark DD, et al: High-resolution surface-coil imaging of lumbar disk disease. *AJR* 1985;144:1123–1129.

8. Flannigan B, Schneideman G, Watkins R: Correlation of MRI and discography in the evaluation of patients undergoing spinal fusion. Submitted to *Radiology.*

Chapter 10

Myelography

Paul M. Duchesneau, M.D.

CONTRAST MEDIA

There are currently only two contrast media available for myelography that have been approved by the U.S. Food and Drug Administration. These are iophendylate (Pantopaque, Lafayette) and metrizamide (Amipaque, Winthrop).

Iophendylate

Iophendylate is often referred to as "oil based" because of its oily appearance and high viscosity. It has an iodine content of 30 percent, which renders it readily visible at fluoroscopy and on x-rays even in large patients or when traversing thick parts such as shoulders and pelvis. Since it does not mix with the spinal fluid, the iodine concentration, and therefore the visibility, are unchanged when the contrast material is moved from one region of the subarachnoid space to the other.

Another advantage is its very low neurotoxicity. The passage of iophendylate is usually not appreciated by the patient, even if it is allowed to enter the posterior fossa. If the contrast material is inadvertently spilled into the anterior fossa, however, most patients will experience retro-orbital pain.

It has also been frequently noted that the passage of iophendylate through the subarachnoid space is not only felt but complained about in patients with active demyelinating disease of the cord.

The major disadvantage of iophendylate use is the risk of late development of arachnoiditis, a crippling disease with no cure. In 1978 the records were reviewed of all patients who came in for repeat myelography in the prior 36 months for various complaints. Ninety-one patients in this series had previous myelography with iophendylate and repeat myelography with metrizamide. All 22 patients who had had surgery in the interim, and whose dura had been opened, had developed epidural scarring and arachnoiditis (Figure 10–1).

It has been demonstrated repeatedly, in animal experiments and human subjects, that there is a very high incidence of arachnoiditis development when iophendylate is mixed with blood in the subarachnoid space. It might be tempting to assume that it would be safe to use this material if the cerebrospinal fluid (CSF) were seen to be clear at the time of lumbar puncture for myelography. Unfortunately, too often the blood does not appear until near the end of the iophendylate removal; by then, it is too late.

For many years, steroids (Depo-medrol, Upjohn) were given intrathecally as prophylaxis against development of postmyelographic arachnoiditis, even when no blood was present. In several review cases, it was found that all such patients who underwent repeat myelography had in fact developed mild to moderate arachnoiditis, in spite of the use of steroids (Figure 10–2). On the contrary, those who had had no bleeding, and who were given no steroid (16 patients), were the only ones who had not developed any arachnoiditis whatsoever. It appears that anything at all mixed with iophendylate and spinal fluid will incite development of arachnoiditis, whether blood, steroids, or even air (open dura).

A more minor disadvantage of the use of iophendylate is that the high viscosity requires the use of fairly large gauge needles for ease of injection and removal. This requires close attention to prevention of postspinal puncture headache. Most myelographers are convinced that the severity and duration of

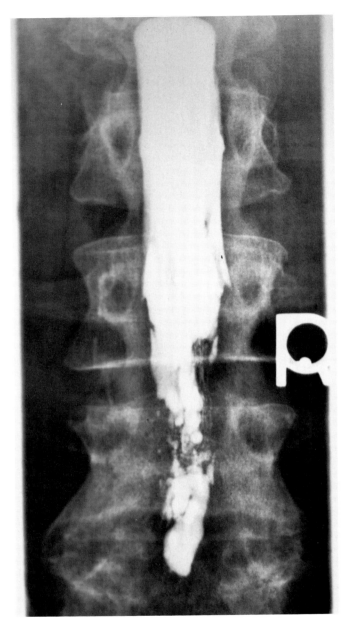

Figure 10–1 Epidural scarring—dura was opened at the time of surgery.

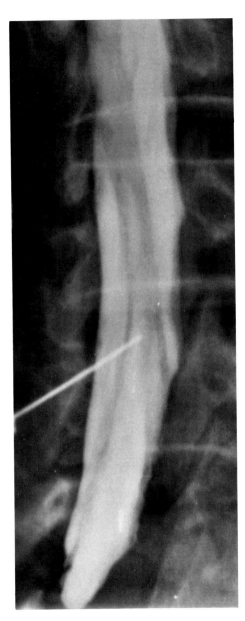

Figure 10–2 Arachnoiditis—nerve roots adherent to each other, without epidural scarring. "Prophylactic" Depo-Medrol given at time of normal atraumatic myelogram.

these headaches are directly related to the total amount of spinal fluid lost during and after myelography. If the patient is allowed to be upright before most of this fluid has been replaced, "spinal" headaches will develop.

The amount of fluid removed at the time of myelography should be limited to the minimum required for those laboratory examinations deemed necessary. The lumbar puncture needle should be oriented with its blade along the long axis of the body, so that it slips between the longitudinal fibers of the dura, rather than cutting across them. This will ensure that the

needle hole in the dura closes promptly after withdrawal, thus reducing subsequent leakage of spinal fluid.

One further minor disadvantage that is sometimes attributed to iophendylate is its very high opacity to x-rays. It is more difficult to see cord, nerve roots, and other structures through the iophendylate column than through a column of water-soluble material. This drawback can usually be eliminated by using a higher kilovoltage for penetration and tight coning of the x-ray beam to prevent underexposure due to scatter from surrounding structures.

Metrizamide

Metrizamide is a water-soluble nonionic contrast medium of low viscosity, freely miscible with spinal fluid. It is used in concentrations of 17 to 30 percent. The low viscosity permits the use of a very small needle for injection into the sub-arachnoid space. This reduces the incidence of spinal head-aches resulting from postpuncture leakage; the amount removed for laboratory tests should still be kept to a minimum.

The water solubility of the medium allows free absorption into the blood stream and excretion by the kidneys. Adequate hydration before and after myelography will help reduce the concentration in the blood, which will minimize systemic effects via the blood stream. Toxic effects, resulting from direct contact with the brain, follow promptly after diffusion up the subarachnoid space because of recumbency and phys-ical activity. Both direct contact and blood-borne effects are definitely dose-related, with fewer and milder side effects, the smaller the amount used.

The most common side effects are headache, nausea, and vomiting, which in most series occur in nearly half of the patients when the maximum dose of three grams is used. These side effects usually occur from one to six hours following the myelogram, after the patient has returned to his or her room. Seizure activity, although rarely observed, usually occurs even later, often the morning after the myelogram. Computed tomography (CT) of the head done at this time is striking in its demonstration of enhancement of the cerebral cortex by the metrizamide (Figure 10–3).

Side effects can be reduced to nearly zero with small enough doses of metrizamide. Side effects are almost nonex-

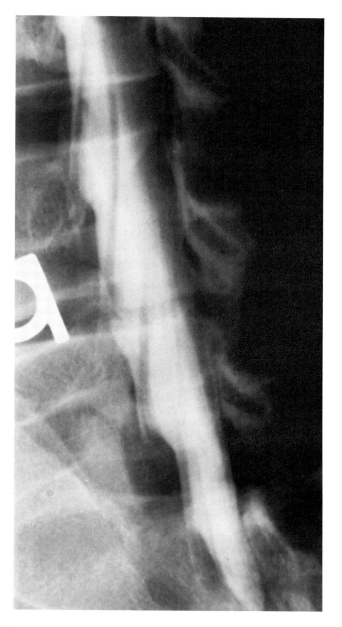

Figure 10–4 Cross-table lateral with small bottle of metrizamide.

istent when the amount used is just enough to opacify the subarachnoid space for CT of the cord or posterior fossa (4 ml of 190 mg/ml). If the clinician needs to see only which nerve root is involved by a disc protrusion, a *radiculogram* rather than a myelogram may suffice. The radiculogram can be performed with little more than the above dose in a cooperative patient. It is done by slow injection to prevent mixing, and with cross-table oblique views. These views will demonstrate the emerging nerve roots on the dependent side as they extend down in the most concentrated portion of the metrizamide (Figure 10–4).

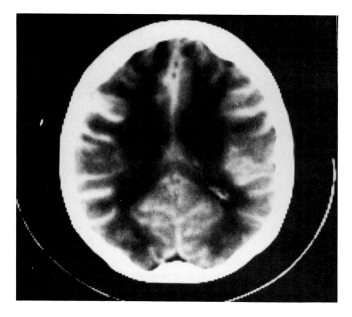

Figure 10–3 CT head 18 hours after myelogram with large bottle of metrizamide.

A minor advantage of metrizamide over iophendylate is its low iodine content. It is thus easier to "see through" the contrast material to demonstrate cord, nerves, and other structures. This same low concentration can be a disadvantage, however, in trying to demonstrate the metrizamide column in heavy patients or through thick parts such as the pelvis or shoulder. The fact that the metrizamide mixes readily with the spinal fluid also makes the examination technically more difficult. All required images must be obtained before the metrizamide mixes and becomes too dilute to be seen. This is especially difficult if a "complete" myelogram involves moving the contrast to the neck following lumbar puncture (or the reverse).

Two more minor disadvantages of metrizamide are the high cost and the fact that it must be freshly mixed prior to each use. The newer water-soluble media, soon to be available, will be heat-stable, and can be marketed in ready-mixed forms. The cost will be considerably less then metrizamide. Most important, of course, is that nearly all of the new media now undergoing clinical trials appear to have neurotoxicity of only one-half to one-third that of metrizamide.

Inevitably, the subject of "contrast allergy" arises in patients who have a history of reaction to contrast material. Most often, reactions occur after intravenous injections for urogram. Sometimes the clinician has told the patient he or she cannot have a myelogram. Other times the radiologist is asked whether the patient should have a "steroid prep" prior to the myelogram because of the previous "allergic" episode. Fortunately, such reactions do not occur with myelography with either iophendylate or metrizamide. In many thousands of myelograms performed at the Cleveland Clinic over the past 24 years, a reaction to the contrast material has never been observed that could be considered "allergic," regardless of a prior history of reaction to an intravenously administered contrast agent.

X-RAY FINDINGS IN LUMBAR DISC DISEASE

Most patients sent for myelography for lumbar disc disease are referred because of sciatica or at least back pain plus some symptoms in a lower extremity. It is good practice to review the lumbar spine films and the patient's chart prior to myelography. This will help decide whether the x-ray findings and the clinically abnormal levels coincide, or whether more than one level may be involved. The x-rays may show evidence of a lesion, other than disc disease, not previously suspected. Tumors of bone, whether primary or metastatic, are often found in this manner (Figures 10–5 and 10–6).

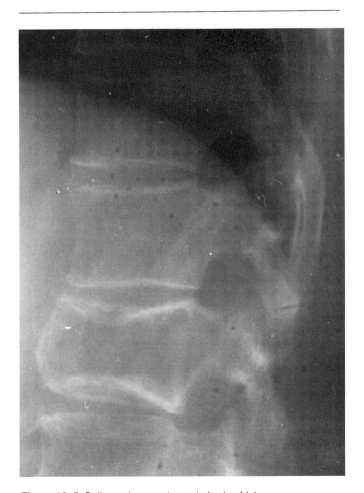

Figure 10–5 Solitary plasmacytoma, in body of L1.

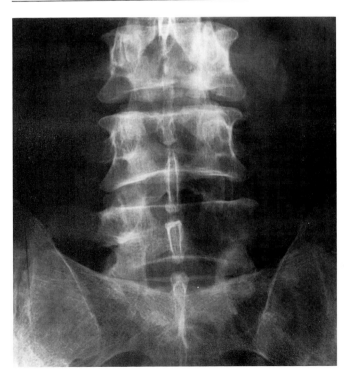

Figure 10–6 Lytic metastasis to left side of L5.

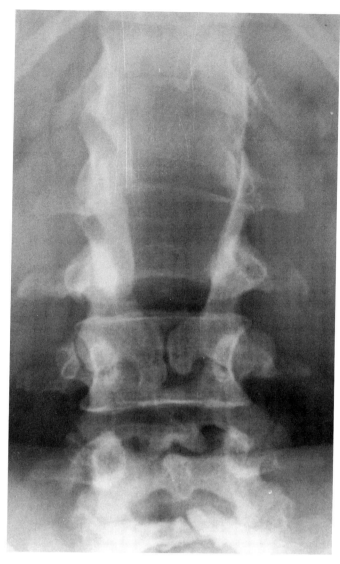

Figure 10–7 Enlarged posterior arch with concave medial borders of pedicles resulting from intraspinal lipoma.

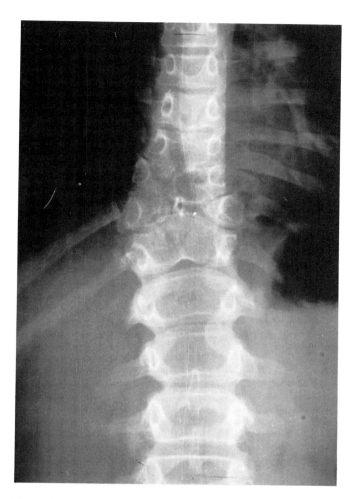

Figure 10–8 Wide separation of normally shaped pedicles at level of diastematomyelia.

Also, because lesions presenting as sciatica may occur above the lumbar region, review of the thoracic spine films may sometimes be of benefit. The films may show the scalloped posterior vertebral bodies of an intraspinal tumor (Figure 10–7) or the classic widely spaced pedicles at the level of a diastematomyelia (Figure 10–8). Review of the x-rays before myelography may show a level or levels to be avoided by the needle. In a severely degenerated spine, it may show the only gap between spinous processes or laminae where a needle can be inserted (Figure 10–9).

Inspection of the lateral view of a normal lumbar spine will show increasing height of each intervertebral disc space beginning at L1 and going downward. A line through the posterior margins of the vertebral bodies will describe a smooth arc; each disc space is also wider anteriorly than posteriorly. Loss of disc substance because of degeneration, protrusion, or any other cause will usually cause three changes to be seen in the disc space. There will be a loss of height, loss of anterior divergence, and the body above will seem to slide posteriorly in the body below as the upper body pivots down and back on intact posterior articular facets (Figure 10–10). If these posterior facets are degenerated, this ''retrolisthesis'' will not be seen; if they are markedly degenerated or spondylolysis is present, the upper body will slide forward on the lower (spondylolisthesis—Figure 10–11). Any of these changes can be present at one or more levels and in various combinations.

Bony lipping around the margins of the vertebral bodies bordering a protruded disc will become apparent after several months to a year. However, this may not be present in a more acute disc protrusion, such as might be seen in a young person following a recent motor vehicle accident or sports injury.

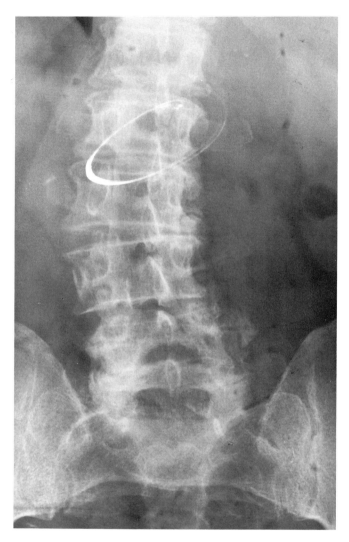

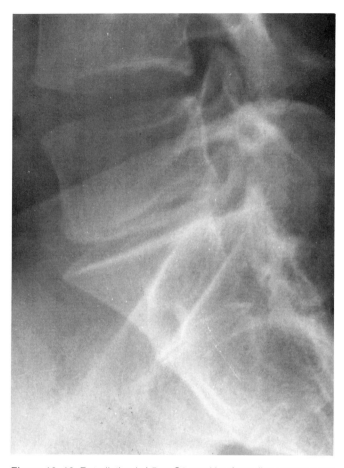

Figure 10–10 Retrolisthesis L5 on S1 resulting from disc collapse with intact posterior joints.

Figure 10–9 Extensive hypertrophic changes—small space between laminae to left of spinous process at L2–3 is only safe aiming point.

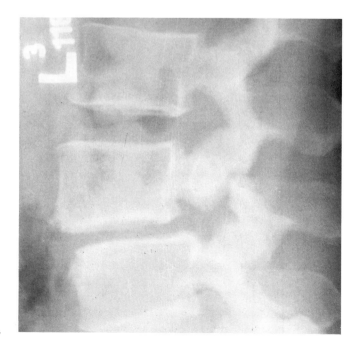

Figure 10–11 Spondylolithesis—bilateral defects pars interarticularis.

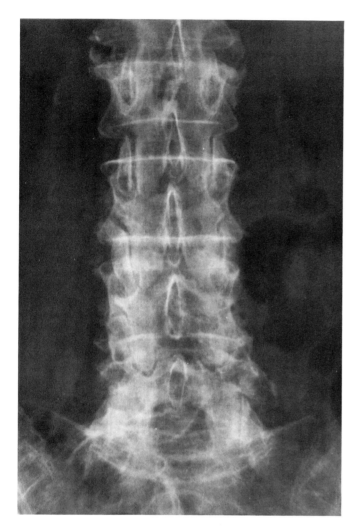

Figure 10–12 Lumbar canal stenosis—tall but narrow posterior bony arch.

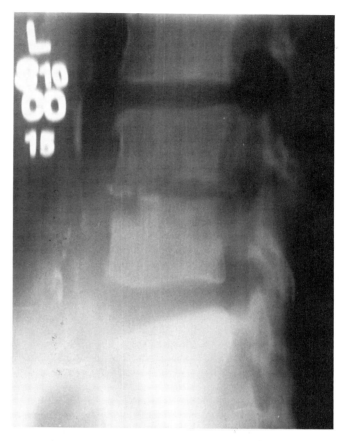

Figure 10–13 Disc space infection—lateral tomogram.

Patients with the clinical diagnosis of lumbar canal stenosis will often have disc narrowing and osteoarthritic lipping at multiple levels. Measurement of the anteroposterior (AP) diameter of the posterior arch on the lateral projection is not usually helpful, except at the level of the lipping. However, inspection of the posterior elements in the AP view can suggest a tight posterior neural arch. The width between the facet joints may be quite narrow compared with the height of the posterior arch from the top of the superior process to the bottom of the inferior process of the same vertebra (Figure 10–12).

Patients with disc space infection most often present with severe back pain rather than typical sciatica. However, these patients do present problems in imaging and confirmation of the diagnosis. On plain films, the end plates of the vertebrae adjacent to the involved disc at first appear only somewhat indis-tinct; the erosive changes may be better appreciated with lateral tomography (Figure 10–13). Radioisotope scanning shows abnormality earlier than x-rays, but the findings are not specific, as they can be mimicked by degeneration or neoplasm.

Probably the most specific imaging method available is magnetic resonance imaging (MRI). The involved disc and the adjacent portions of the vertebrae will have low signal intensity on T1-weighted images (TE 50/TR 500). These same areas will show markedly increased signal intensity (Figure 10–14) on T2-weighted images (TE 120/TR 1500). High resolution CT may also be of value, mainly in identifying any paraspinal abscess in contact with the involved disc space. Myelography has nothing to offer in the diagnosis of disc space infection; it may be needed to demonstrate posterior extension of inflammatory process as an epidural abscess.

Myelographic demonstration of lumbar disc protrusion is usually simple. If the protrusion is in contact with the sub-arachnoid space, the margin of the protrusion will cause a concave indentation on the column of contrast material (Figure 10–15). If it impinges on a nerve root, this nerve root will

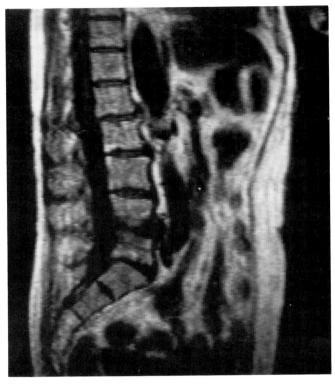

a

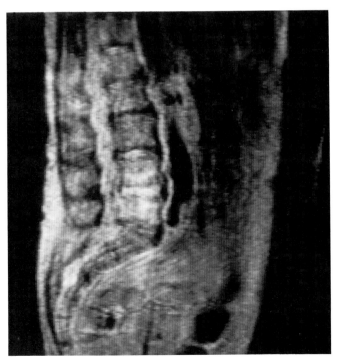

b

Figure 10–14 Discitis L4–5. (a) Low signal from disc on T1-weighted image. (b) High signal from disc and adjacent vertebrae on T2-weighted image.

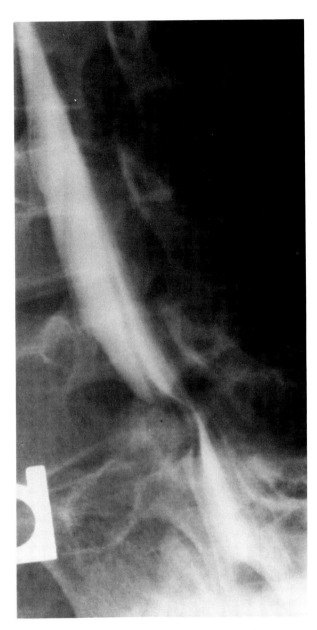

Figure 10–15 Large disc indents radiopaque column, flares, and cuts off nerve root.

be deviated medially and posteriorly; it will be flared as it approaches the protrusion, and may be cut off at the level of the protrusion. Retrograde swelling of the nerve above the level of cut-off can also be present. If the protrusion is large enough, all of these changes will be obvious; if small, the films may have to be inspected more carefully to find the changes affecting the nerve root in question. The nerve impinged upon by a small protrusion may show only medial and posterior deviation, and may not be totally cut off (Figure 10–16).

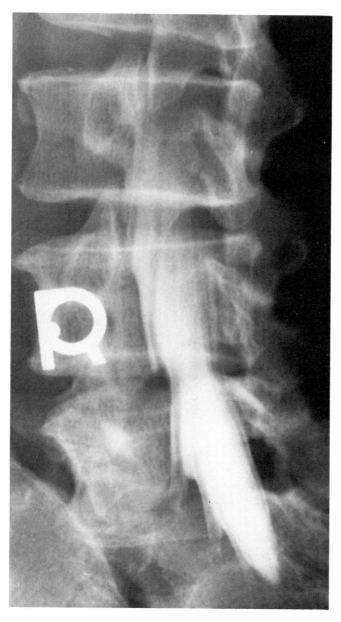

Figure 10–16 Small L4–5 disc only deviates L5 root without cut-off.

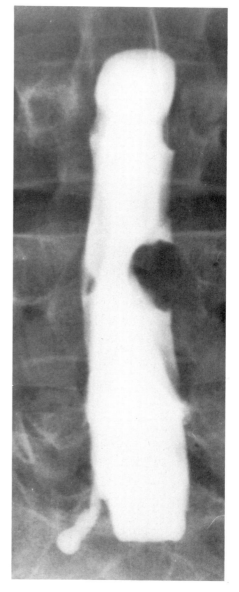

Figure 10–17 Neurofibroma of nerve root intradurally.

OTHER CAUSES OF SCIATICA

Using Lumbar Myelography

Lesions other than disc protrusion that cause sciatic type pain may be demonstrated at lumbar myelography. Intradural or extradural tumors (Figure 10–17) involving the nerve roots may be seen. These tumors mimic the symptoms of disc protrusion. In a patient with prior disc surgery, a recurrent disc may be found, at the same or a different level. Epidural scarring may also be found, which affects the nerve roots outside the dural sac, or arachnoiditis can be present, which involves the roots inside the subarachnoid space (Figures 10–1 and 10–2). In patients with canal stenosis, the narrowing may not be sufficient enough to compress the cauda equina and cause pseudoclaudication. However, a small disc protrusion may

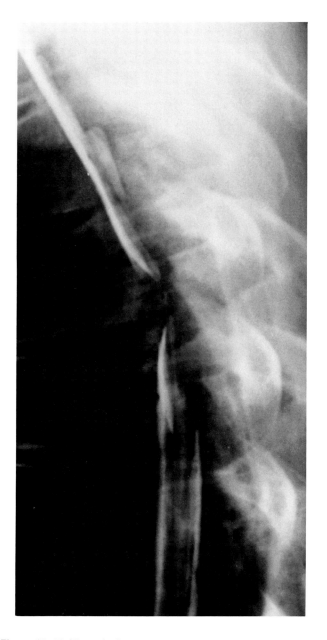

Figure 10–18 Thoracic disc protrusion.

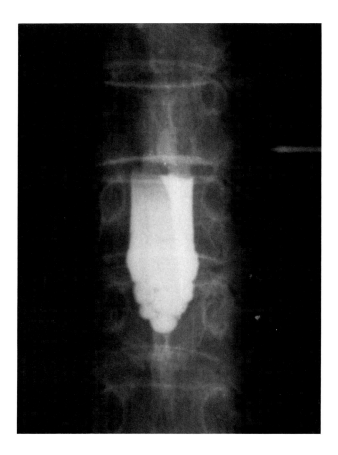

Figure 10–19 Thoracic intradural meningioma.

cause an inordinate number of symptoms because the constricted space is insufficient for both the nerve roots and a disc protrusion.

Using Complete Myelography

Disc protrusions are not limited to the lumbar region; even thoracic discs (Figure 10–18) may present with sciatica before

any long-tract signs develop. These, of course, will not be demonstrated on a lumbar myelogram. With iophendylate, it is common practice to run the contrast medium up to the foramen magnum in all patients, so as not to miss any abnormality higher up, even when the diagnosis was lumbar disc protrusion. There is a tendency to eliminate this practice when using metrizamide because of the technical difficulties involved in keeping a column of water-soluble contrast medium visible above the lumbar region. Undoubtedly, some lesions will be missed. The patient's best interest is obviously not served if he or she is told that the myelogram was normal, when only a lumbar myelogram has been performed and the pathology was in fact higher up.

These lesions that require myelography at higher levels include not only thoracic discs but also such tumors as meningioma (Figure 10–19), neurofibroma, lipoma (Figure 10–20), and ependymoma (Figure 10–21). Some of these can initially present with leg symptoms, especially if they lie

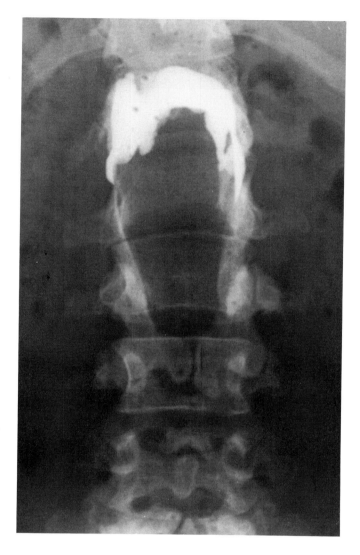

Figure 10–20 Intraspinal lipoma L1–2.

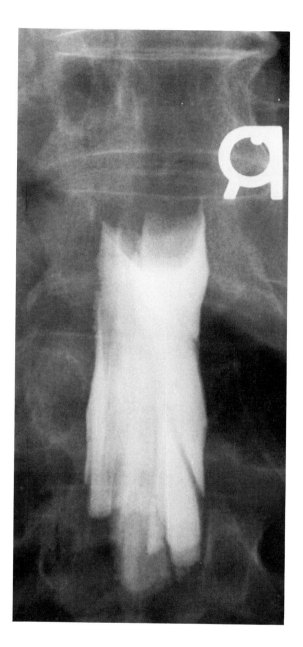

Figure 10–21 Ependymoma of conus.

lateral or posterior to the cord. Rarely, a patient with thoracic arteriovenous malformation (Figure 10–22) will present in this fashion. Epidural deposits of lymphoma (Figure 10–23) or epidural bulging from metastatic lesions of vertebrae may present with similar findings, and may occur in thoracic as well as lumbar levels. Some patients with diastematomyelia (Figure 10–8) can present with unilateral leg symptoms. All of these conditions demand myelography at levels higher than lumbar. A thoracic lesion presenting with sciatic symptoms has been a meningioma as high as T6.

Lesions Not Demonstrable by Myelography

Finally, there are lesions causing sciatic type symptoms that cannot be demonstrated by myelography. The lumbar root sleeves extend only a limited distance beyond the outer margins of the subarachnoid sac, as outlined at myelography. Any

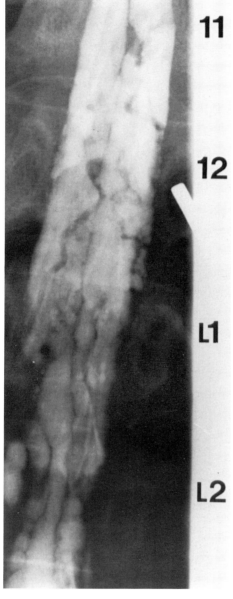

a

Figure 10–22 Arteriovenous malformation of cord. (a) AVM defects at myelography. (b) Angiogram same case.

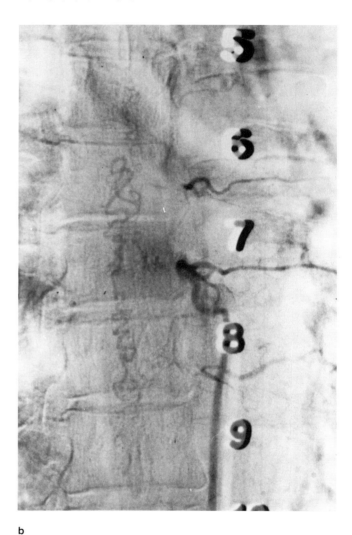

b

lesion distal (lateral) to this will be totally missed by the myelogram. The most common of these are the laterally placed disc protrusions (Figure 10–24), which encroach on the space for the nerves far out in the intervertebral foramina. These involve the nerve root at the same level as the affected disc; i.e., a lateral L4 disc will encroach on the foramen for the L4 nerve root.

Similarly, the compressive lesion in spondylolisthesis is often a compromise of the nerve root foramen in its vertical dimension; that is, the upper posterior corners of the body of S1 can project up into the L5 foramina (Figure 10–25) and compress the L5 (same level) nerve roots. Likewise, tumors such as neurofibroma (Figure 10–26) growing in the region of the nerve root ganglion may not be seen at myelography but

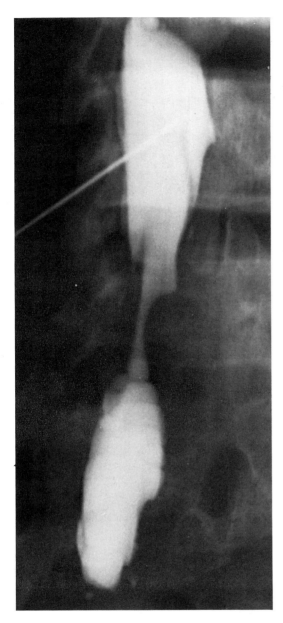

Figure 10–23 Epidural lymphoma.

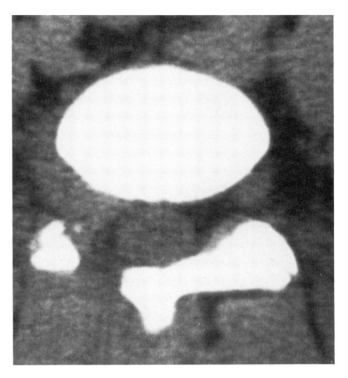

Figure 10–24 Lateral disc protrusion with normal myelogram.

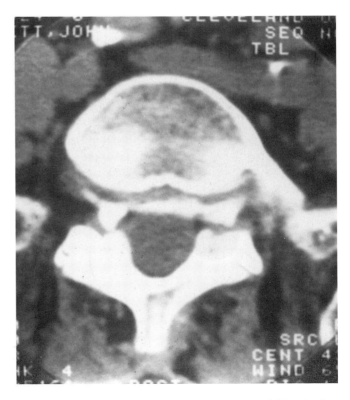

Figure 10–25 Spondylolisthesis—posterior corners of S1 extend up into the foramina to cut into L5 nerve roots.

can be readily demonstrated by CT. A metastatic lesion in the bone (Figure 10–27) extending back into the foramen can also compress the nerve but may be seen on CT and not by myelography. This is commonly seen in lesions involving the sacrum (Figure 10–28), which are below the distal end of the subarachnoid sac. Finally, lesions of the sacral plexus distal to the sacral foramina can be missed by myelography but are readily demonstrated by pelvic CT or MRI.

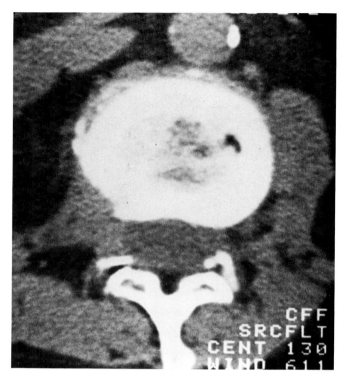

Figure 10–26 Neurofibroma in foramen—normal myelogram.

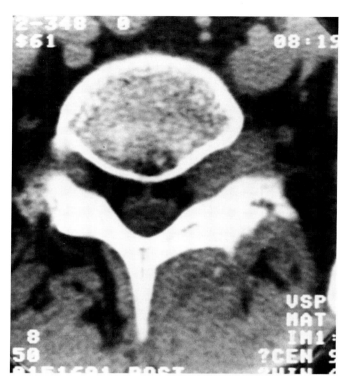

Figure 10–27 Metastatic tumor in foramen from prostate primary.

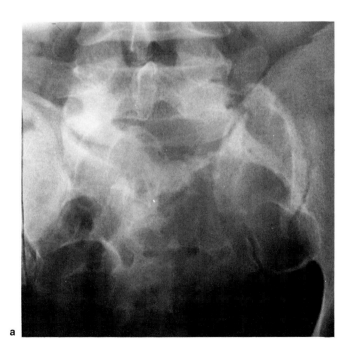

a

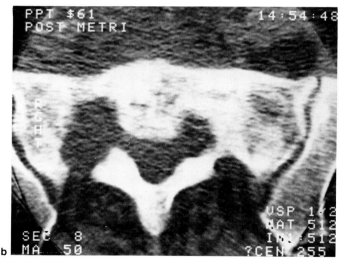

b

Figure 10–28 Lytic metastasis in sacrum from colon primary. (a) Plain x-ray. (b) CT of sacrum (myelogram normal).

Chapter 11

Lumbar Discography

John S. Collis, Jr., M.D.
Young Kim, M.D.
Cesar Rojas, M.D.

In 1962, after analyzing 1,000 consecutive cases, Collis and Gardner[1] concluded that lumbar discography was an extremely valuable test. Lumbar discography[2] has continued to be used effectively. It is recommended that this diagnostic method be used by clinicians who treat patients suffering from low back pain and lumbar disc disease.

The procedure has not been popular because problems related to improper techniques and incorrect interpretations can reduce its value. However, proper technique will avoid producing unnecessary pain and will ensure correct diagnosis in most instances. The ideal table (see Figure 11–1) to perform lumbar disc puncture will soon be available commercially.

PREPARATION AND PREMEDICATION

One hour before undergoing lumbar discography, the patient is requested to urinate. Then the patient receives an intramuscular injection of 10 mg of morphine (or 100 mg of Demerol) and 2 mg of atropine. The anesthetist starts an intravenous solution and can administer medications to the patient as needed.

The lumbar discography table (see Figure 11–1) is a vital part of the equipment. Without a discography table, the clinician will find lumbar discography difficult to perform. The top of the table is radiolucent, and the knee rest is adjustable to accommodate the patient. All roentgenograms are made before needles are removed from the discs, in order to avoid artifacts.

NEEDLE INSERTION: MIDLINE OR OBLIQUE APPROACH

Because image intensification greatly reduces the entire duration of the procedure, it is strongly recommended. All lumbar discograms are performed in the operating room. The anesthetist can use intravenous medication to allay anxiety or relieve pain, if needed.

The fourth and fifth discs are examined routinely. If a herniation of the third disc is suspected, or when the fourth and fifth discs are found to be normal at discography, then the third lumbar disc is also examined. The first or second lumbar disc can also be examined.

A lumbar discography tray should be fully equipped (Table 11–1). The skin and subcutaneous tissues are infiltrated with 1 percent xylocaine, through a 26-gauge needle attached to a 10 ml syringe. Needles can be introduced in the midline. However, a posterolateral approach, the oblique approach, is also recommended. The oblique approach is quicker now that image intensification is available. This approach permits the needle to be directed into the disc without penetration of the subarachnoid space.

Midline Approach

If the midline approach is used, then the 2-inch, 21-gauge, spinal needles are inserted through the interspinous ligaments. After the 2-inch needles are in the correct position (directed toward the interspaces, confirmed by portable image inten-

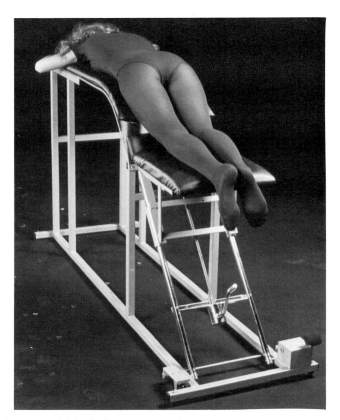

Figure 11–1 The Collis Discography Table allows proper positioning.

sifier), then the 4-inch, 26-gauge spinal needles are passed through the 21-gauge needles into the center of the intervertebral discs.

Oblique Approach

If the oblique approach is used, a 5-inch (or 7-inch if the patient is very large), 22-gauge spinal needle is inserted directly into the center of the disc. The pathway is first visualized on the image intensifier. *The pathway should be the center of the disc that is located immediately ventral to the facet.* The oblique technique is a quick and simple method that is especially advantageous for enzyme application, since this route completely and positively avoids the subarachnoid space. The end of the needle may be cautiously bent into a gentle curve in order to pass around the pelvic rim or transverse process, which is frequently encountered at the L5 space when using the oblique approach.

The "rubbery" resistance of the annulus fibrosis is quite characteristic. The image intensifier will verify that proper position of the needle tip is within the middle one-third of the interspace, and not touching a cartilaginous plate.

From 1½ to 2 ml of 50 percent Hypaque is firmly injected into each disc. A 3 ml Luer-lok syringe is advisable as considerable pressure may be required. Another 2 ml of contrast

Table 11–1 Lumbar Discography Needle Set

Items	Number
26-gauge 1½ in needle	1
10 ml syringe	1
2 in, 21-gauge spinal needles (midline approach)	3
4 in, 26-gauge spinal needles (midline approach)	3
5 in, 22-gauge spinal needles (oblique approach)	1
7 in, 22-gauge spinal needles (oblique approach)	1
3 ml Luer-lok, finger-guard syringes	2
Caps, masks, gloves	
50 percent Hypaque	
1 percent xylocaine	

medium is injected if the discogram reveals initially only degeneration. After every disc injection, usually only a lateral roentgenogram is made. At the conclusion of the last injection, an anteroposterior roentgenogram is also made, showing all injected spaces.

RESPONSE OF PATIENT TO DISC INJECTION

After each injection the patient is asked whether or not pain was felt and, if so, to describe its precise location. When the pain response is unusually severe, an injection of 1 ml of 1 percent xylocaine will almost *instantly* alleviate the pain. A separate 3 ml Luer-lok syringe with 1 percent xylocaine should be readily available for this purpose.

When the discogram indicates that the disc is either normal or herniated, the pain response is of minimal, or confirmatory value, and may be disregarded. However, when the discogram indicates that the disc is degenerated, then reliance is placed on the pain response; in this instance, the response of the patient can determine whether or not an additional portion of the disc is actually protruding but simply not opacified by the contrast medium.

When the patient's response to the injection consists of pain that includes the "clinically symptomatic limb" or represents an exacerbation of the original complaint, then the pain response is positive and is helpful in evaluating the lesion. This positive pain response, combined with a discogram that shows only degeneration, indicates that a disc herniation may be present but just not outlined by the contrast medium.

Relief of pain following intradiscal xylocaine, and/or cortisone, can be of both diagnostic and therapeutic value.

LUMBAR DISCOGRAM

A discogram will indicate one of the three following states of the disc: normal, degeneration (i.e., without herniation), or herniation. Figure 11–2 shows a normal L3 disc, a degenerated L4 disc, and a herniated L5 disc.

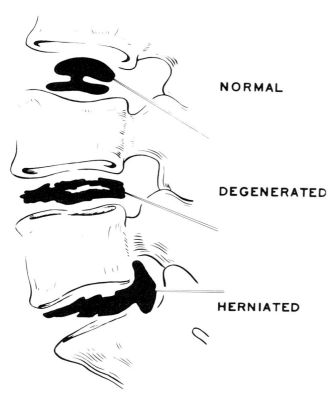

NORMAL

DEGENERATED

HERNIATED

Figure 11–2 Lumbar discography may demonstrate a normal disc, a degenerated disc, or a herniated disc.

When the discogram shows a normal disc, then, despite any pain response, the interspace in reality *is* normal. Usually the injection of a normal lumbar disc produces no pain.

When the discogram indicates posterior herniation, then the intervertebral disc is usually herniated, and the pain response will only reconfirm the presence of a herniated disc. When, however, the discogram shows degeneration, then reliance is placed on the pain response of the patient. In other words, degeneration shown on the discogram, plus a positive pain re-

sponse, indicates a herniated disc; whereas degeneration without a positive pain response indicates only that the disc is degenerated and with no herniation.

CONCLUSION

Experience with lumbar discography over several years has led to the following conclusions:

1. Lumbar discography demonstrates a disc to be (a) normal, (b) degenerated, or (c) herniated.
2. Lumbar discography is a safe procedure. Clinically, lumbar discography has not been harmful to intervertebral discs. Complications of lumbar discography are rare.
3. Lumbar discography is accurate.
4. A good, uncompromising technique and the use of the lumbar discography table are essential. A poor technique will produce poor results.
5. Herniated lumbar discs can be more accurately located with lumbar discography than myelography.
6. Pain response to lumbar disc injection is of clinical significance.
7. Normal discs can be proven so with lumbar discography; a normal lumbar discogram definitely excludes the presence of disc disease.
8. Surgical scarring of healthy nerve roots and unnecessary surgical exposure may be avoided when lumbar discography is used.
9. Arachnoiditis never occurs after lumbar discography.
10. Myelography can never prove a disc to be normal; myelography cannot prove that a disc herniation is not present. Myelography is occasionally associated with arachnoiditis.

REFERENCES

1. Collis JS Jr, Gardner WJ: Lumbar discography: An analysis of one thousand cases. *Neurosurgery* 1963; 19:452.

2. Collis JS Jr: *Lumbar Discography*. Springfield, Ill, Charles C Thomas Publisher, 1963.

Chapter 12

Comparative Use of Myelography, Computed Tomography, and Discography

Scott Kingston, M.D.
Gary Schneiderman, M.D.

The diagnostic evaluation of patients with back pain or sciatica begins with a careful physical examination. Based on the information obtained from the initial history and physical exam, patients may be divided into four basic symptom complexes. These are:

1. Nonmechanical back pain, with or without leg pain—pain generally unrelated to activity
2. Mechanical back pain, with or without leg pain—typified by pain that is provoked by activity and relieved by rest
3. Radicular pain—pain in the lower extremities along a radicular nerve pattern
4. Neurogenic claudicatory pain—lower extremity pain that occurs with ambulation and is relieved with relatively short periods of rest

Based on the particular symptom complex, the diagnostic studies ordered are designed to confirm the source of the patient's complaints. It is important to determine which level is involved, which nerve is irritated, and what pathology is present.

The morphological changes seen on the diagnostic exams must correlate with the patient's clinical presentation in order for them to be considered as the origin of the patient's pain. In this regard, computed tomography (CT) and myelography are the standard modalities used for patients with purely radicular pain. However, discography, when used in conjunction with these studies, can be helpful as a diagnostic study, particularly in those patients presenting with mechanical back pain with or without leg pain. Discography may also be helpful in patients with pure sciatica when CT or myelography do not demonstrate any specific anatomical findings that can be correlated to the patient's clinical presentation. This chapter's purpose is to delineate the situations where discography, CT, and myelography may be of benefit in the diagnostic acumen of the spinal surgeon.

All diagnostic studies have their pitfalls. The myelogram is no exception. The inherent nature of the myelogram necessitates penetrating the dura, with the potential for side effects such as headache, nausea, and vomiting. The water-soluble contrast used may also result in toxic side effects. Myelography is also limited in that it requires the herniated nucleus or other space-occupying lesion to be in direct contact with the opacified dural sac or adjacent nerve root sleeve (Figure 12–1). In cases with lateral herniation or wide epidural spaces, a herniated nucleus pulposus may go undetected on the myelogram because of the lack of continuity between the dural sac and the lesion (Figures 12–2 and 12–3). Myelography does demonstrate an overall view of the spinal canal and also visualizes the thoracolumbar junction.[10,24,28]

Some of the limitations of myelography have been resolved with the advent of the computed tomographic scanners. With high resolution CT, the epidural fat within the spinal canal, dural sac, nerve roots, and bone structures are easily demonstrated (Figure 12–4) and inspected for herniations, stenosis, and other anomalies that may account for the patient's symptoms.[2,3,6–12,17,20,28–31]

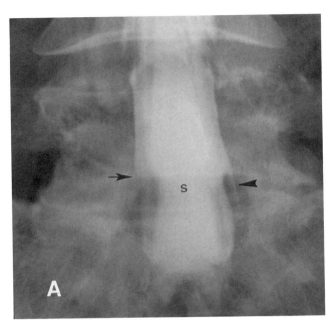

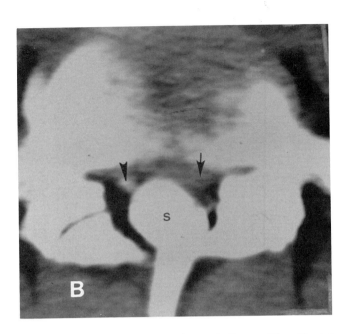

Figure 12–1 Nonfilling of nerve root sheath resulting from herniated nucleus pulposus. (a) Metrizamide myelogram demonstrating nonfilling of the left nerve root sheath (arrow). Note filling of the normal nerve root sheath on the opposite side (arrowhead). There is no significant deformity of the dural sac (S). (b) CT scan following the myelogram reveals a herniated nucleus pulposus (arrow) obliterating the epidural fat with minimal flattening of the dural sac (S). The normal nerve root sheath on the contralateral side enhances with metrizamide (arrowhead).

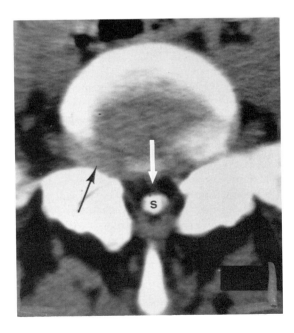

Figure 12–2 Lateral disc herniation (black arrow) on CT does not distort the dural sac (S) because of the posterior position of the sac within the spinal canal and abundancy of epidural fat (white arrow). The myelogram was normal.

However, CT has its limitations. Although the peripheral contour of the lumbar disc and the disc-thecal sac interface can be displayed with clarity, the integrity and internal architecture of the disc is not demonstrated. Occasionally, focal bulges or diffuse bulges in patients with sciatica do not clearly show nerve root impingement. Also, the CT, with its high sensitivity, may demonstrate abnormalities at multiple levels. These abnormalities may lead to problems with the identification of the symptomatic level in patients who do not present with clear-cut neurological findings.

Discography enables the clinician to evaluate the internal architecture of the disc. Assessment of the disc level as a source of pain can also be achieved with discography.[16,18,21,25] This assessment requires careful evaluation of the pain pattern identified by the patient upon injection of contrast.

Discography is considered positive when injection reveals internal disruption of the annulus or leakage of contrast, a low resistance to injection, and reproduces the patient's exact clinical pain pattern. Conversely, discography is considered normal or nondiagnostic if there is a normal-appearing nucleus, a high resistance to injection, no pain, or an atypical pain pattern.[4,5]

CT discography adds a different perspective when used as a supplementary exam to the conventional discogram. The axial

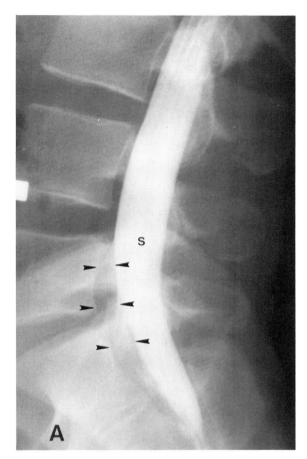

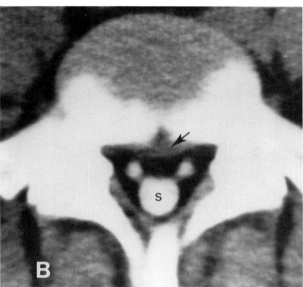

Figure 12–3 Central disc herniation undetected on myelography. (a) Normal lateral view of a myelogram reveals a wide space between the ventral border of the dural sac (S) and the posterior margins of the vertebral bodies (arrowheads). (b) CT scan reveals a central disc herniation (arrow) that was not suspected on the myelogram because of the wide anterior epidural space.

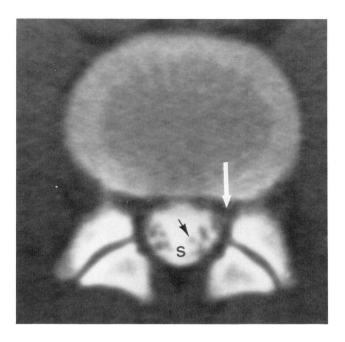

Figure 12–4 CT scan through an intervertebral disc space following metrizamide myelography demonstrates a normal round dural sac (S) with the individual nerve roots (arrow) surrounded by contrast within the subarachnoid space. Epidural fat (white arrow) surrounds the dural sac.

images that are created further delineate annular tears and herniations. The images can also be correlated with the initial CT and can demonstrate the degree of annular disruption and the exact location of a herniated nucleus pulposus, which adds to the definition of the pathological process (Figure 12–5).

The advantages of discography are the test's ability to demonstrate the internal structure of the disc rather than just its periphery and to recreate the patient's symptomatology. On the other hand, the test is invasive and carries a small risk of infection, nerve injury, and reaction to contrast.

The greatest criticism of discography relates to the question of diagnostic accuracy. Holt's study,[14] commonly cited by detractors of discography, found a 37 percent false-positive rate with discography in asymptomatic penal volunteers. However, Hitselberger and Witten[13] noted false-positive lumbar myelograms in 37 percent of four asymptomatic individuals. Weisel et al[27] found the false-positive rate of CT to be 35 percent. Multiple studies have shown discography to be accurate in about 80 percent of the surgically confirmed cases of herniated discs.[5,16,18,21,25]

Bell, Rothman et al[1] compared myelography and CT and found them to be accurate in 83 percent and 72 percent of the cases, respectively. Others have shown CT to be equal to or more accurate than myelography.[10,19,26] It appears that no single diagnostic entity will provide an answer in all cases. Each exam has its place in the spectrum of diagnostic tests for

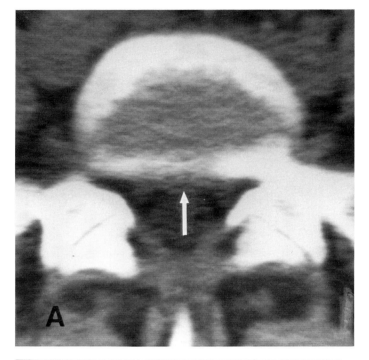

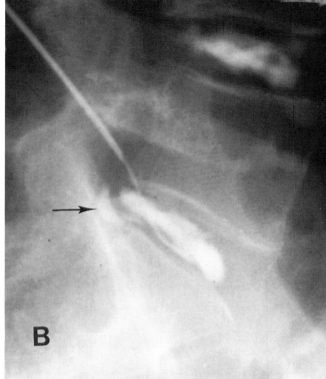

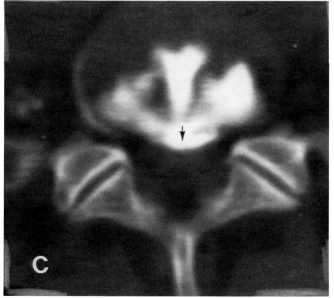

Figure 12–5 CT, discogram, and CT discogram of a central posterior disc herniation. (a) Chronic history of low back and leg pain in a middle-aged male with history of trauma to his back many years ago. Note a small central posterior soft-tissue mass (arrow) compatible with a herniated nucleus pulposus. (b) During discography, there was little resistance to injection and contrast was noted to flow posteriorly (arrow) into the spinal canal. The patient experienced his clinical pain during the disc injection. (c) CT scan following the discogram shows central herniation (arrow) beyond the periphery of the normal lumbosacral disc and correlates well with the plain CT scan (a).

lumbar disease and must be evaluated with regard to the patient's clinical presentation.

In order to study the ability of discography to determine the abnormal disc level, and to compare this ability with myelography and CT, a retrospective study was undertaken at St. Vincent Charity Hospital.[23] A total of 122 levels in 46 patients were studied. The patients were symptomatic with back and leg pain, although the percentage of back pain to leg pain varied. All patients underwent myelography, CT, and discography. Myelography was performed in a routine manner under sterile technique using water-soluble contrast (Amipaque). Each myelogram was then analyzed with a quantitative assessment regarding any defect on the dural sac or nerve roots (Figure 12–6) for each of the three lowermost lumbar disc levels.

All CT scans were obtained on the Picker Synerview 1200 SX Model. A routine CT scan of the lumbar spine included sequential 5 mm thick slices obtained every 4 mm from the was premedicated prior to arrival in the radiology suite. Aseptic technique was utilized, with the examiner wearing a surgical gown, mask, and gloves.

A modified lateral approach was used for several reasons. First and most important, the dural sac was avoided. This reduced the incidence of headache and other side effects that are frequently encountered during myelography. Second, with the lateral approach, extravasation seen in the epidural area indicative of annular or ligamentous disruptions was not confused with the potential leakage of contrast through needle tracks transversing the epidural space. In patients with clinical radicular pain, the approach used was the side opposite to the leg pain in order to avoid any confusion that might occur if the lumbar nerve was encountered with the needle.

The patients were placed in the prone, semi-oblique position with the bolster under the abdomen to open up the disc spaces. After sterile preparation, local anesthesia was employed in the skin and deep muscle tissues. The patient, therefore, remained awake and could relate any pain response upon injection. Using fluoroscopy, the patient was obliqued so that the "Scotty-dog" appearance of the posterior arch was visible (Figure 12–7). An 18-gauge spinal needle was then inserted down to the midpoint of the disc until contact with the annulus fibrosis was achieved. If the nerve was accidentally encountered by the needle, the patient related this to the radiologist, who subsequently repositioned the needle. A 22-gauge chiba needle (20 cm in length) was then passed through the 18-gauge needle after the stylette from the 18-gauge had been removed. In some patients, a small curve at the tip of the 22-gauge at the L5–S1 level was required to enter the disc space. The chiba needle was advanced until its tip was within the center of the disc space. This was confirmed in two planes

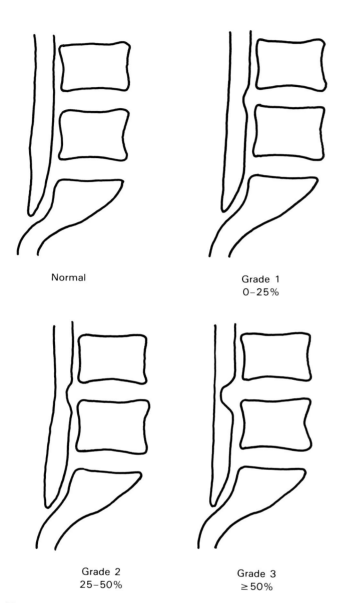

Normal

Grade 1
0–25%

Grade 2
25–50%

Grade 3
≥50%

Figure 12–6 Myelographic grading—Quantitative assessment of each myelogram was achieved by assigning various grades of defects depending on the width of the extradural defect produced on the dural sac. Although only lateral diagrams are shown here, similar criteria in the A-P view were also applied.

midbody of L3 caudally to the first or second sacral segment. Angled CT scans were made of the L5–S1 disc, when necessary, in order to be parallel to the disc space. Reformatted images in the sagittal and coronal planes were routinely done. CT scans were classified as normal, symmetrical bulge, focal bulge, or herniation.

The discograms were all performed under direct fluoroscopic guidance in the radiology department. The patient

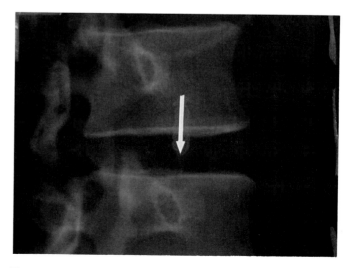

Figure 12–7 Desired appearance of the vertebrae and their posterior elements in performing discography using the modified lateral approach. The needle is inserted at the midpoint of the disc (arrow).

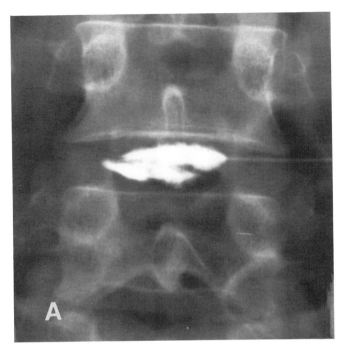
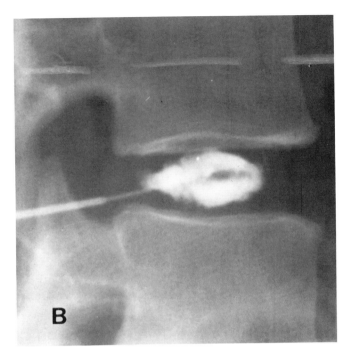

Figure 12–8 Normal lumbar discogram. (a) Anteroposterior view demonstrates the needle within a normal-appearing nucleus pulposus. Note the bilocular appearance of the nucleus. (b) Lateral view also demonstrates the normal nucleus. Although the discogram needle appears to transgress the spinal canal, the AP view confirms the true lateral course of the needle. This approach is desired in order to avoid penetrating the dural sac.

by either turning the patient or by rotating the C-arm so that the disc and needle were visible in both planes. Contrast material was then carefully injected under fluoroscopy and the patient's pain response noted.

With a normal disc, between 0.5 and 1 cc of contrast could be administered, whereupon there was resistance to further injection (Figure 12–8). Herniated or degenerative discs sometimes accommodated up to 4–5 cc of contrast with little or no resistance (Figure 12–9). Injection was stopped with increased resistance to injection, frank annular rupture with extravasation of contrast, or with reproduction of the patient's clinical pain.

Finally, prior to the removal of the needle, intradiscal xylocaine or marcaine was injected for symptomatic relief and to avoid confusing pain responses at different levels. With this technique, there was little morbidity or discomfort to the patient. The complication rate was limited to one case of disc space infection. Following discograms, some patients were sent to CT. Two or three axial scans parallel to the disc space were then made (Figure 12–10). Four basic CT discogram patterns were observed, although combinations were not infrequent (Figure 12–11).

The last three mobile lumbar disc levels were categorized as to the type of defect noted on myelography, the shape of the disc on CT, and anatomical configuration of the disc at discog-

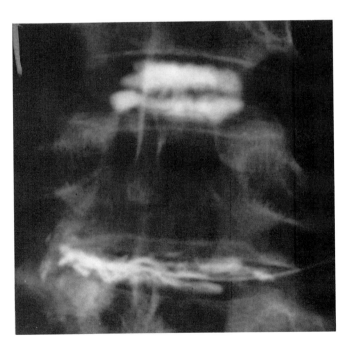

Figure 12–9 A degenerated lumbosacral disc reveals total disorganization with no distinction between nucleus and annulus. There was little resistance to injection of this disc, which easily accommodated 3-4 cc of contrast. Note the normal disc just above.

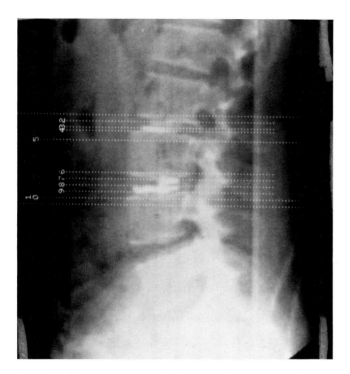

Figure 12–10 Lateral computed radiograph obtained on the CT scanner shows where several axial scans are acquired following discography. These CT discograms are often helpful in correlating the radiographic discogram with the peripheral contour of the disc on plain CT.

raphy. The reproduction of the patient's clinical pain noted on discography was also evaluated.

Discography was compared with myelography. Thirty-four of the 122 levels studied demonstrated abnormal disc morphology on discography despite normal myelography. The majority of these levels were asymptomatic. However, in nine patients, clinical pain was recreated upon injection of the disc space, including sciatica in seven patients. Surgical confirma-

tion of root impingement by a herniated disc at the appointed level was possible in five of the six patients who underwent surgery for persistent sciatica. The sixth patient was found to have nerve root impingement by the pseudoarthrosis of a spondylolisthesis.

Discography was compared with computerized tomography. Eighty-five percent discs read as abnormal on CT were noted to have abnormal morphology on discography. Reproduction of the patient's typical clinical pain occurred at 35 percent of these levels. Although 10 percent of the levels in the study had a normal CT but abnormal disc morphology on discography, of these levels 25 percent had clinical reproduction of pain. However, 40 levels were noted to have diffuse annular bulges on CT. Twelve of these levels in 11 patients had re-creation of their typical pain upon injection. Six had reproduction of sciatica. Five of these patients underwent surgery, and all had the diagnosis of a herniated disc confirmed.

Finally, there were three patients for whom neither CT nor myelography could demonstrate a definitive anatomical reason to explain sciatic symptoms. All three had diffuse annular bulge at one level and normal myelograms. Discography demonstrated herniations in all three associated with reproduction of the patient's sciatica (Figure 12–12). All three herniations were confirmed at surgery.

In this review, discography was able to provide further information on the origin of pain in some patients with radicular symptoms. The exam was found to be particularly useful in patients with sciatica who had normal myelograms but where CT failed to demonstrate significant compressive pathology. The question of fusion for back pain based on discography was not addressed although some patients had back pain only on injection of the disc.

Discography was unable to identify the painful level in 22 percent of the patients despite an abnormal CT and/or myelogram, and more than one level was identified as the origin of clinical pain in 15 percent. No patient had reproduction of typical pain with injection of a normal disc.

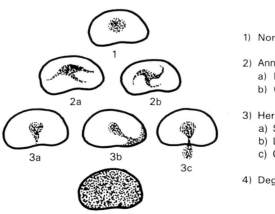

1) Normal

2) Annular Fissures
   a) Radial
   b) Circumferential

3) Herniated Nucleus Pulposus
   a) Subannular/Contained
   b) Lateral protrusion
   c) Central extrusion

4) Degenerated Disc

Figure 12–11 Basic patterns seen on CT discography.

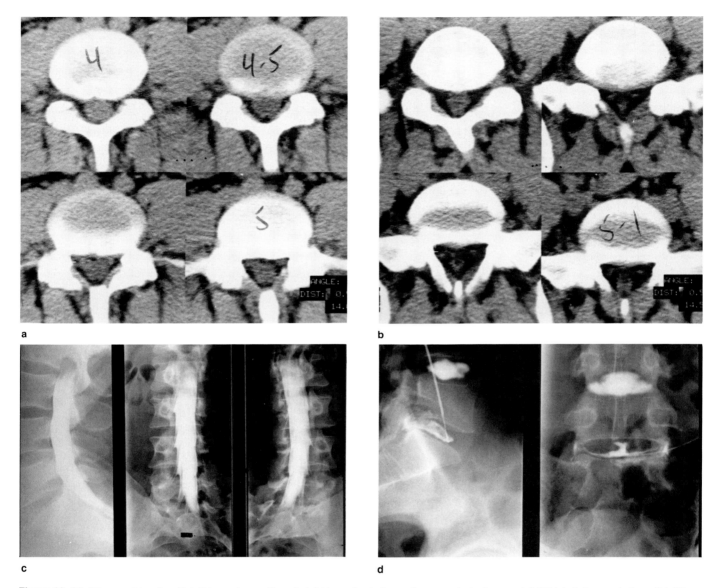

a

b

c

d

Figure 12–12 30-year-old male with left leg pain, positive straight-leg raise but negative neurological exam. (a) CT L4–5 demonstrates mild diffuse annular bulge. (b) CT L5–S1 demonstrates mild diffuse annular bulge. (c) Normal myelogram. (d) Discogram showing herniation at L5–S1 and a normal L4–5 level. Sciatic pain recreated with injection. A herniation at L5–S1 was confirmed at surgery.

SUMMARY

Discography has an advantage over CT and myelography in that it can demonstrate the morphological changes of the intervertebral disc and supply additional information with regard to the patient's pain response. However, many patients do not require discography. Myelography or CT should be performed first. If an unequivocal lesion compatible with the patient's pain is found, discography is rarely needed. In cases where CT and myelography fail to completely explain the patient's symptoms, discography may help delineate the pathological process. Since not all abnormal discs are symp-

tomatic, it is important to carefully evaluate the functional portion of the exam. Exact reproduction of the patient's pain associated with annular disruption or herniation helps to identify a particular disc as the possible source of the patient's pain.

High resolution CT is highly sensitive and accurate in diagnosing lumbar radicular disease. There is generally good correlation between a focal disc herniation on CT with the extradural impression on the dural sac during myelography in the absence of a wide anterior epidural space compartment (Figure 12–13). The advantage that CT has over myelography is that CT will demonstrate the lateral herniations or other

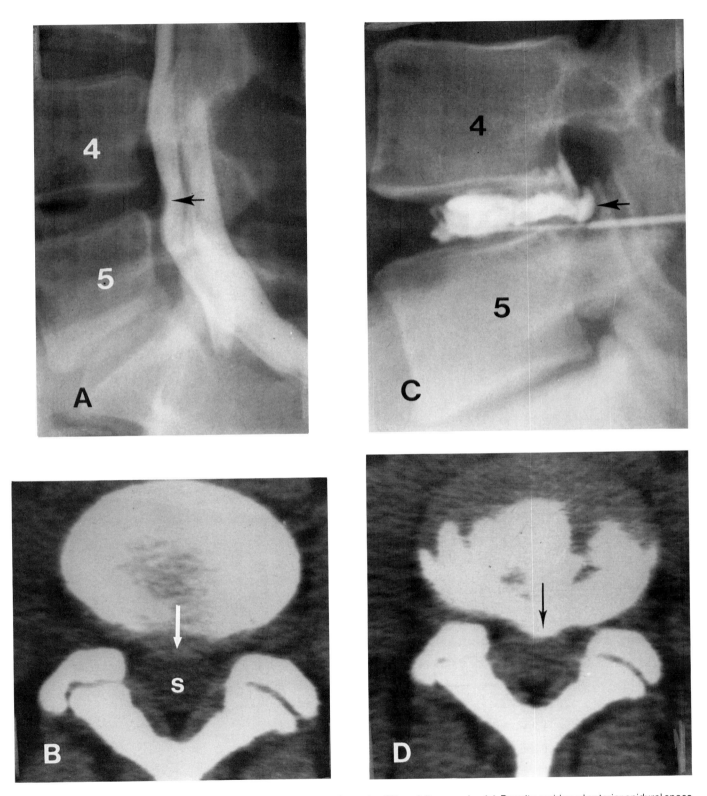

Figure 12–13 Small herniated nucleus pulposus demonstrated on myelography, CT, and discography. (a) Despite a widened anterior epidural space, there is a small extradural impression on the dural sac at the L4–5 disc level. (b) The CT scan shows a focal soft-tissue mass (arrow) having disc density impressing on the dural sac (S). (c) The discogram confirms a central posterior herniation (arrow). (d) A CT discogram shows the focal disc herniation (arrow) as well as extensive fissuring of the surrounding annulus and correlates well with the myelogram and plain CT scan.

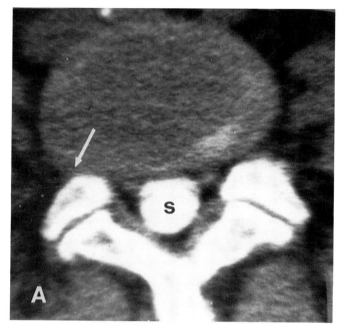

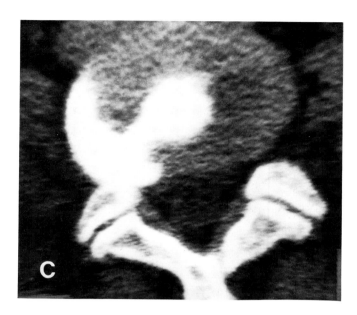

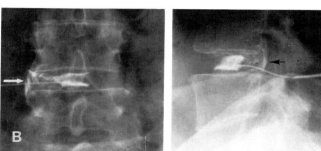

Figure 12–14 Lateral disc herniation appearing as an eccentrically bulging disc on CT. (a) There is a diffusely bulging annulus with a more focal bulge (white arrow) extending into the right neural foramen. The dural sac (S) is normal. (b) Anteroposterior and lateral views of the discogram reveal a lateral herniation (arrow). The patient complained of severe right leg pain mimicking his clinical pain. (c) The eccentric bulge on CT is clearly shown to represent the patient's disc herniation. Such herniations may go undetected on plain CT by the inexperienced observer.

space-occupying lesions that do not deform the dural sac. However, CT is not without its limitations. An eccentrically bulging disc on CT may indeed represent a contained nuclear herniation that is still confined within the outermost annular fibers or beneath the posterior longitudinal ligament (Figure 12–14). This is easily demonstrated on discography. The benign-appearing diffuse annular bulge on CT may also have more significant disc pathology leading to nerve compression (Figure 12–12). The discogram clearly distinguishes between a normally bulging annulus and a contained nuclear herniation or disrupted annulus with internal degeneration. Without the discogram, the referring physician may be unable to diagnose the etiology of the patient's back or leg pain.

CT discography can be used as a supplementary examination to the conventional discogram. The images can then be directly correlated with the initial CT scan and demonstrate the degree of annular disruption, circumferential or radial fissuring, and exact location of a herniated nucleus pulposus (Figure 12–15).

Figure 12–15 Various appearances observed on CT discography. ▶ (a) Normal central nucleus pulposus. (b-c) Radial fissures extending into the annular periphery. (d) Normal nucleus with circumferential fissuring of the annulus. No evidence of herniation. (e) Posterior herniation in the left paramedian location. The nuclear contents have extruded through the peripheral annulus and posterior longitudinal ligament and are impressing on the dural sac and ipsilateral nerve root resulting in left sciatica. (f) Degenerated disc with contrast evenly distributed throughout the disc. There is a focal herniation (arrow) as well, extending into the spinal canal just to the left of the midline.

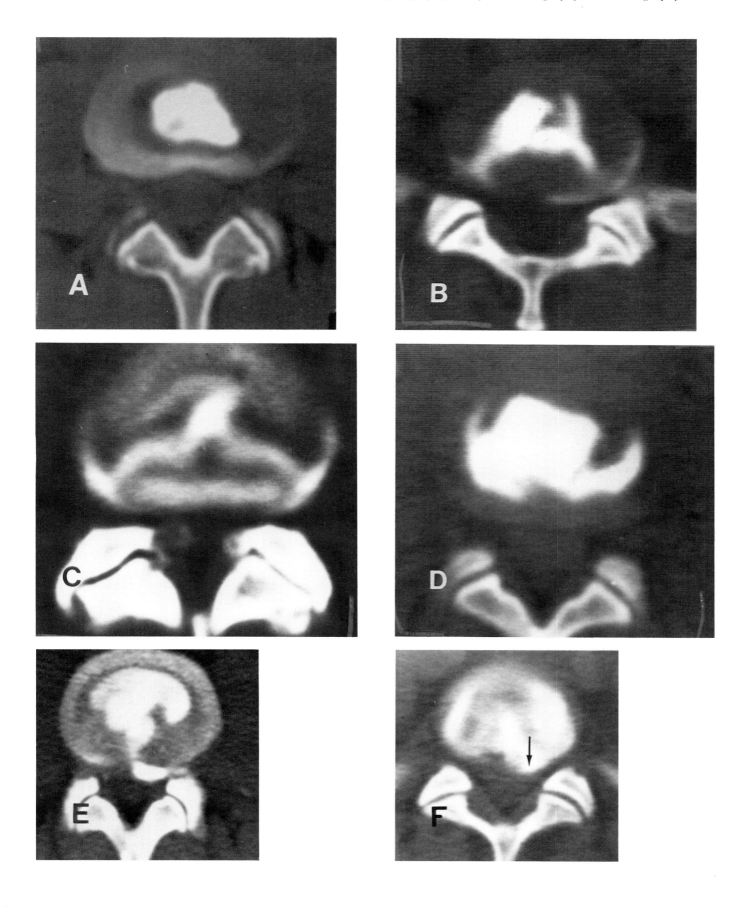

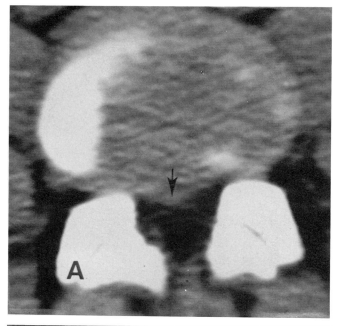

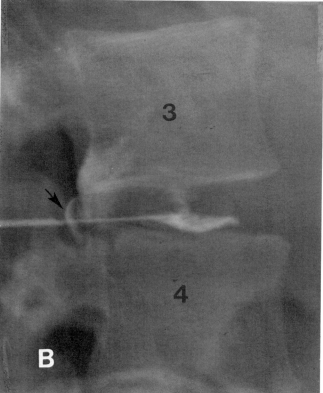

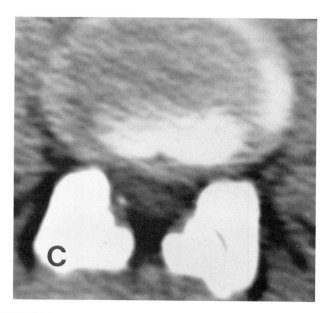

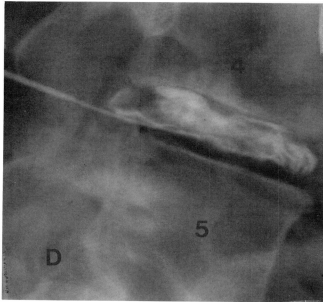

Figure 12–16 Isolating the symptomatic level in patients with multilevel disease. (a-b) The CT scan and discogram at the L3–4 level reveal a small central herniation (arrows). The patient experienced no pain on injection. (c-d) A bulging and degenerated L4–5 disc is demonstrated on CT and discography, respectively. Despite the degree of degeneration, the patient was asymptomatic at this level. (e-f) Reproduction of the patient's clinical pain occurred at the L5–S1 disc level. A degenerated and herniated disc (arrow) is noted on both the CT scan and discogram.

Frequently, the CT scan or myelogram demonstrates multiple levels of abnormality. In these patients with multilevel disease, the functional aspect of discography may help to determine which spinal level is the source of the patient's pain (Figure 12–16). The findings of multilevel disease may also help to rule out surgical intervention.

Discography is useful in evaluating levels adjacent to a segment being considered for fusion. This is particularly true in adult spondylolisthesis where the symptomatic level may be the level adjacent to the slip, secondary to disc degeneration (Figure 12–17). The presence of symptomatic pseudoarthrosis can also be evaluated with discography.[15]

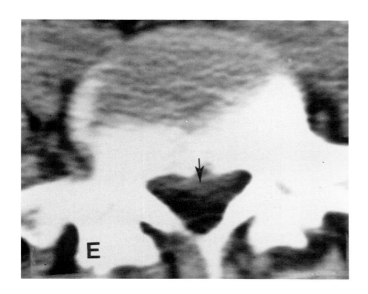

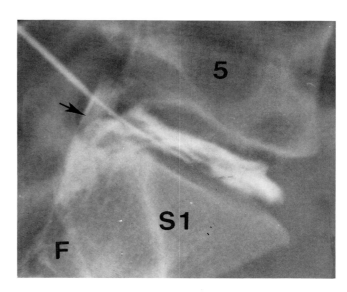

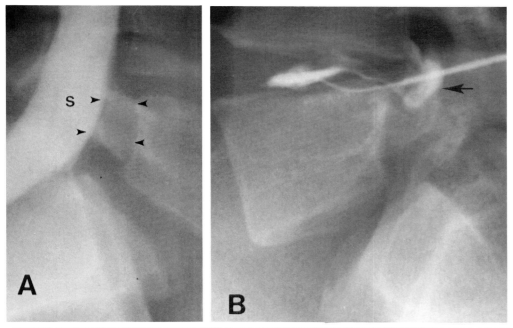

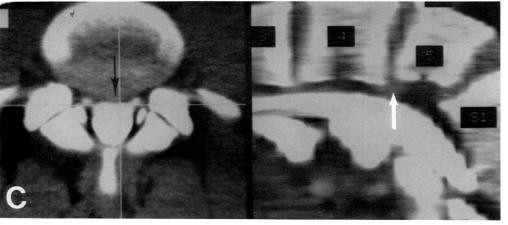

Figure 12–17 Disc herniation above spondylolisthesis. (a) Normal lateral view of a myelogram with a spondylolisthesis of L5–S1. The anterior migration of the L5 vertebral body has created a wide anterior epidural space ventral to the normal appearing dural sac (S). (b) The discogram reveals a large posterior herniation (arrow) at the L4–5 disc space extending slightly below the disc level. (c) Axial CT scan and sagittal reformation demonstrates the large disc herniation (arrow) that does not distort the dural sac because of the widened epidural space produced from the listhesis.

In conclusion, most patients with sciatica do not require discography. Myelography and/or CT should be performed first. If a lesion compatible with the clinical presentation is found, then discography is rarely needed. However, in certain instances, discography can be a useful test for evaluating the integrity of the annulus and the pain response of the disc to injection.

REFERENCES

1. Bell GR, Rothman RH, Booth RE, Cuckler JM, Garfin S, Herkowitz H, Simeone FA, Dolinskas C, Han SS: A study of computer-assisted tomography, II. Comparisons of metrizamide myelography and computer tomography in the diagnosis of herniated lumbar disc and spinal stenosis. *Spine* 1984; 9:6,552–556.

2. Carrera GF, Williams AE, Haughton VM: Computed tomography in sciatica. *Radiology* 1980;137:433–437.

3. Coin CT, Chan YS, Keranen V, Pennink M: Computer assisted myelography in disc disease. *J Comput Assist Tomogr* 1977;1:398–404.

4. Collis JS: *Lumbar Discography*. Springfield, Ill, Charles C Thomas, Publisher, 1963.

5. Collis JS, Gardner WJ: Lumbar discography: An analysis of one thousand cases. Presented at meeting of the Harvey Cushing Society, Mexico City, 1961.

6. Genant HK (ed): *Spine Update 1984*. San Francisco, Radiology Research and Education Foundation, 1983.

7. Glenn WV Jr, Rhodes ML, Altschuler EM, Wiltse LL, Kostanek C, Kuo YM: Multiplanar display computerized body tomography applications in the lumbar spine. *Spine* 1979;4:282–352.

8. Gulati AN, Weinstein R, Studdard E: CT scan of the spine for herniated discs. *Neuroradiology* 1981;22:57–60.

9. Hammerschlag SB, Wolpert SM, Carter BL: Computed tomography of the spinal canal. *Radiology* 1976;121:361–367.

10. Haughton VM, Eldevik OP, Magnaes B, Amundsen P: A prospective comparison of computed tomography and myelography in the diagnosis of herniated lumbar discs. *Radiology* 1982;142:103–110.

11. Haughton VM, Williams AL: Computed tomography of the spine. St. Louis, CV Mosby Company, 1982.

12. Hirschy JC, Leve WM, Berninger WH, Hamilton RH, Abbot GF: CT of the lumbosacral spine: Importance of tomographic planes parallel to vertebral end plate. *AJR* 1981;136:47–52.

13. Hitselberger WE, Witten RM: Abnormal myelograms in asymptomatic patients. *J Neurosurg* 1968;28:204–206.

14. Holt EP: The question of lumbar discography. *J Bone Joint Surg* 1968;50:720–726.

15. Johnson RG, McNab I: Localization of symptomatic lumbar pseudo-arthrosis by use of discography. *Clin Orthop* 1985;197:164–170.

16. Keck C: Discography. *Arch Surg* 1960;80:580–585.

17. Lee BCP, Kazam E, Newman AD: Computed tomography of the spine and spinal cord. *Radiology* 1978;128:95–102.

18. McCulloch JA, Waddell G: Lateral lumbar discography. *Br J Radiol* 1978;51:498–502.

19. Moufarrij NA, Hardy RW, Weinstein MA: Computed tomographic, myelographic and operative findings in patients with suspected herniated lumbar discs. *Neurosurgery* 1983;12:2:184–188.

20. Newton TH, Potts DG: Computer tomography of the spine and spinal cord. San Anselmo, Clavadel Press, 1983.

21. Patrick BS: Lumbar discography: A five year study. *Surg Neurol* 1973; 1:267–273.

22. Raskin SP, Keating JW: Recognition of lumbar disc disease: Comparison of myelography and computed tomography. *AJNR* 1982;3:215–221.

23. Schneiderman G, Kingston S, Watkins R: Comparisons of discography, myelography and computerized tomography. Presented at the First Annual Meeting of the Federation of Spine Associations, New Orleans, February 1986.

24. Shapiro R: *Myelography*, ed 3. Chicago, Year Book Medical Publishers, 1976.

25. Simmons EH, Segil CM: An evaluation of discography in the localization of symptomatic levels in discogenic disease of the spine. *Clin Orthop* 1975;57–69.

26. Tchang SPK, Howie J, Kirkaldy-Willis WH, Paine KWE, Moola D: Computed tomography versus myelography in diagnosis of lumbar disc herniation. *J Can Assoc Radiol* 1982;33:15–20.

27. Weisel SW, Tsourmas N, Feffer HL, Citrin CM, Patronas N: A study of computer-assisted tomography: I. The incidence of positive CT scans in an asymptomatic group of patients. *Spine* 1984;9:6, 549–551.

28. Williams AL, Haughton VM, Daniels DL, Thornton RS: CT diagnosis of lateral herniated disc. *Am J Neuroradiol* 1982;3:95.

29. Williams AL, Haughton VM, Meyer GA, Ho KC: Computed tomographic appearance of the bulging annulus. *Radiology* 1982;142: 403–408.

30. Williams AL, Haughton VM, Syvertsen A: Computed tomography in the diagnosis of herniated nucleus pulposus. *Radiology* 1980;135:95–99.

31. Williams JP, Joslyn JN, Butler TW: Differentiation of herniated lumbar disc from bulging annulus fibrosus: Use of reformatted images. *J Comput Assist Tomogr* 1982;6:89–93.

Chapter 13

Clinical Application of Diagnostic Evaluation

Robert G. Watkins, M.D.

The comparative effectiveness of diagnostic studies is intimately interwoven with the clinical examination of the patient. The history and physical examination make up the basis of the clinical evaluation of the patient. The four objectives of the history and physical examination are:

1. to quantitate the morbidity of the patient
2. to delineate psychosocial factors
3. to diagnose tumors, infections, and neurological disasters
4. to diagnose the clinical syndrome

There are four basic clinical syndromes:

1. nonmechanical back and/or leg pain
2. mechanical back and/or leg pain
3. sciatica
4. neurogenic claudication

The objectives of the diagnostic regimen are to determine:

1. which nerve
2. which spinal column level
3. what pathology

The history, physical examination, and morbidity determine the aggressiveness of the diagnostic and therapeutic plan. The aggressiveness of the diagnostic and therapeutic regimen can be divided into nonoperative (a regimen with adequate diagnostic capability to allow safe, effective nonoperative care) and operative (one designed to pinpoint as ex-

actly as possible all parameters of the anatomy and pathophysiology necessary for effective operative care) categories. There is an appropriate time to know the exact anatomic diagnosis and prognosis. Testing should reflect the severity of the patient's problem. Tests should be ordered when their results will change recommended treatment or are mandatory for an accurate diagnosis or prognosis.

Each of the four basic diagnostic categories has appropriate diagnostic tests that guide treatment:

1. Nonmechanical inflammatory back and/or leg pain

   - Objectives: eliminate intradural, intraspinal, and bone malignancies and infections, stress fractures, pathologic fractures, and localized areas of arthritis.
   - Nonoperative tests: bone scan, magnetic resonance imaging (MRI), protein electrophoresis, complete blood count (CBC), SMA12, bone marrow joint aspiration.
   - Operative tests: myelogram, contrast CT scan, spinal needle aspiration, Craig needle biopsy, or open excisional biopsy.

2. Mechanical axial back pain with or without leg pain. This is predominantly a mechanical back pain problem.

   - Nonoperative tests: MRI. The MRI diagnoses levels of disc degeneration and disc herniations and eliminates neurological intradural tumors. A plain CT scan can diagnose spondylolysis, arthritic change in the lumbar spine, and significant disc bulges. CT scan and MRI aid in interabdominal and retroperitoneal causes of back pain. The bone scan diagnoses active stress fractures and localizes areas of arthritis. MRI is preferable to a CT scan for initial diagnostic screening in Category 2.

- Operative tests: *Myelography and contrast CT scan.* Full examination of the spinal canal and dural contents is imperative to diagnose disc herniations, stenosis, intrafocal tumors, arachnoiditis, and congenital anomalies. Myelography and CT scanning in cases of minimum leg signs and symptoms cannot be expected to yield valuable information in regard to the etiology of the pain and can be dangerously misleading when contemplating fusion or decompression. *Discography.* Discography is both a subjective and objective test. It is designed to reproduce pain from an intervertebral disc by injection pressure and irritation of the dye. In this Category 2, discography is of paramount importance.

CT enhanced discography has shown a number of patterns of discographic dye. The dye will frequently outline extruded disc fragments from inside the disc out through the annulus. An annular tear with dye flowing through a radial laceration in the annulus can often be demonstrated. CT discography can demonstrate a herniated disc with sublaminar or extruded nuclear fragments. There are also subannular collections of dye that are indistinguishable from annular nuclear material on discogram. Some cases of subannular dye collection show a meniscus of dye in an intra-annular fissure on CT discography that looks like a herniation on the discogram.

The symptomatology aspect of discography involves pain reproduction of a clinical pain pattern. The patient draws the pain pattern on a pain diagram at the time of the initial visit. The radiologist does the discography and either draws the pain pattern or comments very specifically as to its intensity, character, and location. The radiologist determines if the pain pattern reproduced was similar to prior pain experienced by the patient. Some patients are unable to participate in this symptom reproduction portion of the study. Some are hysterically oriented toward pain either everywhere or nowhere. These human factors must be kept in mind in evaluating the symptomatologic reproduction of pain. To tell a chronic failed back patient that we are going to discover the source of that person's torment is often too suggestive. It is best not to discuss with patients which levels are being done, not to allow them to watch the monitor, and not to inform them when the dye is being injected. The physician can give an informed consent but avoid phrases such as ''find your pain.'' The accuracy of

discography is dependent on the skill and experience of the discographer.

Operative care for predominantly back pain is controversial. If a surgeon does not do fusions for back pain, discography is less important. This is a preoperative invasive diagnostic study only. Fusion for the instability stage of disc degeneration may relieve a patient of symptoms for a socioeconomically very important 5–10 years. Discography is critically important in determining which levels to fuse for back pain.

If a normal morphology discogram fails to reproduce the patient's pain pattern, the chance of success from fusing that disc is rare to nonexistent. An exception may be an acute posterior element fracture. Clinical success of fusion for back pain is decreased if discography demonstrates multiple symptomatic levels. The ideal candidate for selective fusion for predominantly back pain is one in which discography exactly reproduces the pain at one level only, additional intradiscal anesthetic injection at that level totally blocks the pain, and adjacent levels are totally normal and asymptomatic.

Operative care of patients without radiculopathy includes people with spondylolisthesis. It is critically important to examine, with discography and/or MRI, levels adjacent to a spondylolisthetic level. Fusion of a spondylolisthetic level, when the pain is from an annular disruption at an adjacent level, will be met with clinical failure.

In patients with a higher percentage of back pain than leg pain or 50/50 back and leg pain, discography can be helpful in determining which level is the origin of the pain. The MRI is becoming increasingly effective in screening the adjacent levels. In a review of discography and MRI cases, Schneiderman et al found a 99 percent correlation between degeneration on the MRI and degeneration on discography.[1] They have concluded that the MRI can be used to screen for levels of degeneration. If degeneration is present, discography is helpful in determining whether it is symptomatic in that patient.

3. Sciatica. The history and physical examination points to a discogenic origin for the sciatica, with or without neurological deficit.

- Nonoperative tests: MRI is the primary outpatient screening test. It will diagnose disc herniations, intradural tumors, and disc degeneration. The second preference is the CT scan. This will pinpoint more exactly the diagnosis, the location of disc fragments in the canal, and the presence of stenosis and arthritic spurs. In young people, it is preferable to use the MRI as a screening test, as this will accomplish the objectives of a working diagnosis for nonoperative care. In a young person with predominant leg pain from probable disc herniation, the MRI is performed with CT scan as the second test. In older people where stenosis is a more likely diagnosis, the CT scan is used.

- Operative tests: The contrast CT scan with cuts through the conus medullaris is preferred. This allows a better interpretation of spinal stenosis, whether it is central stenosis, lateral recess stenosis, foraminal, or extraforaminal. A determination of the exact size and location of a disc herniation and extruded disc fragments is possible. A full myelogram is not mandatory preparation for operative care in Category 3. Electromyography (EMG), sensory-evoked potentials and selective nerve root blocks, along with the clinical examination, are used to distinguish which nerve root is responsible for the patient's pain. The CT scan and myelogram and discography help determine which level and what pathology at that level. Discography may be of benefit in patients with predominantly leg pain of a discogenic etiology but is not routinely indicated. If there is a question as to the differential diagnosis of a major canal-obstructing lesion, the discography with CT can clearly outline a fragment from the intervertebral disc.

  A major importance of discography may lie in a negative discogram. An asymptomatic, well-contained nucleus should not be the source of true radicular pain from that neuromotor segment. Discography in this case helps eliminate pathology. In cases in which there are bulges and protrusions of intervertebral discs at levels adjacent to a herniation that could be producing radicular symptoms, discography may be helpful. Under these circumstances, discography may very clearly reproduce the patient's exact pain pattern, giving greater indication that this is the spinal column level of pathology. The definitive test is usually the contrast CT scan. The other tests are more supportive. The more tests that point to the same level, same nerve, and same pathology, the more exact the diagnosis and successful the surgery.

4. Older patients with predominantly claudicatory leg pain and no sciatic signs.

  - Nonoperative tests:
    a. Vascular evaluation, i.e., Doppler studies, bicycle test, evaluation by a vascular surgeon.
    b. The plain CT scan. The plain CT scan eliminates bone tumors and metastatic tumors, reasonably common in the older age group, and will show spinal stenosis. The levels for the CT scan are determined from the plain films.

- Operative care: The myelographic patterns of spinal stenosis give a good indication of which levels to decompress. A contrast CT scan follows the myelogram. CT demonstrates foraminal and extraforaminal stenosis. The morbidity of the myelogram is higher in older people, and nausea, vomiting, or mental changes may last several days. The contrast CT scan may soon eliminate the full myelogram. Discography plays little role in evaluation of these patients. Patients in this class are in the stabilization phase of degenerative disc disease and not the instability stage. Soft disc herniations are less frequent in older patients with stenosis. The decision to fuse is primarily based on flexion-extension films demonstrating dynamic instability, not discography. Fusions are to prevent further destabilization from the decompression leading to a return of radicular symptoms, not for back pain.

In summary, the comparative use of myelography, CT scan, and discography in terms of accuracy depends on the condition being diagnosed. Each test has an optimum diagnostic capability, depending on the symptomatology: discography—mechanical back and leg pain; MRI—mechanical back and leg pain; CT scan—radicular pain, claudicatory pain; myelography—radicular pain, claudicatory pain.

Myelography has its limitations. It is still only a shadow on the wall of the cave. CT scanning allows one to determine what is causing a myelographic defect. Myelography is very good for assessment of etiology of leg pain. A normal myelogram is good for eliminating an intraspinal source for radicular pain. Its limitations are the limits of the nerve root sleeve. Significant sources of radicular pain occur beyond the nerve root sleeve. Myelography is of no benefit in evaluation of annular pain.

CT scanning is a very specific look at the static black and white anatomy of the spine. It is imperative for spinal stenosis. Metrizimide-enhanced CT scanning has been found to be of great benefit, encompassing both the nonfilling root sleeve aspect of a myelogram as well as the identification of the exact reason why. Discography is a good test for identifying symptomatic annular pain from a specific neuromotor segment. It is good for identifying radicular pain associated with that neuromotor segment. It has no application in the evaluation of spinal stenosis.

To make a clinical decision on a specific case, the facts in the case are weighted according to the patient's symptoms. The facts are added up to accomplish the objective of determining which level, which nerve, and the cause. The more facts pointing to a specific area, the better the ultimate result of treatment will be.

REFERENCE

1. Schneiderman G, Watkins RG, Flanagan B, Kingston S: Comparison of MRI and discography in disc degeneration. Submitted to *Spine*, August 1986.

Chapter 14

Conservative Care

Arthur White, M.D.

For surgeons, the conservative care of the low back pain patient has classically meant bed rest, medications, and braces or corsets. It is understandable that surgeons have not spent time learning and developing their skills of conservative care. They have been busy surgically treating patients. Conservative measures have been developed by other specialties such as physiatrists, family practitioners, osteopaths, and physical therapists. Each of these specialties has a frame of reference from which they work and each has developed techniques that work. A few orthopedists have subspecialized in conservative care and have helped develop the areas of back schools, injection techniques, body jackets, and pain rehabilitation programs.

Nonspecific low back pain is a vague entity, and spontaneously resolves most of the time. In its treatment, there is little scientific proof that any conservative measure is better than placebo response. The only conservative measures that have some scientific studies validating their successes are back schools, exercises, and epidural blocks. Despite this, there have been conservative treatments such as traction and manipulation that have been used "successfully" for hundreds of years and continue to be used in private practices and spine centers all over the world.

Conservative care for low back pain is generally considered to be back care that is nonsurgical. In reality, sometimes, surgery is the most conservative care for an individual patient. Surgery is sometimes the most efficient, economical, and reasonable way to make a patient better. The vast majority of patients with low back pain, however, get better with time and nonsurgical measures.

It is clear that when someone develops low back pain that does not spontaneously resolve, that person has altered the normal state of anatomy. This usually means that a vertebral segment has lost its usual supportive capabilities. What we see on investigation of individuals with low back pain are various states of disc tears, fissures, herniations, facet overriding, abnormal motion, and alignment. In other words, we see a change in the normal state of affairs of a particular vertebral segment, which, under its current level of use, creates some form of inflammation and pain.

Conservative measures that are most likely to control such low back pain are measures that will alter or improve the support, alignment, or motion of a vertebral segment.

Some pathological change has occurred in the spine and, in order to decrease the pain, we have to change something to make up for the pathological changes that have occurred. We can temporarily realign the spine with some form of manipulation or traction. We can hold the spine in its normal position with some form of corset or brace. We can give medication or injections to reduce inflammation. In the final analysis, however, a permanent change must be made to make up for the pathological condition that is created.

Some of the things that can be changed permanently are a person's strength, posture, and the way the spine is used (body mechanics). Such changes usually require an understanding of the underlying condition and then doing some exercises for strengthening and developing habits to maintain a balanced normal state. Such education and training have come to be known as back school.

All other conservative measures that temporarily correct a pathological state and then return the patient to previous activities and abuses are doomed to failure. Even surgery, with correction of underlying pathological conditions, has a 30 percent failure rate when a patient is returned to previous abusive activities. Postoperative spinal stenosis and recurrent herniated discs occur 30 percent of the time after disc excision. Even when fusion is done on a vertebral segment, the adjacent level of the spine will develop stresses that can create a recurrent pathological condition.

The key, then, to conservative care for low back pain is to "change something" and then not see the patient return to the same abusive activities. All of the other conservative measures are supportive while the patient is undergoing change. Patients need to continue to live as actively as possible. When patients cannot change enough, or when the conservative measures become too burdensome, or when they are just not adequate to allow the patient to live a "reasonable" normal existence, then surgery becomes the next most reasonable conservative measure. The first obligation to all patients is, therefore, education, strengthening, and training.

BACK SCHOOL

Education and exercise have been used for decades in surgical practices. These have taken the convenient form of back schools over the last 20 years. The first back school was probably developed by Dr. Farnhi, in Vancouver, in the late 1950s and early 1960s. By the late 1960s, the back school at the Volvo factory in Sweden was developed, and in the 1970s, back schools began to spring up all over the world. There are now several thousand back schools functioning in the United States.

The back school concept is basically one of giving patients understanding about their condition and how they can take responsibility for it. Patients are taught appropriate exercises (Figure 14–1) to strengthen the muscles necessary to control their condition. They are taught self-manipulation or mobilizations that allow them to control their own condition, and they are taught body mechanics. Body mechanics (Figure 14–2) for back problems is the study of moving the body through space and the activities of daily living with decreased

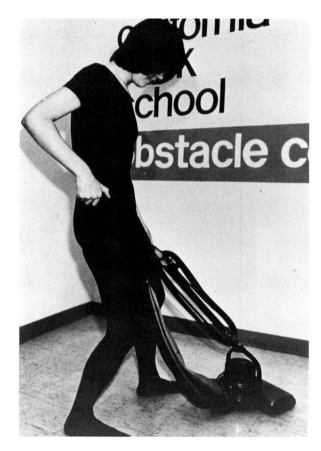

Figure 14–2 Body mechanics for household activities.

utilization of the spine by substituting other joints and muscles to replace spinal movement. Thus, patients are taught to take stress off the spine by learning to bend from the hips rather than from the lumbar spine, and using knees and hips to position themselves to do whatever job is at hand (Figure 14–3). They are taught positions of sleeping, sitting, bending, and lifting that will reduce the wear and tear on the spine, thus reducing inflammation and pain.

Back school can become as complex as the understanding of the therapist and patients can tolerate. Patients may only be given a sheet of exercises and instructions that are safe and valuable for anyone. These include isometric strengthening exercises and range of motion exercises, as long as they are painless. The sheet may include helpful hints about sitting and sleeping. The physical therapist or physician can take a specific diagnosis and select specific exercises and activities that work best for a particular patient. For example, an elderly patient with spinal stenosis will have a totally different set of exercises from those of a young patient with an annulus tear. The back school can serve as a nucleus for community education, industrial prevention and treatment programs, hospital diagnostic and rehabilitation spine programs, and chronic pain rehabilitation programs.

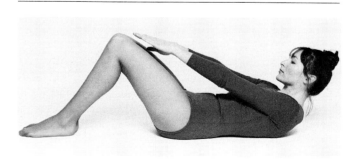

Figure 14–1 The partial sit-up (hold for 3 minutes).

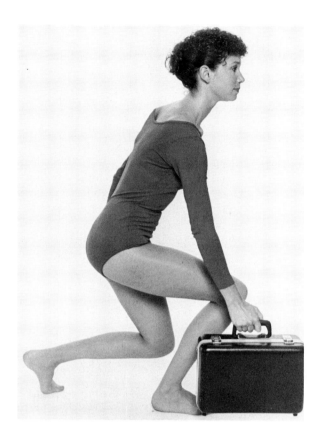

Figure 14–3 Practicing body mechanics.

Back school, in its simplest form, has come to mean just education, with no hands-on modalities, specific diagnostic categories, or exercises. In its broadest form, however, back school has come to mean total conservative management and includes all of the tools we have available to us for conservative care. In this broad form, the physical therapist works hand-in-hand with the orthopedist to come to a specific diagnosis and then select the conservative measures that are most likely to work for a particular patient. The following sections of this chapter represent some of the conservative measures that a teamwork of this type might utilize.

EXERCISE

Exercise in general has been proven to reduce the incidence of back injuries in industry. Exercise in almost any form that keeps the heart and lungs active and healthy and keeps the muscles strong tends to reduce postural deformities and bad habits such as "swayback," "pot-belly," and "widow's hump." General strength and flexibility allows one to use hips, knees, quadriceps, and pelvic musculature for bending and lifting, rather than placing excessive stresses on the lumbar spine. Specific exercises can be given and instruction for proper bending and lifting, so that from a prophylactic

standpoint, people learn how to take care of their backs, just as they learn how to take care of their teeth with dental hygiene.

Exercise programs have been used successfully for centuries. Williams' flexion exercises have proven successful in the clinical setting for decades. The exact reason for their success is not known. They do tend to unload the facet joints, stretch the hamstrings, and shift the spinal load bearing temporarily.

Extension exercises have recently become very popular. They work very well for early disc lesions such as annulus tears (Figure 14–4). They theoretically change the intradiscal pressure and the location and size of annular fissures and nucleus pulposus fragments.

Specific exercises for patients who have back pain with nerve involvement are usually isometric in nature. Patients can be taught how to do isometric or partial sit-ups, wall slides, or squatting exercises and hamstring stretching exercises, which do not cause pain. As inflammation and pain subside, exercise and activities are increased and monitored closely.

In more chronic forms of back pain, more extensive exercise and strengthening is necessary to change the individual's body and patterns of bending and lifting in order to compensate for the internal damage that has occurred to the spine. These individuals usually have chronic degenerative disc disease (Figure 14–5), some form of arthritis, early spinal stenosis, or possibly small herniated lumbar discs. They have created enough permanent damage to their spines that they have pain whenever they exceed a certain level of activity. By changing their strength and habit patterns and flexibility, they will be able to increase their level of activity before they create

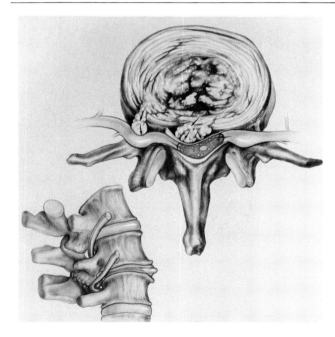

Figure 14–4 Herniated nucleus.

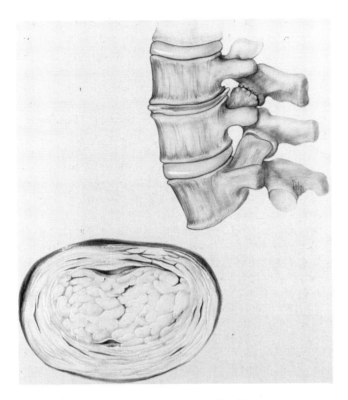

Figure 14–5 Chronic lumbar degenerative disc disease.

enough stress and inflammation to cause pain. More specific and extensive exercises are necessary in such a case. This requires fairly close monitoring by a therapist or physician. Too much exercise, too fast, will create pain and force the patient to abort the attempted exercise. In a closely monitored back school setting, patients can overcome many conditions that would otherwise lead to surgery. As with other forms of athletic training, ''the sky is the limit.''

Once patients have mastered exercise at home and in the office, they can progress to a gym, spa, pool, or athletic field.

Nautilus gyms and other forms of weightlifting equipment (Figure 14–6) can be used to position the patient's spine comfortably, while heavy exercise is done with the extremities.

Endurance can be developed on bicycles, in swimming pools, and on treadmills. Stress on the spine is reduced by body mechanics techniques, ergonomics, or altering the working environment.

TRACTION

Traction is one of the most popular therapeutic measures for patients with low back pain. It is used in patients in bed and in the physical therapy department with intermittent loads of horizontal traction. For the last 20 years, several forms of gravity traction have been popularized. In the early 1960s, Victor Steele developed the gravity gym, which is an inversion

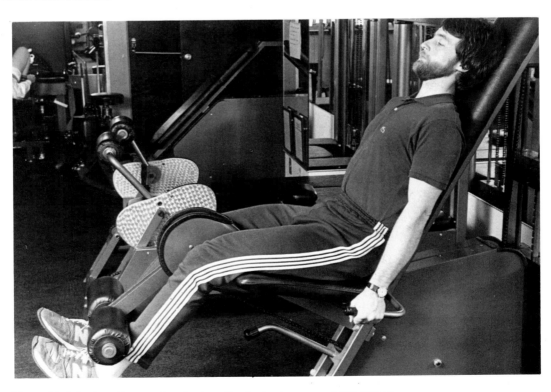

Figure 14–6 Back and lower extremity strengthening is of paramount importance.

form of gravity traction in which patients' knees are bent. In the late 1960s, inversion traction was developed with the patients' legs straight, using gravity boots. Gravity traction in the upright position with the individual suspended in a chest harness obviates the theoretical problems of hanging upside down with regard to blood pressure changes, intolerance in the upside down position, aneurysms, and ophthalmological problems.

A variety of apparatus for gravity has been developed from these basic principles. There is every size, shape, and expense. There are doorway models, free-standing models, hospital bed models, and some that fold up as small as an umbrella. The principle, of course, is that of producing traction on the lumbar spine, which theoretically reduces interdiscal pressure and places the spine in a position of greatest volume and least trauma. Weightbearing frequently aggravates low back pain conditions, and therefore, theoretically, the reverse of weightbearing (traction) will at least temporarily relieve back pain. This, by clinical experience, is true in many cases. The exact reason is not totally understood.

There is much argument whether traction should be done in a bent-knee or straight-leg position or whether it should be inverted or upright. In the final analysis, it is a matter of what works for the particular patient. One can use a trial-and-error method with various types of traction that can be found in a "back store" or spine center. One can experiment by hanging from doorways, schoolyard jungle gyms, etc. One can do exercises in the inverted position, either flexion exercises or extension exercises, depending on which is the most beneficial. Hypothetically, conditions such as annulus tears and those that are improved with extension of the lumbar spine would be better with a straight-leg position, and conditions that improve with slight flexion such as spinal stenosis should improve with the bent-knee inversion position. When extended periods of traction are needed, the upright position will be best tolerated, as long as the chest halter is not too irritating.

Complicated programs have been developed for the use of every form of traction device. Many who have attempted to use all the various types and follow the programs as closely as possible have not found that there is really one type of traction that is superior to another. As with other forms of conservative care, when one understands the underlying pathophysiology, one can select the appropriate conservative measure or specific type of traction that will work best.

CORSETS, BRACES, AND BODY JACKETS

When a patient, for some reason, is unable to strengthen and learn how to control his or her condition, an external support might be of some advantage. There is no scientific evidence that these devices are of clinical value. Placing patients in elastic corsets, however, does give them a reminder not to bend. They can still bend as far as they could without the corset, in most instances. In a flexion body jacket, one is limited in motion and the position of the spine is slightly changed. Theoretically, a flexion body jacket tightens the posterior longitudinal ligament and increases intra-abdominal pressure, thus giving more support to the spine. Any given patient with a specific disease of the lumbar spine could theoretically do more activity with a perfect support or postural training device. Determining and obtaining the perfect support is a complex science in itself.

A simple elastic corset seems to give some patients a feeling of security, although many doctors have labeled these as simply a badge of disability. Weightlifters have used supportive belts for years as an aid in increasing their ability to lift. More formidable corsets of canvas with pulls, stays, and buckles do seem to be used regularly by certain types of patients. They use them on a daily basis while working and have several available. They renew their prescriptions for these corsets over the years. Some football players and other athletes use corsets during play and find they have less pain when they do so. If nothing else, these types of garments act as a reminder to keep the back straight and give the wearer something to push against with the abdominal musculature. Perhaps this makes them more able to develop greater intra-abdominal pressure at important times of peak performance.

The flexion body jacket is more difficult to fit and use than a corset. It is also much more expensive. A patient has to be fairly serious about its use before it is ordered. It works best for patients who have demonstrated that they do improve in a position of pelvic tilt and slight lumbar flexion. Such patients usually have spinal stenosis and bulging or herniated discs that are behind the posterior longitudinal ligament. Flexion body jackets are especially valuable for patients who are unable to, or will not learn to, use good body mechanics in the form of pelvic tilt, abdominal tightening, and straight back bending. Patients are tested to determine if they need this type of garment by the back school physical therapist, who works with the patient on using pelvic tilt under various circumstances of lying down, standing, walking, and daily activities.

Flexion body jackets need to be fitted properly by an orthotist and their use monitored clinically by a therapist or physician to be sure that the fit is proper and instructions are given and followed. Close observation is needed for pressure points, especially at the groin area, where neurological compression can cause some lateral thigh numbness or circulatory compression.

INJECTIONS

Injections allow medications to be placed at the exact site of a pathologic process in order to give maximal benefit. A physician can quickly learn to place the needle, especially with the use of fluoroscopy, into a facet joint or over a specific nerve root, disc, or other vertebral structure (Figure 14–7). Diag-

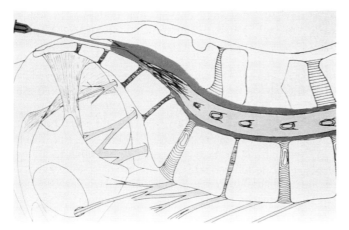

Figure 14–7 Injection section.

nostic information is also delineated by the placement of needles and medications in and around pathological entities.

TRIGGER POINTS

For centuries, needles have been placed into painful areas and tender areas of the back in order to control pain. The exact mechanism of pain relief is still not known. Dry needles have as much effect as saline, which has as much effect as local anesthetics, which have as much effect as cortisone. There are studies on all of these entities demonstrating each one to be more effective than the other. It probably depends on the particular entity that creates the pain.

If a painful trigger point is created by referred pain from a distant site, the response is likely to be different than if the trigger point is actually the site of an inflammatory process. Trigger point injections do not cure patients but they certainly alter the painful response temporarily. As long as there is not an allergic reaction to the medication injected or not too much cortisone given, there is little danger associated with such trigger point injections. One needs, of course, to be quite familiar with the anatomy and where the needle is being placed.

EPIDURAL BLOCKS

Second to back school, epidural blocks are the most valuable conservative measure in the treatment of low back pain. Their great value is in the immediate and dramatic change that epidural blocks can make in most acute low back pain syndromes. Even though these blocks do not cure most low back pain problems, they reduce the pain and increase the patient's function. This allows the patient to go home comfortably rather than being hospitalized. The patient gains confidence in

his or her doctor and is able to start back school immediately, which brings about the ultimate cure of the condition.

Another value of epidural blocks is in sorting out the severe from the not so severe conditions. If an epidural block does not work, then we know we are dealing with a relatively resistant and probably more severe condition. If the block works immediately to relieve positive straight-leg raising and leg pain, and temporarily reproduces that leg pain as the injection is made, one has confirmed the diagnosis of nerve root irritation. Thus, epidural blocks give diagnostic information, help with the prognosis, provide temporary good relief, and facilitate rehabilitation.

The theoretical reason that epidural blocks work so well is that the injection includes both an anesthetic and cortisone. The anesthetic partially anesthetizes the epidural space, which is the site of many low back pain problems. The cortisone is then directly in contact with the inflammatory process that is creating the pain. Inflammation in the epidural space, which develops from herniated lumbar discs, can come from mechanical irritation of neurological structures, chemical irritation, or autoimmune phenomena. All three of these forms of inflammation can be counteracted quite readily with steroids that are in contact with that inflammatory process.

It is well known that oral and intramuscular injections of cortisone will also decrease many low back pain problems. The systemic effects of cortisone in high enough doses can reduce inflammation anywhere in the body. Injections of cortisone in the epidural space will also have a systemic effect even if the cortisone does not get to the exact source of the inflammation. The effects, however, will not be as rapid as they are when the anesthetic and steroid come directly in contact with the source of the inflammation and pain. A lower dose of cortisone is also another great benefit of epidural blocks as compared with the large amounts of cortisone that are required orally.

Since epidural cortisone works best on acute inflammation, it is best to do the epidural block early rather than late. After several weeks of rest or nonsteroidal anti-inflammatories, much of the acute syndrome has subsided. Chronic ''mechanical'' back pain of degenerative disc disease, spinal stenosis, or herniated discs is not changed significantly with cortisone. Recurrent episodes, however, of acute nerve root inflammation because of these conditions will respond each time to the epidural steroids.

Some individuals feel that repeating the epidural block three times has more benefit. Of course, there are greater amounts of cortisone given with the three injections, and the location of the ultimate resting site of the cortisone will vary with each injection. It is for this reason that all epidural blocks should be done under x-ray control with a small amount of contrast medium, usually in the form of Conray. One can see the path that the cortisone is going to take and ensure that the needle is accurately placed. In controlled studies, it was found that needle placement was done incorrectly 25 percent of the time when the needles were placed "blindly," even in the hands of an anesthesiologist. It was interesting to note that the needle placements were intravascular 6 percent of the time.

Epidural blocks can be placed through the sacral hiatus or between any two lumbar spinous processes. Needles placed by the lumbar route are more likely to penetrate the dura and can create postinjection headaches and cerebral spinal fluid leak. The dangers of ultimately having a spinal anesthetic are obvious under such circumstances. Otherwise, the lumbar route does offer a more accurate localization of the placement of the injection at the site of inflammation.

The technique of epidural blocks through the sacral hiatus involves simply palpating the hiatus, anesthetizing the skin over the hiatus, and then "walking" a 22-gauge spinal needle into the sacral hiatus. Air acceptance technique (Figure 14–8) might be of some value but a few drops of contrast medium is the best way to confirm adequate localization. The contrast medium travels in a rivulet-type fashion proximally into the lumbar epidural space. If the contrast stays in a localized globule or in a straight line, the needle is in a fascial plane and not in the epidural space. Via the lumbar route, an 18-gauge Crawford or Thoey needle is used because of their more blunt tips. A needle is advanced with the hanging drop or air acceptance technique. Less anesthetic is necessary from the lumbar route. Two to three cubic centimeters of depository cortisone are used by both routes. The longer-acting anesthetic, such as Marcaine, can give one a longer period of temporary relief and a better opportunity to evaluate the results of the block for diagnostic purposes.

MEDICATION

Medication is probably the least valuable tool in the treatment of low back pain. Medication does not change the underlying condition, nor does it change the abusive factors that have led to the condition. It "covers up" the symptoms rather than encouraging the patient to accept responsibility for the symptoms. With the symptoms covered up, the underlying condition continues on unabated and becomes a more severe condition.

There are times, however, when medication can be of value in allowing the patient to stay out of the hospital or train to a new level of strength, flexibility, and self-responsibility.

The treatment of chronic pain patients is an intricate specialty that requires balancing psychological and behavioral factors with addictive medications and drugs that act on the central nervous system. Since the specialized form of medical management is not within the scope of the average orthopedic surgeon, no further time will be spent in this section on that type of medication.

The most common medications in orthopedic management of low back pain are nonsteroidal anti-inflammatories, steroidal anti-inflammatories, muscle relaxants, and analgesics.

Since most forms of low back pain emanate from an inflammatory source, it seems reasonable to use some form of anti-inflammatory agent. Cortisone is the most potent of the anti-inflammatories and carries with it the most complications. It should not be used indiscriminately. However, when one is faced with hospitalization, two weeks of bed rest, surgery, or other invasive procedures, the risks of cortisone become much less worrisome in comparison. Cortisone should be used only in the more extreme cases, specifically where there is nerve root irritation. A small amount of cortisone placed at the location of the inflammation of the facet joint or over an inflamed nerve root is the preferred treatment rather than giving it orally. But when injections are not acceptable for one reason or another, a two-to-six-day course of cortisone (Medrol DosePak) can be used. Single intramuscular injections of cortisone can also have dramatic effects on inflammation and pain. Because of the side effects of cortisone, it should not be used for any one patient more than once or twice a year. Patients who find great relief from cortisone will sometimes continue abusive activities and expect their pain to be relieved each time with pills or injections. They need to be educated and controlled.

Nonsteroidal anti-inflammatories have fewer complications but are much less effective. Most of them have both pain-relieving effects as well as anti-inflammatory effects. There

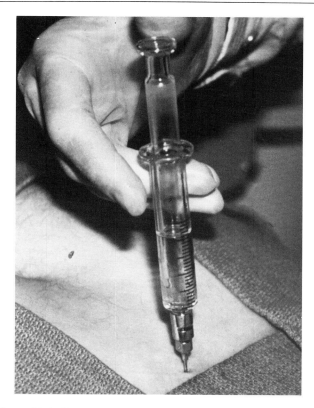

Figure 14–8 Air acceptance technique of "lumbar epidermal."

are several chemical families of nonsteroidal anti-inflammatories with different sites of action. When one family does not work, another is likely to. For the semi-acute back condition, or chronic recurrent inflammatory back condition, it is well worth trying a trial or two of these various nonsteroidal anti-inflammatories. There are various complications and side effects from anti-inflammatories. The major problem is gastrointestinal intolerance. Aspirin, it should be remembered, provides an immediate available anti-inflammatory with good analgesic properties.

Analgesics relieve the pain from low back conditions but again have little or nothing to do with the source of the pain. There is danger in relying on pain medications, rather than treating the cause, and developing addiction and side effects from the medications that can be worse than the original condition. It is best to use analgesics only when patients are at rest. If they are going to be active they should not take analgesics. When patients are active more inflammation can be created, which requires more analgesics. If a patient has overdone and developed significant pain, he or she should rest and take an analgesic or two until the pain subsides. It is then up to the patient to return to activity painlessly. There is one thing that is worse than an undiagnosed chronic low back pain patient and that is an addicted, undiagnosed chronic low back pain patient.

The strengths of analgesics and their addictive properties are well known. There are no known nonaddicting analgesics that are much better than aspirin. There may be social and psychological reasons to select a particular brand of analgesic. In general, however, pain medication is just not in the best interest of the patient.

Presumably, muscle relaxants are used because the users assume that the pain is coming from the muscle spasm. However, muscle spasm is a protective mechanism that is a response to an underlying, more significant spinal abnormality. Muscle spasm is better treated by rest, manipulation, bracing, injections, or other more specifically aimed modality. It has not been proven that muscle relaxants do make a significant difference in a patient's clinical course for low back pain. If there is any significant effect on the patient's symptoms, it is likely to be a central nervous system effect. As in the case of analgesics and anti-inflammatories, if the patient has improved symptomatically and is taking responsibility for his or her condition, there will not be a need for the medication for very long and there is probably little harm in a short course of muscle relaxants.

Chapter 15

Anesthesia for Spinal Decompression Surgery

Irv Klein, M.D.

This chapter focuses on those clinical aspects of anesthesiology that facilitate successful surgical decompression of the spine. These methods are routinely incorporated while making modifications as the patient's pertinent medical history or physical habitus dictates.

First, decompressive spinal surgery can best be facilitated by utilizing methods that ensure as "bloodless" a surgical field as is possible. The lower the systolic blood pressure during surgery, the less the bleeding encountered. Dramatic decreases in surgical field bleeding are often observed as the systolic blood pressure is lowered from a range of 115–125 to a range of 85–95.

Blood pressure lowering is accomplished by a combination of patient positioning and pharmacologic methods. For the past several years, almost all patients undergoing posterior spinal decompression surgery at Centinela Hospital Medical Center were placed on an Andrews' frame in a prone kneeling position rather than the more conventional straight prone position on either a Wilson frame or chest bolsters. It is remarkable how often by just positioning the patient on an Andrews' frame the patient's blood pressure can be lowered to the desired level without additional pharmacologic manipulation. Also, by allowing free excursion of the abdominal contents by positioning the patient in such a manner, the epidural venous pressure may also be lowered, further contributing to a dryer surgical field.

Occasionally, pharmacologic interventions must also be employed so as to lower the systolic pressure to the desired level. Often, by just increasing the inspired concentration of isoflurane—the inhalational anesthetic agent most commonly utilized—to a level greater than that necessary to provide for an adequate depth of anesthesia, this can be easily accomplished. In those instances use of a hypotensive agent such as nitroprusside is necessary.

When utilizing nitroprusside, radial arterial monitoring is the rule because of the rapid fluctuations in blood pressure that can ensue. Use of nitroprusside is far more common in those procedures in which spinal cord evoked-potential monitoring is performed. This is because inhalational anesthetic agents such as isoflurane are contraindicated since they interfere with the equipment's capacity to perform the task at hand. As such, a narcotic anesthetic technique must be chosen. The blood pressure tends to run higher with narcotic anesthesia; hence, utilizing nitroprusside becomes more commonplace.

During longer procedures, efforts are made to keep the total dose of nitroprusside administered to a minimum. This is to avoid the possibility of cyanide toxicity—cyanide being a metabolite of nitroprusside. This is done by incrementally administering doses of either propranolol, hydralazine, or droperidol, which have the net effect of limiting the nitroprusside dose requirement.

In patients with treated hypertension, cerebrovascular disease, or cardiovascular disease, the systolic pressure should not be lowered to less than 95 to maintain adequate tissue perfusion. Performing surgery on untreated hypertensive patients possessing marked elevations of the blood pressure is discouraged unless there is impending spinal cord compression. In patients with angina pectoris, nitroglycerin may be chosen as the hypotensive agent rather than nitroprusside in order to capitalize on nitroglycerin's ability to increase coronary artery blood flow.

During posterior spinal decompression surgery extreme vigilance must be maintained with regard to ensuring adequate padding of all dependent body surfaces so as to avoid pressure injury. The head should be maintained in as near neutral position as is feasible to minimize the possibility of carotid artery kinking and prevent nerve root compression in the intervertebral foramen. The eyes are routinely lubricated with sterile ophthalmic ointment and taped closed. Use of a Foley catheter is recommended in those procedures lasting longer than several hours.

Nondepolarizing muscle relaxants are generally administered at the start of the procedure prior to patient positioning. However, marked degrees of muscle paralysis should be avoided so that surgical colleagues can detect proximity to neural tissue while utilizing electrosurgical devices.

In those patients with coexistent cervical spine disease it is mandatory that this be communicated to the anesthesiologist prior to the induction of anesthesia. Occasionally, fiberoptic intubation techniques are necessary to adequately visualize the vocal cords. Forewarning allows for adequate preparedness and avoids undue delays in initiating the surgical procedure.

Though not routine at present, the administration of preservative-free morphine in the epidural space at the time of spinal surgery may become more commonplace in the future. This technique is considered to provide excellent analgesia of a superior quality and longer duration than conventional systemic analgesics.

Myelographic procedures are often performed as part of the diagnostic evaluation prior to surgery. A significant percentage of patients in whom such procedures are performed will develop signs of a "spinal" headache within several days because of a persistent leak of spinal fluid through the dural puncture site. When these troublesome symptoms do not abate with more conservative measures, epidural blood patches can be performed. After the administration of approximately 15 cc of autologous blood aspirated from an antecubital vein following prior needle localization of the epidural space at the level of the original dural puncture site, significant amelioration of symptoms usually occurs within 12 hours.

Anesthesiologists may also be helpful in treating symptomatic patients with lumbar spine pathology causing nerve root compression or irritation and in whom the decision has not yet been made to proceed directly with surgical decompression. A course of lumbar epidural steroid injections has proven beneficial in a subset of these patients.

Chapter 16

Spinal Instruments

William H. Dillin, M.D.
Gary Schneiderman, M.D.

The purpose of this chapter is to review the commonly used spinal instruments in the performance of decompressive lumbar laminectomy for spinal stenosis and lumbar disc excision. The indications for surgery and methods of patient selection have been reviewed elsewhere. We have divided the operative procedures for lumbar disc excision and decompressive laminectomy for spinal stenosis into three main categories. The instruments that are utilized in each of these categories fulfill specific functions.

The first step is the exposure of the spine. The instruments reviewed are designed to remove the soft tissue from the bony spinal elements. The principle of this step is to provide a bloodless exposure of the spine. The second step is canal entrance. The instruments reviewed are specifically designed to safely enter the spinal canal and to expose the neural elements. The final element in the procedure is neural decompression. With the appropriate use, the instruments presented are designed to decompress the neural elements with minimal retraction of the neural tissues.

Regardless of the type of instruments employed, the principles of lumbar spine surgery remain the same. Adequate exposure, proper magnification and illumination, a bloodless field, leading to a safe neural decompression remain the hallmarks of the surgical techniques employed.

EXPOSURE OF POSTERIOR BONY ELEMENTS

After the skin and subcutaneous tissue have been incised down to the lumbar fascia, an incision made in the lumbar fascia at the appropriate level is completed with the electrocautery just lateral to the spinous processes. At this point, a variety of retractors can be placed in the skin and subcutaneous tissue to allow for exposure of the fascia and to allow for continued dissection. These may be the Gelpi-type retractor, the Wheatlander, or cerebellar retractors. If deeper exposure is required in a patient with excessive subcutaneous fat, the Beckman-Adson retractor might be useful with its deeper blades.

Dissection of the muscle and ligamentous attachments off the posterior bony elements is accomplished utilizing soft-tissue elevators (Figure 16–1). Single and double instrument techniques can be utilized. In part, the instrument utilized is determined by the depth of the wound. In cases with a small amount of subcutaneous fat and muscular layer, a single instrument type technique can be used, utilizing Key or Langenbeck elevators. The elevator is placed against the spinous process medially against bone. The soft tissue is then swept off the posterior elements, moving from medially cephalad to laterally caudad. The Cobb elevator can be used singly or doubly. If two Cobbs are used, one is used for cutting and a second Cobb for retracting. Initially, the cutting Cobb is turned with the flat head portion medially under the bulbous tip of the spinous process. The subperiosteal dissection is begun. When bone is exposed, the Cobb can be diverted laterally. The tissue is dissected off bone, sweeping medial to lateral and the tissue held back with the second Cobb whose flat portion is turned laterally. This affords good exposure throughout the dissection and also helps the assistant to control bleeding with packing and cautery. The Cobb can also be utilized as a single

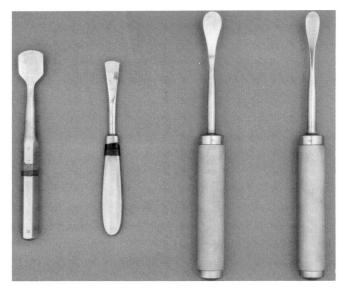

Figure 16–1 Key elevator, Langenbeck elevator, Cobb elevators—large and medium.

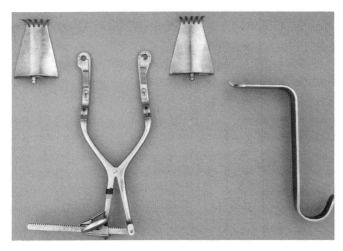

Figure 16–3 Cloward and Taylor retractors.

instrument as described for the Key and Langenbeck dissectors.

Exposure of the bony elements through the remainder of the operation is facilitated by a second set of retractors. The type used is determined by the depth of the wound and by the amount of exposure of the posterior elements desired. If limited exposure is required in such procedures as single-level unilateral discectomy, a smaller retractor that affords unilateral retraction with limited soft-tissue disruption is beneficial. The Williams-type retractor (Figure 16–2) is ideally suited for this purpose. The single-pronged portion of the retractor is placed medially against the spinous process. The blade portion of the retractor retracts the lateral muscle and fascia. This retractor affords excellent exposure of the lamina while avoiding dissection lateral to the facet capsule. The Taylor retractor (Figure 16–3) can also afford unilateral

exposure. The tip of this retractor is placed lateral to the facet and generally requires greater soft-tissue dissection than does the Williams retractor. It is more useful in the patient with bulky muscle or significant subcutaneous fat.

When bilateral exposure is required, double-bladed retractors allow for the required exposure. Again, the Taylor-type retractors can be placed bilaterally, but if more lateral exposure of the facets is required, such as in a transverse process fusion, these retractors will generally interfere with exposure of these elements. The Cloward retractor (Figure 16–3) is useful for smaller wounds and can be used proximally and distally for excellent exposure. However, Cloward retractors are somewhat limited if a wide, lateral retraction is required. In cases requiring exposure of the transverse processes or sacral ala, heavier duty retractors with a wide excursion can be used. The Watanabe retractor (Figure 16–4) and the Collis retractor have a variety of detachable blades that allow the tip to be placed deep to the paraspinous muscle. The variety of depth also allows for the retractor to lie flat on the skin margin, therefore not interfering with the surgeon's use of

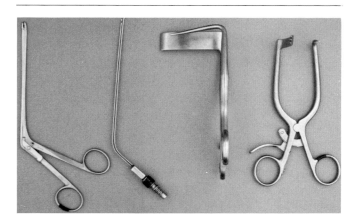

Figure 16–2 Williams microdiscectomy instruments, microlumbar discectomy forceps, nerve suction retractor, soft tissue retractor.

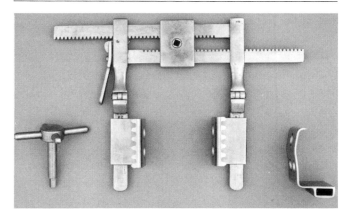

Figure 16–4 Watanabe retractor: wrench, retractor, blade.

other instruments in the remainder of the procedure. The placement of these blades is easily accomplished by first retracting the subcutaneous tissue and muscle with a Cobb retractor laterally and then placing the blade with teeth facing outwards behind the Cobb.

CANAL ENTRANCE

After the exposure of the bony elements has been completed, the canal may be entered by either a laminotomy approach or by an interlaminar approach. Again, the type of approach will dictate which instruments are utilized. In the laminectomy approach, the superior lamina is resected from caudal to cephalad to the insertion of the ligamentum flavum on the undersurface of that lamina. The instruments required are curved and straight curettes (Figure 16–5), Penfield dissector (Figures 16–6, a–b), a dental tool (Figure 16–7), and 90-degree and 40-degree Kerrison-type rongeurs (Figure 16–8). It is beneficial that the curettes, in particular, have a long handle. This allows for better control of the instrument, particularly in a patient with a deep wound.

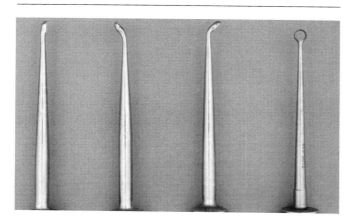

Figure 16–5 Curette: straight, bent back, curved, ring.

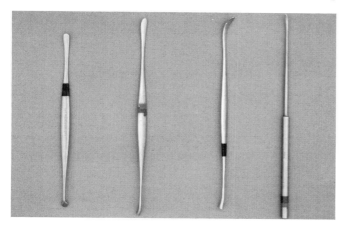

Figure 16–6a Penfield dissectors #1, #2, #3, #4.

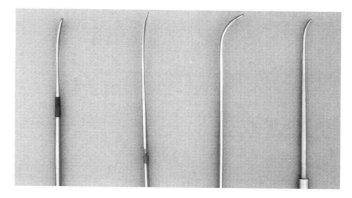

Figure 16–6b Profiles of Penfields #1, #2, #3, #4.

In this approach, the straight curette is used initially to expose the ligamentum flavum. The curved curette is then placed underneath the cephalad lamina. Care is taken to keep the cutting surface against bone. A sweeping maneuver commencing from medial to lateral is then utilized to expose the inferior edge of the cephalad lamina, dissecting away ligamen-

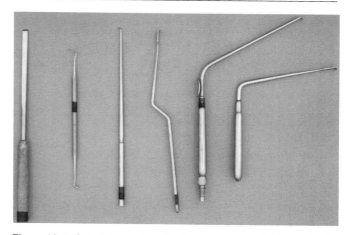

Figure 16–7 Spinal chisel, dental tool, nerve hook, straight hove, Smith with suction, Scoville angled nerve root retractors.

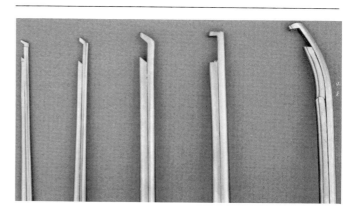

Figure 16–8 Kerrison-type rongeurs: micro 40-degree, 40-degree, large 40-degree, 90-degree, custom curved.

tum flavum. After the ligamentum has been dissected away from the superior lamina, the 40-degree Kerrison rongeur is inserted, again taking care to maintain the cutting surface of the instrument against bone. An appropriate amount of bone is resected to the point where the ligamentum attaches at its most superior attachment to the lamina. The degree of bone resection is determined by this superior attachment of the ligamentum flavum and can be assessed during exposure with either a #4 Penfield or with a dental tool. These instruments are again placed under the lamina with care being taken to keep the instrument against bone. Entrance into the canal can be determined by feel using these instruments.

After the superior portion of the ligament has been removed from the undersurface of the cephalad lamina, it can be retracted back utilizing a ligamentum flavum clamp and then carefully dissected off the inferior lamina with a curved curette. At all times, the cutting edge of the curette is directed against bone and moved away from the dural sac and neural elements when dissecting. A dental probe and Penfields are used to probe the area of dissection throughout the procedure to help determine if there are any adhesions to the dura and if there is any tension or pressure under the neural elements that could lead to injury during dissection with the sharp curette or Kerrison rongeur. The Kerrison rongeur is placed under the lamina and the cutting edge of the tool is kept parallel to the bony surface to be cut. This helps prevent trapping of the dura between the bone and the instrument. The dura can also be carefully packed away utilizing cottonoids if there is not a significant amount of pressure under the dura. The amount of pressure is determined with the Freer elevator or dental tool. The cottonoid is inserted with the bayonet forceps and positioned with the dental or sucker tip.

If the interlaminar approach is chosen, the superficial portion of the ligamentum flavum is first dissected away from the deep portion. This approach requires a 15-blade, in addition to the instruments noted above for the laminotomy approach. Only the lateral third of the superficial ligamentum flavum is incised longitudinally. It is important to avoid puncturing the deeper level. The superficial ligamentum flavum is then dissected from the deep portion, sweeping from lateral to medial with the straight curette. After the deep portion of the ligament has been exposed, one can still proceed with the laminotomy approach, utilizing the instruments in the steps noted above. However, to continue with the interlaminar approach under magnification control, an incision is made longitudinally in the lateral third of the deep ligamentum flavum. The undersurface of the ligamentum flavum is then explored with care freeing up the dura from ligament with either a dental tool or #4 Penfield. The lateral ligamentum flavum is resected with the 40-degree Kerrison elevator or dissected off the superior and inferior lamina with a curved curette.

In the case of total laminectomy, a bone cutter (Figure 16–9) is utilized to remove the spinous process. Care must be taken when using this instrument to cut only at the base of

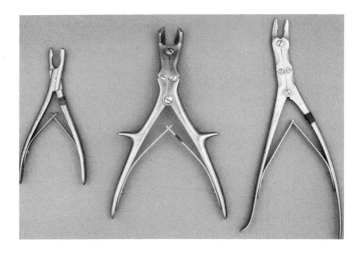

Figure 16–9 Luck bone rongeurs, Horsley bone cutters, Leskell double-action rongeur.

the spinous process and not into the lamina. Cutting into the lamina itself may lead to entering the canal and possibly injuring the dura. The Midas Rex and double-action rongeurs (Figure 16–9) may be used to pare down the bone posteriorly to allow use of the angled Kerrison rongeurs in the canal itself.

NEURAL DECOMPRESSION

Decompression of a compressed nerve root from disc herniation embodies a variety of principles. It is important that the nerve root be approached from a lateral position. This facilitates judgment of the tightness of the nerve root, eliminates the possibility of mistaking a conjoined nerve root for a herniated disc, and minimizes nerve root trauma during removal of disc material. Whether a surgeon employs an interlaminar technique or a traditional technique of hemilaminotomy with medial facetectomy, the end result should be a position lateral to the nerve root before the disc material is addressed and nerve decompression initiated. This will minimize the amount of retraction of the nerve root itself.

At this point a decision has to be made regarding the degree of nerve root compression. If the nerve root is retractable over a protruded disc, then the use of a series of nerve root retractors, such as the Williams' retractor, may allow displacement of the nerve root, gaining further exposure of the disc. With significant compression of the nerve root, retraction of the nerve root will only result in its injury. Thus, if a lateral position is established, bipolar cautery can be used to cauterize the epidural venous plexus over the disc space and disc material. If the nerve root is extremely tight because of a huge amount of disc herniation, whether contained or as a free fragment, use of a William's nerve root retractor (Figure 16–2), which is a combined suction device and nerve root retractor, may facilitate the exposure. This is not used at this step to retract the nerve root, but merely to block the access of the surgeon's knife to the nerve root.

An incision would then be made in the annulus laterally to attempt to excise the disc material prior to the retraction of the nerve root if the nerve root is significantly tight. In the case of free fragments, a nerve hook (Figure 16–7) may be passed superior to the disc space, sweeping material from the medial aspect of the nerve root toward the lateral aspect of the nerve root. This can also be accomplished with a Woodson, a small dental instrument, or a Frazier (Figure 16–10).

The purpose of using all of these instruments is to facilitate the removal of disc material in the severely compressed nerve root without retraction of the nerve root, thereby giving maximum protection to the nerve root. The free fragments are frequently removed with a pituitary disc rongeur (Figure 16–11) or they may be teased from the position medial to the nerve root with the nerve hook, Frazier, or dental instrument. An incision will be made in the annulus to evacuate the disc space. This may be done in quadrangular fashion with a small wedge of annulus excised or in an annular splitting fashion where the annular ligament is split along its fibers and blunt entrance into the disc space may be accomplished. The straight pituitary, the angled up-biting pituitary, and angled down-biting pituitary are all used to evacuate the disc space of free disc material. The technical requirements are that the pituitary remain in the disc space and not be placed greater than 1⅜ inches in terms of its depth.

After all free disc material is removed with the use of the pituitary rongeurs, the ringed curette (Figure 16–5) is frequently used to generate any further loose material from the space. Once this has been accomplished to the satisfaction of the surgeon, it is important to make a decision about the

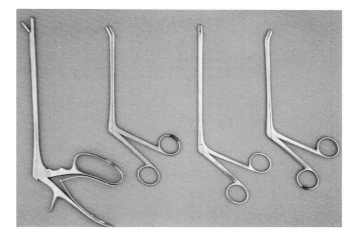

Figure 16–11 Pituitary rongeurs, Hodgson rongeurs, upbiting rongeurs, straight rongeurs, downbiting rongeurs.

complete neural decompression of the nerve root. This is done in two ways. Judgment of the medial-lateral freedom of the nerve root is accomplished with the use of a #4 Penfield and judgment of its freedom in the remaining subarticular gutter and in the foramen is accomplished with the use of a Frazier or Woodson. Some surgeons prefer the use of gall bladder dilators to make a decision in terms of graduated size of the foramen.

The same principles of neural decompression apply in the patient with spinal stenosis. Spinal stenosis encompasses such a wide variety of pathology that the judgment of freedom of the nerve root is related to the adequacy of analysis of the pathology and the experience of the surgeon. Stenosis frequently involves a number of pathologic elements, including hypertrophy of the lamina, hypertrophy of the posterior vertebral body, infolding and perhaps overgrowth of the ligamentum flavum, degeneration and bulging of the lumbar disc, and hypertrophy of the facet joints with the forming of spurs not only in the foramen but in the subarticular gutter. Thus, the technical requirements for addressing the pathology will, of course, vary.

In general, the principle of neural decompression is the removal of intervening tissue with minimal retraction and minimal surgical trauma to the nerve root. The purposes of decompression are the resolution of lateral entrapment phenomena by the resection of the subarticular gutter and/or foraminotomies. Some surgeons prefer to use the double-action rongeurs to perform the foraminectomies and medial facetectomies. Others use graduated sizes of Slesinger instruments or the 40-degree angled Kerrisons after thinning the facet joints and lamina and foramen from above. More recently, there have been more and more surgeons who have employed power instruments such as the Midas Rex or the air drill to thin the medial aspect of the facet joint and the area of the foramen so that the Slesingers or 40-degree Kerrisons can

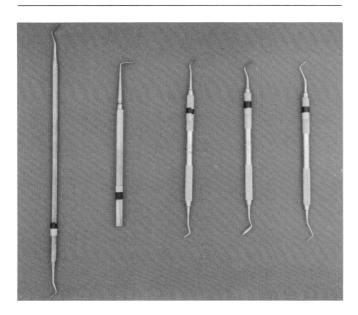

Figure 16–10 Woodson, Frazier, small dental instrument.

then be used appropriately to remove bone without nerve root compression.

After the surgeon has decided that the pathology has been adequately addressed, it is important to determine the degree of freedom of the nerve root. The instruments that are frequently utilized are the Penfield in a medial lateral direction. The angled Frazier or Woodson may be passed both above and inferior to the nerve root out into the foramen to determine the degree of freedom. Some surgeons prefer the use of graduated dilators to make an assessment of the total degree of foraminal freedom.

Since the hallmark of a successful lumbar disc surgery is the adequate decompression of the neural elements, the appropriate use of the instruments presented here will facilitate that goal. Of course, there are no instruments that can obviate the problems of poor patient selection or of poor surgical judgment.

Chapter 17

Posterior Approach to the Lumbar Spine

Robert G. Watkins, M.D.

The proper method of positioning the patient for a posterior approach to the lumbar spine should allow full chest excursion, maintain the neck in a safe position, and allow the abdomen to hang completely free of pressure. The hips and knees should be flexed enough to relieve nerve root tension but not so much as to obstruct arterial flow to the legs. The Andrews frame is recommended.

To set up this frame, connect the Andrews frame to the operating table and check all the connections to make sure they are tight. Position the patient prone on the operating table with his or her knees at the level of the knee pad of the frame. Place a steri-drape just across the top of the gluteal crease to cover the buttocks. Flex the knees and check the pulses. Put the right angle kneeling pad on the frame and insert the safety pin. Place the 90-degree kneeling pad on the table. Put the booties on the patient's feet and fix the straps on the booties to the clips on the frame. Next lower the distal half of the table. Approximately halfway down insert the buttocks pad and post. Continue to lower the distal half of the table to 90 degrees.

At this time, after alerting the anesthesiologist to maintain the tube properly, the patient is pulled back onto his or her knees with the knees and hips at approximately 90 degrees. Adjust the tilt of the buttocks pad to fit the patient. The table at the time of the positioning is in slightly reversed Trendelenburg to keep the buttocks back on the buttocks pad. Squeeze the lateral thigh posts to the patient's thighs and tighten the cranks to hold those posts in place. The Bovie pad can be placed on the patient's anterior thigh. Position the arms at 90 degrees to the trunk and the elbows at 90 degrees with

ulnar notches carefully padded. The Wiltse adjustable chest pad is used or foam rubber pads (4–8 inches) are placed under the chest. Raise the buttocks with the positioning crank to an appropriate level. Recheck the pulses. At times, there is an increase in lordosis in a patient with extreme flexibility. This should be compensated for by alternating the amount of hip flexion and building the chest pads up higher than the buttocks adjustment. A Betadine prep and paint can be used. Next, a wet sponge is used to wipe the superficial Betadine off, followed by a dry sponge and a Betadine impregnated Bi-drape.

Get a skin marker x-ray by inserting two 20-gauge spinal needles perpendicular to the skin approximately three finger breadths lateral to the spine. The objective is to position the needles in the transverse plane of the disc. Do not insert the needle into the spinous process. Inserting the needle at the level of the disc space is a more appropriate skin incision than with a spinous process marker. (See Figure 17–1.)

Use a skin marking pencil to draw the skin incision relative to the two needles over the disc space. Only a dermal skin incision should be made. The average length is 3.2 cm for a one-level microscopic discectomy, longer for a more extensive decompression; 25–50 cc of 1 to 500,000 epinephrine is injected through the dermal incision into the subcuticular tissue and directly down to the lamina into the paraspinous muscle mass. Cut with a scalpel through the dermal incision directly to the fascial layer. The lumbodorsal fascial attachments to the spinous process, the interspinous ligament, and the supraspinous ligaments are preserved by making a paraspinous fascial incision that can be sutured at closure without

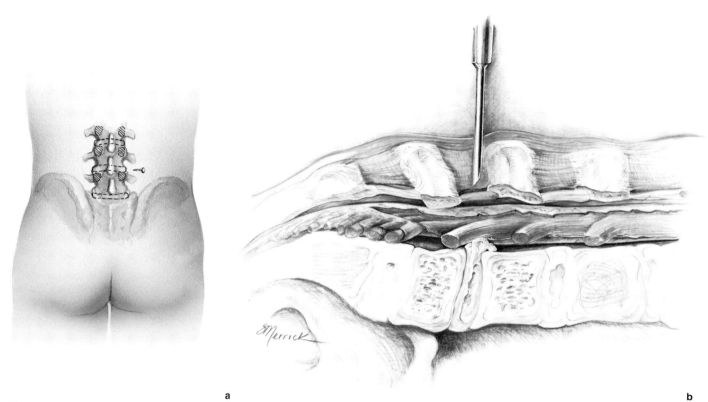

a
b

Figure 17–1 (a) Place the needle lateral to the spine at the approximate level of the disc space. The spinous process is not used as a marker because of its varying relationship to the disc space. For an operation on the disc, the skin incision is best placed directly over the disc. (b) Three dimensional thinking is very important. You must understand the relationship of the spinous process, the lamina, the interlamina area, the facet joints, and the transverse processes to the disc space. The interlaminar area leads to the disc space.

tension. This is preferable to removing all soft-tissue fascial attachments from the spinous process, unless a total laminectomy is to be done.

The lumbodorsal fascia is critical for spine stability. Maintaining the fascial attachments to the spine is important and should be done when possible. The abdominal, trunk, and gluteal muscles contract and tense the lumbodorsal fascia. The fascia attaches to the spine and allows muscle strength to stabilize the spine. The effect produced is much like a circus tent in that one pulls on the sides of the tent to stabilize the pole in the middle and provide a true tracking pattern for the spine. Contracting the trunk musculature to increase intra-abdominal pressure produces a larger, more rigid cylinder with an increased cross-sectional area, which includes the entire trunk rather than only the spinal column. This larger cylinder is better able to resist loading and bending stresses.

Using a slightly paraspinous incision and sewing the lumbodorsal fascial leaves together after the surgery retains more potential spinal stability. Make an incision into the lumbodorsal fascia just lateral to the bulbous tips of the spinous processes (see Figure 17–2). Lengthen the fascial incision. Insert the Cobb elevator, turned up, onto the spinous process just under its bulbous tip to begin the subperiosteal dissection (Figure 17–3). Then turn the Cobb bevel down. In dissecting

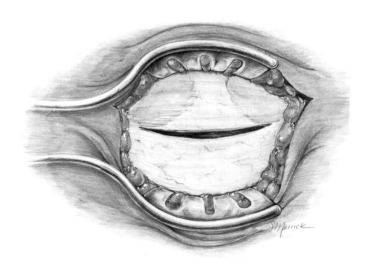

Figure 17–2 After incision of the skin, dissection proceeds in the midline directly to the fascial layer. The Cobb elevator is used to sweep the subcutaneous fat off the fascial layer for a 2 cm distance from the midline. A knife then opens the paraspinous fascia just off the lateral border of the bulbous tip of the spinous process.

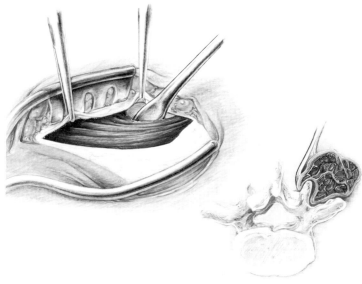

Figure 17–3 After incising the fascia, Ellis clamps are used to open the leafs of the fascial incision. A Cobb elevator is inserted with the blade pointing dorsally, under the bulbous tip to the spinous process. A subperiosteal dissection is begun, the bone of the midspinous process is dissected clear with the Cobb. The Cobb is reversed with the blade pointing laterally and the muscle is dissected off the cephalad and caudad lamina, exposing the interlaminar space. The Cobb is very careful not to injure the facet joint capsule and stops medially to the facet joint capsule. Holding the muscle laterally, the Williams self-retaining retractor is inserted. The Williams self-retaining retractor is inserted directly over the interlaminar area and is opened to extend just over the facet joint capsule laterally. The fascial incision is elongated cephalad or caudad as needed to provide proper self-retaining retractor placement.

the cephalad and then the caudad lamina must be identified by touch and cleared, taking care not to cut through the outer cortex of the lamina. Sweep the superficial soft tissue off the interlaminar area laterally out to the facet joint capsule. Do not damage the capsule. Protect the facet joint capsule and sweep the tissue laterally over the capsule. Remember that the interlaminar area is the only area that need be exposed for an operation on one intervertebral disc.

With exposure of the intralaminar area, the Williams self-retaining retractor is placed with the blade retracting laterally over the facet joint capsule and the pointed tip placed medially (Figure 17–4). For larger, bilateral exposures the Watanabe or the Collis retractor can be used and both sides exposed similarly. The superficial ligamentum flavum blends laterally into the facet joint capsule. Incise with the 15-blade or electrocautery into the lateral third of the intralaminar area or at the junction of the superficial ligamentum flavum and the facet joint capsule. Feather the blade as it cuts so that you can see the knife cutting edge as it goes through the ligamentum flavum. Use a curette to elevate lateral to medial the superficial ligamentum flavum from the deep ligament. Remove the superficial ligament with a pituitary. The vertical striations of the yellow deep ligamentum flavum can be seen in the depths of the interlaminar area. Use the angled curette to clear under the caudal edge of the cephalad lamina and a straight curette to define the ligamentum flavum attachment to the caudad lamina. Expose the deep portion of the ligamentum flavum's vertical striations.

Figure 17–4 The exposed right side interlaminar area. The superficial layer of the ligamentum flavum can be removed by gently cutting the attachment of the superfical ligament to the facet joint capsule and dissecting this out with the curette. This will expose the yellow longitudinal fibers of the deep portions of the ligamentum flavum.

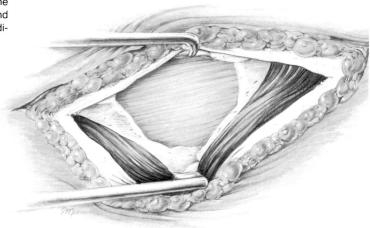

Several aspects of the anatomy of the ligamentum flavum are important:

1. The ligamentum flavum has a deep and superficial portion.
2. The ligamentum flavum blends with the facet joint capsule laterally.
3. It inserts over the caudal 50 percent of the undersurface of the cephalad lamina.
4. It inserts on the cephalad edge of the caudad lamina.
5. The undersurface of the ligamentum flavum is the ideal dural covering.
6. There is a vertical, parasagittal orientation of the ligamentum flavum deep in the lateral recess under the superior facet that may contribute to lateral recess stenosis.
7. It is the main stabilizing ligament of the posterior column and preservation of as much of the ligamentum flavum as possible will benefit ultimate spine stability at that neuromotion segment.

THE LAMINOTOMY

Perform as much of the lateral wall resection and laminectomy as possible prior to opening the ligamentum flavum. Estimate the size of the interlaminar area that will be needed for correcting the present pathology. A portion of the caudal edge of the cephalad lamina can be removed if it is felt that exploration of the spinal canal will require greater cephalad exposure. The walls of the interlaminar area may be the pathology to be removed. Progressing from dorsal to volar, the lateral wall of the interlaminar area is the facet joint capsule, the inferior facet, the intra-articular space of the facet joint, the superior facet, deep capsule and ligamentum flavum, the nerve root, blood vessels, and the floor of the canal. The preoperative CT scan should determine the amount of lateral recess stenosis and how much of a medial facetectomy is needed. Remove as much bone as necessary. For a standard L5–S1 discectomy bone removal is seldom necessary. At L3–4 a centimeter of cephalad lamina is often removed. Evaluate the CT scan for cephalad migration of a disc fragment that would require more lamina removal. To allow a more lateral approach to a larger extruded disc fragment, a small portion of the medial facet is removed. More extensive exposure may be required, depending on the pathology.

For a discectomy, make an incision with a 15-blade into the deep portion of the ligamentum flavum, approximately 50 percent of the width of the interlaminar area (Figure 17–5). Incise the ligamentum flavum by feathering the knife blade, allowing the surgeon to see the cutting edge of the knife into the ligamentum flavum. Make the incision by long cuts into the ligamentum flavum reaching from lamina to lamina watching for any sign of the white undersurface of the ligamentum flavum, followed by the bluish hue of the dura. Once the

undersurface is reached, the handle of the knife or a #4 Penfield is used to open the last few underlayers of the ligamentum flavum. The #4 Penfield is used to complete the entire length of the ligamentum flavum opening. Under the ligamentum flavum is usually a layer of epidural fat over the dura, but with a large space-occupying lesion in the canal, the dura may be immediately adjacent to the undersurface of the ligamentum flavum (Figure 17–6). Pass the #4 Penfield under the lateral leaf of the ligamentum flavum and retract the dura medially away from the lateral leaf of the ligamentum flavum (Figure 17–7). A cottonoid may be placed under the lateral leaf of the ligamentum flavum. With a 40-degree angled Kerrison rongeur in the right hand and the #4 Penfield in the left, pass the Kerrison rongeur under the lateral ligamentum flavum and remove the lateral ligamentum flavum (Figure 17–8). The epidural fat, the dura, the nerve root, and the longitudinal blood vessels in the lateral recess can usually be identified after removal of the lateral half of the ligamentum flavum.

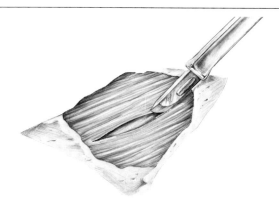

Figure 17–5 The ligamentum flavum is incised in its mid to lateral third portion. The #15 blade is feathered so that the cutting surface of the knife is seen clearly during the incision process. The blade is never sunk deeply into the ligamentum flavum for fear of lacerating the dura. Open the ligamentum flavum throughout its full length from lamina to lamina. If any laminotomy is to be performed, it is done prior to opening the ligamentum flavum by inserting the Kerrison under the caudad edge of the cephalad lamina and resecting a portion of the cephalad lamina.

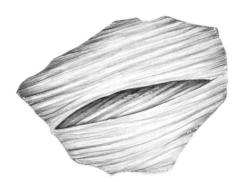

Figure 17–6 The #15 blade eventually reveals a whiter undersurface of the ligamentum with a bluish hue of the dura showing through.

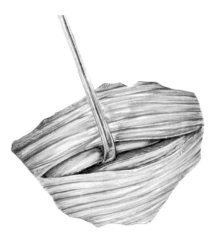

Figure 17–7 The lowest levels of the ligamentum flavum are opened with the #4 Penfield. The Penfield is used to extend the opening of the ligamentum flavum to its full cephalad and caudad extent. The #4 Penfield is safe for use near the dura in this manner.

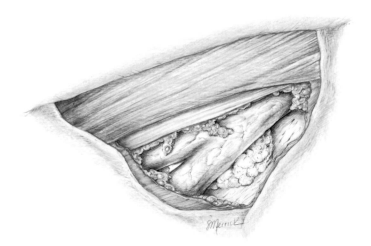

Figure 17–9 After removal of the lateral leaf of ligamentum flavum, the nerve root is well visualized as well as the suggestion of nuclear fragments under the root. Gently inserting the #4 Penfield lateral to the nerve root, assess the tension in the nerve root and its ability to be retracted. If the tension in the nerve root is too great, remove more of the lateral ligament and medial portion of the facet joint. For a tight nerve root, initially go laterally. If the nerve root is unretractable, then removal of the cephalad lamina is begun as well as the caudad lamina over the critical angle. The pedicle is identified and dissection continues laterally, removing the lateral wall of the interlaminar space until the facet is resected to a point just lateral to the medial wall of the pedicle. Over a large space occupying lesion under the nerve root, with considerable tension in the nerve root, resection of a portion of the cephalad lamina, the medial facet, allows one to expose the shoulder of the nerve root and to insert the #4 Penfield lateral to the medial wall of the pedicle in an area where there will be no traversing nerve root. If this extreme lateral position is needed, it must be used.

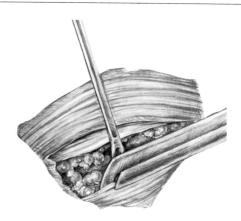

Figure 17–8 The #4 Penfield is then inserted under the lateral leaf of ligamentum flavum, between this lateral leaf of ligamentum and the dural sac and gently retracts the dura away from the lateral leaf of the ligamentum flavum. This allows insertion of the small 40-degree angle Kerrison rongeur. The Kerrison rongeur removes the lateral leaf of ligamentum flavum.

The deep portion of the ligamentum flavum runs vertically in the lateral recess and attaches to the facet joint capsule. Position the cottonoid or #4 Penfield between this portion of the ligament and the underlying nerve root. This stage of entering the canal is often an anxious one because of fear of bleeding and damaging the nerve root. The more delicate the approach, the less bone that is cut, and the less vigorous the lateral ligamentum flavum removal, the less bleeding there will be. (See Figure 17–9.)

Magnification is of tremendous value in identifying vessels and allowing safe, accurate retraction and, when needed, bipolar coagulation. Removal of fat causes bleeding and later scarring. Bleeding often starts when exposing the disc or nerve root. With the microscopic dissection technique, the magnification allows exposure of the disc with the #4 Penfield and micro retractor. Bleeding is seldom encountered. For those instances in which bleeding is encountered, lateral exposure is obtained out to the pedicle, and the longitudinal vessels lateral to the root can be identified and cauterized with the bipolar. Cottonoids, used only when necessary, placed laterally at the cephalad and caudad extremes of the exposure can collapse the vessels and allow work in the area between the cottonoids. There is a transverse or horizontal supply exiting each intervertebral foramina. The most consistent vascular leash is found just caudad to the nerve root exiting in the caudal portion of the intervertebral foramina at the cephalad portion of the disc.

For large exposures, when the dural sac needs to be retracted to the midline, the leash is identified, bipolarized, and cut. The more electrocautery that is used, the more scarring there will be. Use of cottonoids, SurgiCel, and thrombin-soaked Gelfoam retard bleeding. It is preferable not to leave Gelfoam and SurgiCel packing in the spinal canal. Cottonoids remove epidural fat and should be used judiciously.

The surgeon needs to know where the disc and root are without undue exploration. The key to intracanal anatomy is the pedicle (see Figure 17–10). The pedicle is deep to the caudad third of the inferior facet. After the ligamentum flavum removal, a nerve hook or dental tool is used to palpate into the canal. Often the pedicle is lateral under an overhanging roof of superior facet. In fact, the superior facet may be mistaken for the pedicle. To remove the roof of the lateral recess and to relieve lateral recess stenosis, with the Kerrison remove the facet joint medial to the parasagittal plane of the medial border of the pedicle.

Knowing the location of the pedicle tells you:

1. The disc space is less than a centimeter cephalad to the pedicle. Often it appears to be immediately cephalad to the pedicle.
2. The intervertebral foramina cephalad to the pedicle is for the exiting nerve root and the intervertebral foramina caudad to the pedicle is the foramina for the transversing nerve root.

3. Dorsal and immediately cephalad to the pedicle is the superior facet. The superior facet is the roof of the intervertebral foramina for the exiting nerve root and the A portion of the roof of the lateral recess for the traversing nerve root.
4. Just medial to the pedicle is the traversing nerve root.

Often it is imperative to expose the disc space. The disc is a raised, white, soft structure that may be covered by epidural fat, veins, and the nerve root. Feel for the disc using the #4 Penfield (Figure 17–11). It causes little bleeding and allows for palpation of the disc with the tip of the instrument.

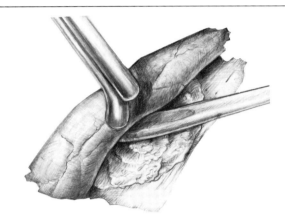

Figure 17–11 Whether from this lateral position or a much more medial position in a less critical situation, the #4 Penfield is inserted with the right hand the Williams microsucker retractor is inserted in the left.

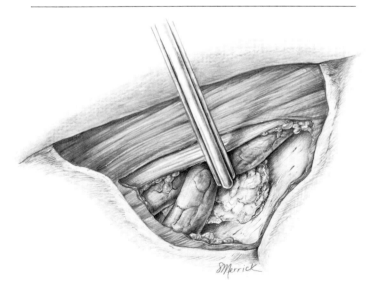

Figure 17–12 The microsucker retractor is used to gently retract and elevate the nerve root. This is a very benign process and seldom causes bleeding.

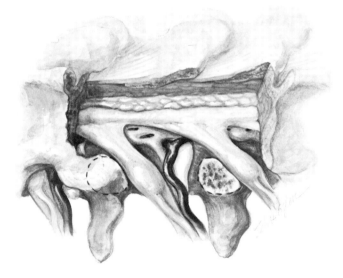

Figure 17–10 The relationship of the pedicle to the disc and the nerve root are shown in Figure 17–3. By knowing the pedicle, one can identify the disc less than a centimeter cephalad to the pedicle, the nerve root is immediately medial to the pedicle and the nerve root in the intervertebral foramina is immediately caudal to the nerve root. By identifying the pedicle with a dental or nerve hook, the relationship of these structures is known. Also, the transverse process is immediately lateral to the pedicle. To identify the pedicle from the transverse process, you simply bisect the diameter of the transverse process and this leads directly to the pedicle. The vascular leash is caudal to the nerve root, slightly cephalad to the disc space or over the disc space for large exposures of the spinal canal. The vascular leash should be identified and coagulated with the bipolar.

Reach out laterally, feel for the floor of the canal, gently retracting medially with the #4 Penfield and feeling for obstruction to this medial retraction. Do not retract against a major obstruction. Retracting gently, insert the microsucker retractor (Figure 17–12). Lift the root up and medial with the left hand, exposing the disc with the #4 Penfield in the right hand.

When there is difficulty in finding the disc and or retracting the nerve root, several methods have been used to prevent damage to the nerve root. Knowing the location of the pedicle in the canal is probably the most significant way to avoid major damage to the nerve root. Find the pedicle. The transversing nerve root adjacent medially to the pedicle must be identified. If the root cannot be retracted because it is tightly against the medial wall of the pedicle, proceed cephalad to the pedicle slightly lateral to the medial wall of the pedicle. The transversing nerve root should not be lateral to the medial wall of the pedicle. Exposing the disc cephalad to the pedicle and lateral to the medial wall of the pedicle can avoid nerve damage. The nerve root exiting in this intervertebral foramina cephalad to the pedicle will usually be further cephalad, just under the pedicle above. The exiting nerve root as it runs in an oblique direction will cross the intervertebral disc laterally in the intervertebral foramina.

The further lateral one goes on the intervertebral disc, the more likely one is to reach the cephalad exiting nerve root. A lateral disc herniation may trap the exiting nerve root in the intervertebral foramina. A conjoined root may totally fill the entire foramina from pedicle to pedicle. An exiting conjoined nerve root limits exposure of the disc. It can usually be identified preoperatively on the myelogram and contrast CT scan. The key to avoiding damage to a conjoined nerve root is recognition. This is facilitated by lateral exposure of the traversing root shoulder.

For further exposure of the disc, determine the amount of tension in the nerve root, being careful not to retract the root against a solid obstruction. If it can be retracted easily, it should be retracted medially with the nerve root retractor. If it is tight, it will feel like retracting against a solid wall. There are four common methods of dealing with a tight nerve root:

1. Explore the axilla of the transversing root with the #4 Penfield. The axilla is in the caudal part of the exposure between the root and the dural sac. If a fragment is found, remove it with the nerve hook. Bleeding may be encountered.
2. In obtaining more lateral exposure, be sure you have identified the pedicle and exposure lateral to the medial wall of the pedicle. The traversing nerve root should not be lateral to the medial wall of the pedicle.
3. Enter the disc space lateral to the root and try to decompress the disc and pull disc material from under the root through the disc space.

4. Be sure the root is free cephalad to the disc and that the ligamentum flavum and undersurface of the cephalad lamina is not an obstructing factor. Remove enough cephalad lamina and ligament to expose the shoulder of the nerve root.
5. The nerve root may be tethered caudal in the foramina to the pedicle. Remove the roof (the junction of the caudad lamina and the superior facet) over the transversing root as it exits around the pedicle. A foraminotomy of the foramina below may allow better retraction of the root.

The nerve root is gently lifted and retracted with a sucker retractor in the left hand and the disc area is explored with a nerve hook in the right hand (Figure 17–13). Great care should be taken not to stretch the nerve root. Exploration underneath the dural sac may reveal a large fragment of herniated disc that can be pulled out from under the nerve root with the nerve hook. The lateral exposure allows one to pull this fragment of disc laterally rather than vertically. Removing the fragment laterally from under the nerve root will decrease the nerve root tension and allow better visibility and protection for the nerve root. Large dilated vessels will often decrease in size and not bleed when the fragment is removed, relieving vascular distention.

Expose the annulus with the #4 Penfield and determine the texture of the annulus, amount of bulge, presence of herniation, or presence of a hole in the annulus. If an existing hole can be entered, sweep out free fragments with the nerve hook and insert the pituitary (Figure 17–14). If the hole is too medial, then extend the opening laterally. If there is no hole, open the annulus, making either a square annular window, a cruciate incision, or puncturing the annulus with a micro Penfield #4. The hole is expanded with increasing sized pituitaries (Figure 17–15). The size of the hole in the annulus is determined by one's philosophy concerning how much of the disc is to be removed (Figure 17–16). Most surgeons make a large incision and remove all disc material that can be freed by moderate curetting. From a technical standpoint, the bigger the hole, the more disc material should be removed. If you make a large hole in the annulus and fail to remove a substantial portion of the nucleus, it is more likely to reherniate (Figure 17–17).

Preserving as much functional annulus as possible, while removing the portion of the disc causing the intracanal obstruction and other loose nucleus material, is a good approach. If disc removal can be accomplished through a small hole in the annulus, the annulus potentially can heal if protected and retain more of its important mechanical function. When the entire annulus is to be removed, use a discotome, ¼ inch osteotome, or scalpel to cut a square hole. Make the medial and lateral cuts first, then the cephalad and caudad cuts. The cephalad and caudad cuts can include a portion of the cartilagenous end plate.

The weight of the specimen of intervertebral disc has little to do with the patient's symptoms or ultimate outcome. The

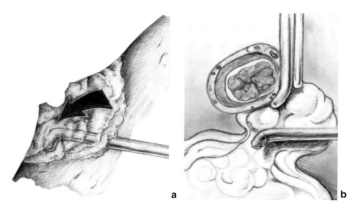

Figure 17–13 The retraction of the nerve root allows a nerve hook to be placed under the nerve root and to remove free fragments of the intervertebral disc. Skill in use of the nerve hook is imperative in microscopic lumbar discectomy. The nerve hook must be used not only to identify extruded fragments, but also to identify the hole in the annulus, to retrieve sequestered fragments by hooking them with the nerve hook and pulling them out laterally under the nerve root and undue bleeding should be avoided. When the annulus is not open, the micro #4 Penfield is used to puncture the annulus; a larger #4 Penfield is inserted and then the micropituitary is inserted through the puncture wound in the annulus. Rarely, a knife cruciate incision is used.

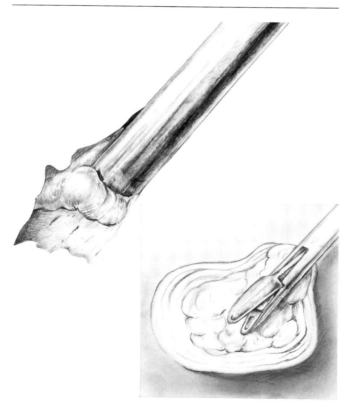

Figure 17–14 The micropituitary is inserted into the annulus fibrosus or into the puncture or opening in the annulus fibrosus. The pituitary should not be inserted deeper than the joint of the pituitary and by maintaining retraction of the nerve root in the left hand, the major bulk of the disc herniation is removed with the micropituitary in the right hand.

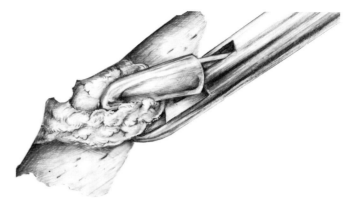

Figure 17–15 Remove larger intervertebral disc pieces laterally from under the nerve root and avoid direct, vertical extraction of the fragment and also avoid nerve root injury.

weight of any intradiscal specimen can be increased by the amount of cartilagenous end plate and bone that is removed from the vertebral body. Bone removed from the vertebral body is seldom required for clinical success. The surgeon retracts the nerve root with the small sucker retractor with one hand while cutting the annulus and using the pituitaries with the other hand. Avoid having the assistant on the other side of the table retract the nerve root. It is difficult for the assistant to retract with the proper amount of tension, and nerve root damage may result, especially if the assistant is trying to see the annular hole. When the surgeon needs both hands, position the retractor for the assistant, being aware of the angle of the pull, the amount of retraction time, and some idea of the tension. A cruciate incision is usually made, and through that incision loose disc material is removed with gradually increasing sized pituitary rongeurs.

The end plates are curetted. One of the greatest dangers is to use an angled curette and to pull upward in the disc space. An angled curette angled medially can cut the nerve root if the curette slips out of the disc space. To avoid cutting with the curette on the edge of the end plate near the nerve and to avoid the tendency to pull up under the nerve, two things should be done. The first is to use a ''00'' straight curette with two hands and lever the handle caudally while putting the cutting surface on the cephalad end plate. A windshield wiper motion is used. Then, reversing the hand, levering against the cephalad bone, curette with a windshield wiper motion on the caudad end plate, avoiding an up/down in/out motion, which can cause the curette to fly out of the disc space cutting the nerve. This windshield wiper motion frees plenty of disc material.

The second step is to carefully insert the reverse-angled curette into the opening in the annulus and push down to remove material from the outer edge of the end plate. After it has been freed, remove it from the disc space with a pituitary. A depth of 2 cm at any time within the disc space is the absolute maximum for an instrument. While there usually is a

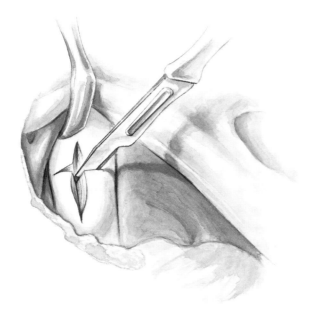

Figure 17–16 After removal of the lateral ligamentum flavum and retracting the nerve root centrally, the annulus of the disc is incised. A cruciate incision of this type can be used, or rectangular, complete excision of the annulus is used.

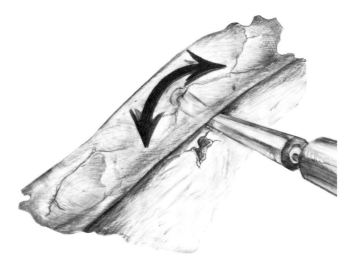

Figure 17–18 A variety of Frazier and Woodson dissectors are used to explore the entire spinal canal under the nerve root. This is both with and without nerve root retraction. The intervertebral foramina is explored and the disc space is explored underneath the central annulus, underneath the lateral annulus and outside the annulus laterally in the exiting intervertebral foramen. The back of the vertebral body above and the back of the vertebral body below are palpated and any raised area of disc herniation at the disc space level is assessed compared to the level of the vertebral body.

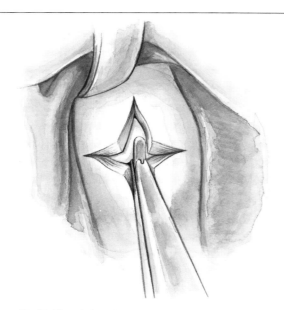

Figure 17–17 The pituitary is advanced into the annulus. It is seldom extended beyond the joint on the pituitary, and loose portions of the nucleus are removed.

safe 3 cm of depth in the midline, if the 2 cm of area is maintained, there will be little chance of anterior penetration of the annulus. All instruments can be permanently marked at 2 cm.

When does one stop attempting to remove the disc? When there is no more free material or easily freed material. A great amount of time is often inappropriately spent removing the

frayed edges of the annulus. If the decision was made to use the cruciate annular incision, then time should not be spent removing the incised edges of annulus. It is much faster to use the osteotome initially and remove the annulus in one piece with a portion of the end plate, if that is planned in advance. There will be scar under the nerve root whether edges of the annulus or an empty hole remains. Nature abhors a vacuum and will fill the hole with scar up to the nerve root. Leaving a healed, decompressed annulus is the protection against a volar scar under the root. For significant spinal stenosis, central, lateral recess, or foraminal stenosis, more exposure is needed. Explore the canal with the nerve hook, dental tool, or Frazier dissector (Figure 17–18).

TOTAL LAMINECTOMY

When a total laminectomy is needed for central stenosis, the fascia is removed entirely from the tip of the spinous process bilaterally. The bone cutters remove the spinous process (Figure 17–19). The Midas Rex AM1 can be used to remove all of the lamina over the ligamentum flavum and down to a 1 mm thin shell over the dura (see Figure 17–20). Alternately, the #1 Luxel rongeur can be used by inserting it under the caudad edge of the cephalad lamina and rotating the instrument cephalad, rolling a bite of lamina off. This allows one to look under the instrument and see a possible inadvertent dura pinch early. It is safe over the ligament. After reaching the cephalad

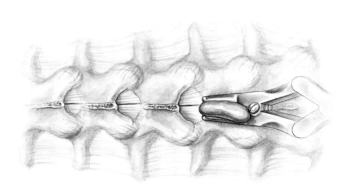

Figure 17–19 The bone cutter is used to remove the spinous process and a significant portion of the midline lamina. The Luxell can also thin down the outer surface of the lamina very quickly by cutting on the removed base of the spinous process.

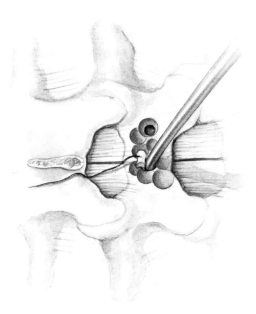

Figure 7–21 A cottonoid can be placed in this hole to push dura away. Often the thin hole allows easy removal of the remaining thin inner cortex of lamina with either a Penfield 4, a curette, or the small Kerrison.

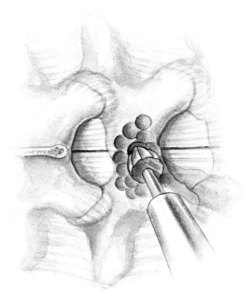

Figure 17–20 The Midas Rex AM1 burr allows one to burr through the outer cortex of the lamina to the inner cortex with excellent control. These acorn shaped burrs allow an excellent feel for cortical versus cancellous bone. The AM1 burr can be used to produce small pox holes that are blended together to send the outer table and cancellous layers of lamina down to a thin inner cortical layer. When the inner cortical layer is violated, the tip of the acorn burr does not cut the dura and allows identification of the dura through the initial small hole into the canal.

extend of the ligamentum, the cottonoids can be used to protect the dura from the Luxel and the entire lamina can be removed. Prior to using the Midas, the pars must be exposed by curetting the caudal tip of the inferior facet. Seeing the articular surface of the superior facet and the pars at each level allows full removal of the lamina and medial portion of the facet without danger of cutting the pars. Identify the pedicle as soon as possible to avoid removing too much facet.

Using the Midas AM1 held with the tip straight down, the lamina can be thinned to 1–2 mm. Even with penetration of the undersurface of the lamina, the dura is protected from damage because the tip of the acorn-shaped AM burr is blunt and does not wrap up soft tissue. The sides of this instrument will, so keep it at 90°. (See Figure 17–21.) Use just enough irrigation to cool it—not so much as to obscure vision. The lamina over the dura can be very thick and deep in stenosis. Once the lower lamina is open and the dura starts ballooning out under tension, be quite careful to use the drill only when the dura is totally protected by Penfields. Cottonoids can be wrapped up by the sides of the drill, so use the Penfields between cottonoids or dura and the drill.

Put the drill in the wound just off the bone prior to turning it on. Do not turn it on while touching anything. Turn it off in the same position. Be sure it has totally stopped moving before removing it from a position in air just off the structure that has been cut. Never remove it from the wound while moving. Be careful to use the drill perpendicular to the dura. Cut with the drill in a horizontal plane side to side rather than in a verticle plane up and down.

The Midas is a higher speed drill than the Hall drill. It provides good control because its speed eliminates the need for pressure and, therefore, it has less tendency to "run." Soft-tissue wrapping and running may also be a problem with the Midas, but the blunt tip AM burrs used perpendicular to the bone serve to avoid this.

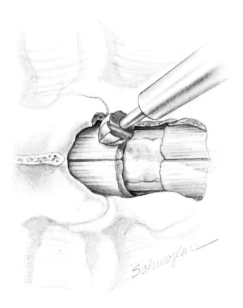

Figure 17–22 The AM1 or AM3 burr is then used to burr out laterally to the approximate level of the pedicle. This removes the overhanging medial portion of the superior facet. The ligamentum flavum can be used as a guide to protect this lateral removal of bone.

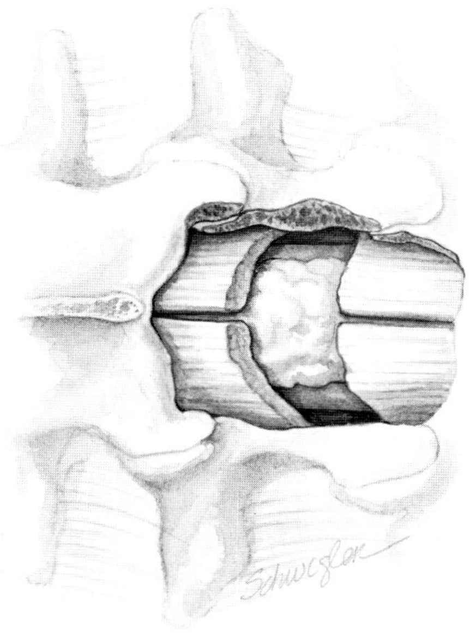

Figure 17–23 Identify the ligamentum flavum as the bone is being removed and stay on the ligament. With the lateral recess removal having been carried out, the ligamentum flavum, and the edges of the cephalad and caudad ligamentum flavum are identified with the fat covered dural sac interval.

After burring down the lamina to a 1–2 mm layer over the dura, the AM3 may be used to cut laterally over the ligamentum flavum to its more lateral extent. (See Figures 17–22 and 17–23.) With the ligamentum flavum exposed, it may be opened with a #3 Penfield and clasped with a ligamentum flavum clamp. Pass a cottonoid between the ligament and the dura. Remove the major portion of the ligament with a large straight curette from the opposite side of the table (Figure 17–24). The lateralmost ligament is removed by undercutting with the angled Kerrison from across the table. The surgeon can position the cottonoid and the assistant on the other side of the table removes the ligamentum flavum with a 45-degree Kerrison (Figure 17–25). The medial edge of the superior facet is removed with the lateralmost ligamentum flavum. Alternately, the assistant on the opposite side of the table also can position this cottonoid very effectively using the sucker and the bayonet. The surgeon uses the 90-degree Kerrison rongeurs to remove this lateral portion of the ligamentum flavum.

The objective is to identify the pedicle and remove all facet medial to the pedicle that is causing compression. Cut with the Kerrison out to the pedicle. The tip of the Kerrison usually first identifies the pedicle. Use the nerve hook to confirm this by finding the medial wall of the pedicle and following it volarly to the floor of the canal (Figure 17–26).

The ligamentum flavum can be detached with a curette from its caudad and lateral attachments, and a curved osteotome can free the cephalad attachment of the ligamentum flavum from

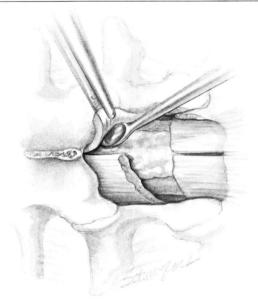

Figure 17–24 The ligamentum flavum can be removed by grasping the ligament with the ligamentum flavum clamp. Insert the curette between the dura and the ligament out laterally onto the undersurface of the remaining facet. A cottonoid can be used between the curette and the dura.

the undersurface of the cephalad lamina. Use a nerve hook to pull the detached cephalad edge of the ligamentum flavum into the intralaminar area. Use a straight curette to detach the

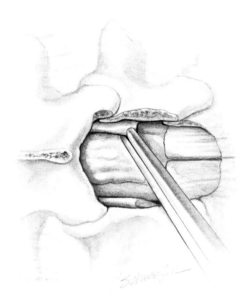

Figure 17–25 Cut the ligament from the undersurface of the facet and remove. The Kerrison can be used to remove additional ligamentum flavum. We often used cottonoids to tuck the folds of dura away from this lateral most portion of ligament during its removal.

caudad edge of the ligamentum flavum from the edge of the caudad lamina and the angled curette to detach the lateral ligamentum flavum. With this detaching method, the ligamentum flavum can be retracted intact with a medial attachment to the ligamentum flavum from the opposite side, allowing access to the spinal canal with retraction—not removal—of the ligamentum flavum. While the ligamentum flavum will shrink from its original attachment because it is an elastic ligament, it will still provide an excellent dural covering when reapproximated upon closing. There is some danger in detaching this ligamentum flavum in the lateral recess because of the nerve root. Great care is needed with the ''critical angle,'' which is the junction of the base of the superior facet and the caudad lamina, as the nerve root exits under the critical angle (see Figure 17–27).

MEDIAL FACETECTOMY FOR LATERAL RECESS STENOSIS

The lateral wall may protrude significantly into the spinal canal, causing lateral recess stenosis. This lateral wall (the inferior facet, joint, and superior facet) is often too thick to remove with the Kerrison rongeur. The medial dorsal portion of the lateral wall (the inferior facet) can be cut back with the Midas Rex AM 3 or M8 or A2. The #3 or #1 Penfield protects the dura when using the Midas Rex in this fashion. If the partial medial facetectomy is to be done, the Kerrison rongeur is a safe instrument to remove the medial facet when

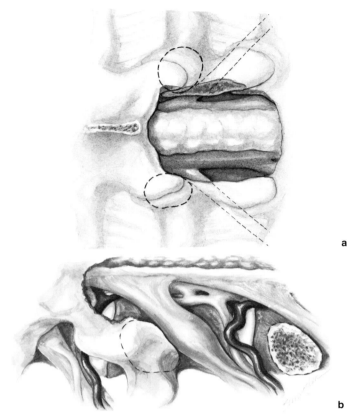

a

b

Figure 17–26 The location of the pedicle must be kept in mind at all times. The nerve root exits medial to the pedicle, the foramina is caudal to the pedicle, and the lateral recess will be removed when the pedicle is easily identified with no overhanging bony obstruction.

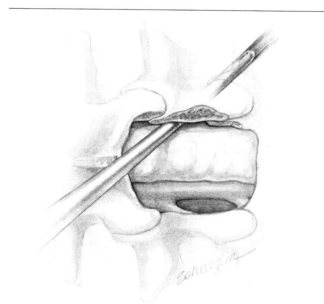

Figure 17–27 The intervertebral foramina is probed with increasing sized gall bladder probes and the dental and Frazier dissectors are used to probe dorsal and ventral to the nerve root to ensure the patency of the intervertebral foramina.

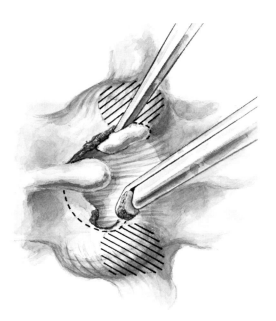

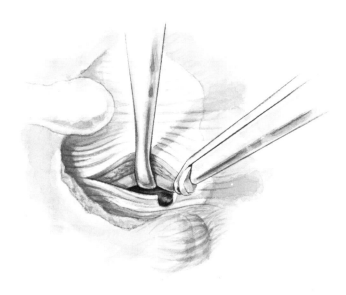

Figure 17–28 After clearing off the superficial ligamentum flavum, the deep ligamentum flavum is separated from the undersurface of the cephalad lamina. The Kerrison can be used to remove the caudal portion of the cephalad lamina and the medial portion of the inferior facet. A chisel seen on the right can also be used to remove the medial portion of the inferior facet to reveal the articular surface of the superior facet.

Figure 17–30 The #4 Penfield is inserted into the opening in the ligamentum flavum and the dural sac retracted medially. The Kerrison is used to remove the lateral portion of the ligamentum flavum.

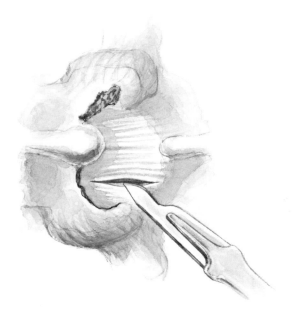

Figure 17–29 Opening the ligamentum flavum can be accomplished either by detaching the ligament from the undersurface of the lamina with the angled curette, detaching it laterally from the facet joint capsule with a straight curette, or, as we show in this illustration, by incising the ligamentum flavum directly in its midportion and then resecting the lateral portion of the ligamentum flavum.

the tip is protected from the dura and when the wall to be removed is not too thick for the instrument to bite properly. Starting medially on the lamina, cut the caudal portion of the lamina and continue laterally out onto the inferior facet (Figure 17–28). The amount of inferior facet removed varies according to the pathology. An alternate method of exposing the lateral recess starts with the Cloward chisel cutting the caudal edge of the cephalad lamina and the medial portion of the inferior facet. Using the bevel of the chisel and twisting it properly are the keys to proper use of the chisel. The chisel is safe on the inferior facet because the superior facet provides a guard from possibly injuring the nerve root. This exposure allows visualization of the facet joint space and the superior facet. The shiny cartilagenous floor is the superior facet. The ligamentum flavum inserts on the superior facet (Figure 17–29). The nerve root may be under this superior facet. Position the #4 Penfield, the #3 Penfield, or the cottonoid under the superior facet to protect the nerve (Figure 17–30). Use the Kerrison to remove the medial portion of the superior facet and the lateral most ligamentum flavum. With skill and experience the superior facet likewise can be removed with a chisel by cutting over the pedicle with the Penfield protecting the nerve. The Midas Rex A2, M8, or AM 3 can be used to remove the medial facet.

A foraminotomy begins after the lateral recess removal and pedicle identification. The root exists around the pedicle. It is the roof over that root as it exits that must be expanded first. The Midas Rex AM 3 or M8 can be used to cut a dome over the root—leaving a thin shell of bone over the root and plenty of

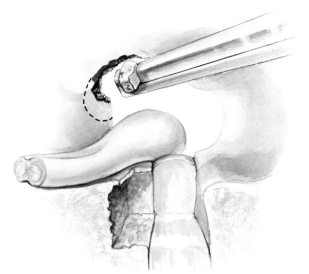

Figure 17–31 A more typical form of foraminotomy is to use the Kerrison to undercut the roof of the foramina, which is usually the superior facet and increase the size of the intervertebral foramina itself by removing a portion of the roof of the foramina.

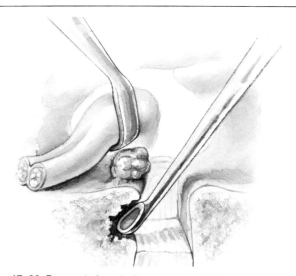

Figure 17–32 Removal of a volar bone spur under the nerve root. The bone spur is approached through the disc space and after incision of the annulus, the curette is used to undermine under the bone spur, cutting into the vertebral body endplate.

undersurface of facet. The Kerrison then is inserted on the root and removes that thin shell of bone and any ligamentum flavum attached to it (see Figure 17–31). Probe the foramina until it is clear. Gall bladder probes up to 5 mm in diameter or a Woodson can be used. Often the tip of the superior facet compresses the nerve root from below. Remove the cephalad tip of the superior facet with the Cloward chisel. The double-angled Kerrison removes more of the roof of the foramina laterally.

Volar spurs arise from the caudal vertebral body, caudal to the pedicle, at the edge of the disc space below. CT foraminal

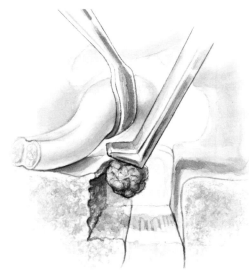

Figure 17–33 This allows one to impact the bone spur down into the disc space, thereby removing the obstruction under the nerve root.

reconstructions show these volar, uncinate spurs. The root can be tented over the spur and tethered laterally by foraminal ligaments. Removing the roof is not enough to relieve this nerve root tension. The spur under the root should be removed. While these spurs can be removed from cephalad to caudad by putting a chisel under the root, it is easier to approach it from the level below. Remember, these spurs are under the annulus of the disc below, covered with soft tissue, making removal with a chisel more difficult. Putting a knife under the root is dangerous.

Expose the disc below. Working from caudad to cephalad, identify the exiting root. Open the disc with a knife laterally. Use the chisel and curette to burrow under the spur and then the end plate of the vertebra. Hollow out a space (Figure 17–32). Use an angled curette inserted between the root and the annulus covered spur and knock the spur into the hole. The spur can be left in the hole or removed. It is a lot safer to remove it after the root tension is relieved (Figure 17–33).

After the discectomy, the delicacy of the approach will determine how much fat is left covering the nerve root. It can be supplemented with a large, free fat graft taken from the layer above the fascia in the caudal portion of the wound. When fat is not available, Depo-Medrol-soaked Gelfoam can be used.

After closing a dead space left by the fat graft, close the fascia with interrupted ''0'' vicryl. When midline fascial structures have been removed from spinous process, reattaching is necessary. The layers above the fascia are closed with multiple layers of interrupted ''00'' vicryl. Close the subcutaneous fat in at least two layers, tacking each layer to the lower layer. Draining both the subfascial and suprafacial layers is recommended. The subcutaneous layer is closed immediately adjacent to the subcuticular layer. The skin is closed with a subcuticular dexon, benzoin, and steristrips. The dexon is retracted and cut off after the steristrips are applied.

Chapter 18

Laminotomy for Lumbar Disc Disease

Donlin M. Long, M.D.

The goal of lumbar disc surgery is restoration of normal anatomy with the least possible tissue disruption. Current techniques have been in use for at least 30 years and are well accepted among spine surgeons.[3,10,12] The most significant recent advance has come, not from a surgical innovation, but through computed tomography (CT) and related techniques. These precise imaging modalities allow accurate localization of the anatomical abnormalities so that the surgical procedure can be planned to correct them. The location of the disc herniation can be clearly defined. The extent of protrusion and any unusual features such as migration of a fragment can be ascertained in advance of surgery.[2,14] There is virtually never a need to explore second interspace now.[9] Both medial and lateral disc protrusions can be identified in advance. The localization of the root with respect to the disc fragment can usually be seen and this greatly helps reduce the risks of the operative exposure.

When the patient has not undergone previous surgery, CT scanning or nuclear magnetic resonance (NMR) can be adequate in diagnosing the disc protrusions without any other adjunctive techniques. In patients with previous operations, particularly when these have been multiple, it is necessary to carry out simultaneous myelography or better to utilize small amounts of dilute intrathecal contrast. The role of NMR in evaluating the patient who has undergone previous surgery is not yet defined.

Before undertaking surgical removal of a protruded lumbar disc, it is important to accurately define the disc protrusion using these techniques. This will allow the surgeon to correctly identify the level, predict the localization and extent of

bone removal, anticipate the location of the disc protrusion, particularly with reference to the root, and appreciate the occurrence of related problems such as spinal stenosis.[15] At one time, lumbar surgery for disc herniation was stylized with a ritual designed to locate the disc and to be certain that protrusion was not present medially or laterally or at another level.[11] Now it is possible to individualize the procedure doing only what is required for an individual patient with resultant reduction in surgical trauma.[5]

PREOPERATIVE PREPARATION OF THE PATIENT

The patient undergoing lumbar surgery does not require significant preparation. Of course, a complete preanesthesia medical evaluation is required, but there is nothing unique in lumbar surgery that requires more than the routine examination. The patients are instructed in the potential postoperative complications, as well as the details of surgery and the expected results. The specifics of what patients are told will vary from surgeon to surgeon and must be individualized according to the patient's personality and ability to understand. Ideally, the operative procedure, including the incision, and the specifics of what is to be done are described in detail and the postoperative course is explained as well, so the patient knows what to expect. The options for therapy are emphasized again so the patient understands that continued conservative care and intradiscal injection are both reasonable treatments in most situations. The patient must be told about the usual potential problems: infection, failure of wound healing, postoperative hematoma, and anesthetic complications. From the psychological standpoint it is clear that this is not the best course of action for many patients, but the current medical/legal situation mandates that patients know about the serious problems that attend disc surgery, even though they are extremely rare. The missed disc fragment, the retained foreign body, injury to nerve roots, injury to the cauda equina, bowel laceration, and injury to great vessels are all subjects that can be discussed.[1,4,7,8]

As a final part of the preoperative preparation, the expected outcome of the surgical procedure is discussed again. Current data indicate that the success rate from surgery with the truly herniated free fragment disc should be 90 percent or greater, that the long-term success rate for all lumbar disc surgery is probably no greater than 70 percent, and that the long-term results of therapy over five and ten years show little difference between those who have surgery and those who do not. This re-emphasizes the patient's option to avoid a surgical procedure.[6]

The timing of surgery is also important. Lumbar disc surgery can easily be carried out on the same day that a patient is processed for admission to the hospital, provided all the necessary preoperative evaluation has been carried out earlier. However, it is not the best practice to carry out lumbar disc surgery on the day of myelography or sometimes even the day following. If a reaction to the water-soluble contrast media occurs, it may greatly complicate the postoperative evaluation of the patient. In the best circumstances, lumbar disc surgery is so safe that it is unwise to do anything that may lead to difficulty in the evaluation of a postoperative problem. It is a good idea to wait a minimum of 24 hours to be certain that no untoward drug reaction has occurred before proceeding to surgery.

PHYSICAL PREPARATION OF THE PATIENT

Special skin care scrubs or showers are not necessary. Most patients shower or bathe utilizing hexachlorophene soap the day before surgery and nothing more specific is necessary.

THE ANESTHETIC TECHNIQUE

It is feasible to carry out lumbar disc surgery utilizing either general or local anesthesia. General anesthesia is preferable. These cases are short and the anesthetic requirements are minimal. It is necessary to utilize agents that provide good muscle relaxation and do not cause venous dilatation. Otherwise, one anesthetic technique does not have great advantage over another and any standard procedure that achieves these twin goals should be adequate.

THE SURGICAL POSITION

If local anesthesia is used, most surgeons utilize either a knee-chest position or place the patient on the side. A variety of positions are available when the patient is to be operated on under general anesthesia. The most common is prone with support from the iliac crest to the acromion laterally. This may be accomplished with soft rolls or one of several kinds of surgical frames or special laminectomy tables. The principles are to provide freedom for chest expansion and avoid abdominal compression. Both of these techniques allow for free venous return and reduce the venous congestion in the epidural plexus. Most of the frames and tables built for this purpose also allow for maximum flexion opening the intralaminar space. The lateral and knee-chest position may also be utilized under general anesthesia. There is no particular advantage of one of these surgical positions over another as long as the abdominal and chest compression are avoided. If the patient is improperly positioned, the distention of the epidural plexus can be extreme and the increase in venous bleeding dramatic.

LOCALIZATION OF THE SURGICAL AREA

Accurate localization allows the surgical incision to be as small as possible. Before it was possible to so accurately delineate the anatomy with CT scanning, it was common to make a surgical incision that would expose the surgical site from the interspace to be entered to the sacrum to ensure that the localization was accurate. Most surgeons still depend upon the anatomy of the area. By careful study of the plain films and an appreciation of the anatomy of the interspace to be entered, it is usually possible to be certain of the position of the skin incision. However, the back should always be prepared so that extension of the incision in either direction is possible if an error in localization has occurred. It is also feasible to obtain a film as soon as the patient is positioned that will accurately localize the interspace to be entered and so guide the surgical incision. If there is any question concerning localization, a film is also indicated during surgery.

THE SURGICAL PROCEDURE

Following the introduction of anesthesia, the patient is rolled from the transport cart to the prone position on a lumbar frame and carefully positioned so that the anterior superior iliac spines and the shoulders are the principle support. The patient's abdomen must hang free and the chest should move easily. The arms may be placed either at the side or over the head. It is important to be certain that the breasts are not compressed, and for the male, that penis and testicles are free as well.

The back is prepared with a ten-minute scrub using an antiseptic soap and the surgeon then applies an iodine solution. Skin towels are applied with enough opening to allow for a single space error in localization in either direction. The potential surgical opening should extend from the spine of S1 to the spine above the interspace to be explored. A skin incision is made to cover the area of the expected herniation. Experienced disc surgeons frequently make incisions of approximately 1 inch. Incisions of 2–3 inches are reasonable when the anatomical localization alone is to be utilized. The skin incision is carried to the spinous processes and lumbar fascia in the midline. Skin towels are not needed and there is no reason to coagulate the small bleeders that occur at the junction of skin and subcutaneous tissue. Hemostasis is obtained throughout the field at each step before proceeding to the next. Self-restraining retractors are utilized to spread the subcutaneous tissue exposing the spinous processes and the broad expanse of the lumbar fascia. The subperiosteal dissection of the muscles from the spines and laminae can be carried out sharply or with the cutting current. The insertion of the lumbar fascia on the lumbar spines is carefully cut in the midline down to bone utilizing a cutting current knife. It is very important to maintain the relationships of the lumbar fascia. Utilizing the cautery knife, the attachments to one-half the spinous process are undercut until the lateral edge of this process is shown. This will allow a truly subperiosteal dissection and will allow closure of the heavy lumbar fascia in the midline restoring virtually normal musculoligamentous relationships.

The dissection is carried down the spines with the knife until the full thickness of the lumbar fascia is divided. As soon as the muscle bundle is clearly seen, osteotomes are utilized to complete the dissection. One inch square osteotomes will fit most lumbar laminae and allow for an accurate subperiosteal dissection. The osteotomes should be very sharp to minimize muscular trauma. When a proper subperiosteal dissection is performed, the longitudinal paravertebral muscle mass is not disturbed. The interspinous and intertransverse process muscles are disrupted, but the integrity of the major paravertebral mass is preserved completely.

The proper use of the osteotomes is also important. The first cut is made with either hand, depending upon the surgeon's preference, directly down the spinous process to the lamina and then out the lamina. This cut should remove muscle out to the medial aspect of the facet. With the muscle retracted by the osteotome, the second osteotome in the other hand is used to scrape the muscle away from the ligamentum flavum and upper or lower edge of the laminae. If the right hand has been used for the initial section, then the left-hand osteotome is utilized to cut muscle from the superior margin of the lamina and the ligamentum flavum of the space above. Then the muscle is retracted with the left hand and the right-hand osteotome is utilized to cut the muscle from the inferior margin of the lamina and the space below. If more than one interspace is to be visualized, the process is then repeated at the spine and lamina above or below, depending on the exposure to be made. It should be possible to completely expose each interspace with three cuts with the osteotome. It is important to avoid trauma to muscles, and the muscle capsule should virtually be intact when this maneuver is complete. Bleeding will often ensue, but if the wound is packed with a sponge, the bleeding will usually stop by the time the retractors are in place.

It is always a good idea to leave a tail of the 4 × 4 packing sponge extending out of the incision. It is quite easy to leave one of these sponges tucked in under the muscle gutter and if one corner is always left out, it will reduce the chance of this happening. The sponges are then removed, the muscle mass retracted with an osteotome, and the laminotomy retractors put in place.

There are many kinds of retractors available. It makes very little difference which one is used as long as one blade adequately retracts the paravertebral muscle and the other is not in the way of the surgeon. The cerebellar-type retractor with one broad flat-toothed blade and a post on the opposite side is a good retractor. The broad blade will expose one interspace effectively and the post can be placed between the spinous processes, where it is out of the way.

The next step is to validate the location of the exposure. The sacrum is usually easily identifiable by its characteristic hollow sound when the osteotome scrapes across it. The first spinous process above should be grasped with a towel clip and an attempt made to move the joint. When no movement occurs, the sacrum is identified. The first movable joint should be L5–S1; this provides the landmark for subsequent space identification. Of course, anatomical variations must be appreciated beforehand in order to be certain about localization. It is easy to be at the wrong space and sometimes very difficult to tell even with two or three interspaces exposed which is L5–S1. When there is any question, the best thing to do is take an x-ray in the operating suite.

It is now time to begin the actual approach to the disc. The first decision that must be made is whether or not bone should be removed.[11] If the interspace is broad and the interlaminar distance adequate, it may be possible to remove only ligament. If there is little room, it is necessary to remove a small amount of the superior lamina exposed. The Adson or Leksell rongeurs are a perfect size. One or two bites with one of these instruments will remove one-fourth to one-third of the lamina, which is usually adequate. It is rarely necessary to remove more than half. The cut edge of the bone is waxed. Operating microscopes are rarely used, except in unusual circumstances, but two and one-half to three power loupes are very helpful.[16] Overhead light is usually adequate, but a head lamp may be employed as well from this point forward.

Next, the ligament is opened medially. There are many ways to do this. The ligament can be opened longitudinally, with a 15-bladed knife, until a small amount of epidural fat is seen in the bottom of the incision. The incision is then enlarged bluntly with a small dissector and the interspace checked to see how close the root is to the ligament. The remaining ligament is then cut away with the knife, creating a window that is virtually the size of the bony removal. The interspace is then carefully explored utilizing suction and a blunt dissector. The epidural fat should not be removed unnecessarily. By blunt dissection, it is usually possible to determine the size of the disc herniation, its general location, and the location of the root.

It is then necessary to decide whether or not more bone should be removed. If the nerve root can be retracted medially or laterally without more bony removal, then disc excision can proceed. If the disc cannot be easily seen and the nerve root is difficult to retract, then utilizing Kerrison-type rongeurs with a 45-degree angle, ligament and possibly bone should be removed in the directions that will give the best access to the disc.

When the disc is laterally placed and the root is very tight, it may be necessary to carry out a foraminotomy before actually approaching the disc. The interspace is now carefully explored and the root must be clearly identified before anything further is done. Epidural fat is swept out of the way carefully so that it is disrupted as little as possible, compatible with good visualization of the root and the disc. The surgeon must now decide whether the disc can best be removed by retracting the root medially or by approaching the disc through the axilla. It depends on the position of the disc and the ease with which the root can be retracted.

When a free fragment is present, generally all that is required is to sweep the root off of the disc so that one corner of the disc fragment can be visualized. The exposed disc is grasped with a disc rongeur and the fragment or fragments gradually teased out. The same disc rongeur is then utilized to enter the interspace, usually through the herniation in the annulus, for removal of all extraneous degenerated materials. When this is complete, the interspace is thoroughly curetted.

The removal of the disc material within the interspace and the curettage are the dangerous parts of this procedure. It is possible to push the instrument through the annulus and anterior longitudinal ligament injuring the bowel, ureter, or a great vessel. This occurs most commonly when the anterior structures are deficient. For the beginning disc surgeon, instruments with measured lengths that allow the surgeon to accurately judge the depth to which the interspace is entered, may be a good idea. For experienced disc surgeons, this is unnecessary. Injury to these retroperitoneal structures is more dependent upon anatomical variation than it is upon some deficiency in surgical technique. It is important for the surgeon to always be aware of the depth to which the interspace is entered to be alert to the feel of the disc material within the interspace, and to be very careful about opening the jaws of the biting instruments.

A good trick is to open the jaws of the disc rongeur as soon as they have been passed beyond the annulus. It is much harder to push the open jaws through the anterior annulus and anterior longitudinal ligament than it is to slip the closed instrument through a small defect. It is important to check laterally out in the foramen and medially to be certain no other small fragments are present. This can usually be done by simply palpating and judging the tightness of the root. The experienced disc surgeon learns immediately when the root is loose and freely movable and when it is tight. It should be possible to gently manipulate the root and move it 2 or 3 mm without any feel of tension.

If this is not the case, then something continues to compress the root. If thorough inspection fails to reveal any offending lesion around the interspace, then the most likely point of compression is laterally in the foramen.[13] It will be necessary to carry out a bony foraminotomy in order to be certain the root is decompressed. This can be done with a Kerrison-type 45-degree angled punch to remove the inferior surface of the superior articular process, so enlarging the foramen. A high-speed drill or small chisels can be used. The pedicle may often have to be reduced in size, as well, until the bony opening is sufficient to eliminate all root compression. Unilateral facetectomy is of little consequence, and if necessary to provide adequate decompression, certainly is permissible, but should be avoided if not necessary.

When the disc is not a free fragment, but simply herniated out of the interspace, still contained by the posterior longitudinal ligament, a slightly different technique is required. Again, the root should be retracted in the direction in which it is most freely movable. When the root and dura are clearly defined and the ligament clearly seen over the bulge, an incision is made through the ligament to gain access to the disc. A small cruciate incision is preferred, though a window is utilized by many. The same techniques are then employed to remove the disc tissue from the interspace.

Handling these tissues in the interspace is very important. If the patient is properly positioned, epidural venous bleeding will be kept to a minimum. In the event that bleeding does occur, it can usually be controlled by packing. The twisted ends of 4 × 4 sponges, rather than cottons or cottonoids, are preferable. This is simply because they are easier to identify and the chance of leaving one in position is lessened. It really does not make any difference what packing material is used, as long as the surgeon is careful not to leave anything behind. The epidural fat and vein should be disturbed as little as possible. However, it is necessary to have perfect visualization and nothing should be done, except with direct visualization of the structures involved, until the interspace is entered. Of course, the removal of material within the interspace must be blind. Once the disc is removed and hemostasis is obtained, the tissues should be allowed to retain their normal configuration.

Hemostasis can best be obtained by taking a small amount of fat from the subcutaneous space and packing it carefully around the root. This also can minimize postoperative epidural fibrosis. Immaculate hemostasis is required. It is not permissible to close a wound that is still bleeding. The rest of the incision is closed in a simple fashion. The muscle is inspected to be certain that no bleeding has occurred and then the lumbar fascia is closed with single 2/0 absorbable sutures. If the wound has been opened properly, these stitches are simply placed in the lumbar fascia and should not enter the muscle at all. Large stitches through the muscle will produce fibrosis and reduce the chance of having a painless, strong, supple back. The subcutaneous tissue is closed with 3/0 absorbable suture and a 4/0 subcuticular stitch utilized in the skin. This means that no stitches will have to be removed and the patient can leave the hospital promptly, with no need for return.

POSTOPERATIVE CARE

The patient can be mobilized immediately. It is routine for the patients to be out of bed on the evening of surgery with adequate analgesia. There is no reason why a patient's incision should be painful and the use of narcotics should be sufficient to virtually totally control pain. Injectable narcotics are usually preferable in the first 24 to 48 hours and should be given on a regular basis rather than p.r.n. At the end of 48 hours, a switch to the regular use of oral narcotics is virtually always possible. Persisting pain that requires the use of injectable drugs signals either a complication or an abnormal psychological response. Patients can be allowed to leave the hospital as soon as they are able to care for themselves.

The psychological response to surgery has not been emphasized enough. There are patients who will remain in bed for a long period of time if allowed to do so and who will continue to utilize narcotics in large doses. When it is certain that no painful complication has occurred, the physician must see to it that the patient is mobilized promptly and that narcotic usage is reasonable. This does not mean limiting narcotics in the first few days after surgery, but it does mean that by the time the patient is ready to go home, the use of narcotics should be reduced. There is little reason to believe that any person who has undergone simple discectomy will require even occasional narcotics for more than two weeks. Patients are allowed to return to white-collar work at the end of two weeks, moderate work at six weeks, and heavy laborers are not allowed to return to work for three months. At the first routine postoperative visit, patients are given an exercise program and instructed to continue it for life.

POSTOPERATIVE COMPLICATIONS

If the patient awakens with a catastrophic neurological deficit that is unexpected, immediate reexploration or radiographic evaluation of the surgical site is required. If the deficit is less serious and commensurate with the findings at surgery, it is not necessary to evaluate the situation. This is a decision that must always be left to the discretion of the surgeon, who best knows the findings.

Prolonged ileus following surgery raises the possibility of a bowel injury and should always be evaluated. Ileus following extensive laminectomy is quite common, but virtually never occurs after simple single-level exploration. Injury to great vessels is rarely apparent in the postoperative state, but is more commonly signaled by a catastrophic fall in pressure during surgery. If such an event occurs during surgery or in the immediate postoperative period, then immediate evaluation and vascular repair is mandatory.

If the patient fails to achieve prompt relief of pain, it is suspicious that a disc fragment may have been missed or that root compression continues. This is particularly true if the pain is actually worsened. Most patients with true disc herniation or clear-cut root compression syndromes will achieve pain relief immediately and certainly within a few days. If this does not occur, reevaluation of the patient may be indicated, particularly if the surgeon is unsatisfied with the findings. Again, this is a decision that cannot be generalized and is best left to the individual surgeon, who best understands the abnormalities found at surgery and what is to be expected.

REFERENCES

1. Dohn DF: Complications of lumbar disc surgery, in Hardy RW (ed): *Lumbar Disc Disease, Seminars in Neurological Surgery*. New York, Raven Press, 1982, pp 165–176.

2. Duchesneau PM: Radiologic diagnosis of lumbar disc disease, in Hardy RW (ed): *Lumbar Disc Disease, Seminars in Neurological Surgery*. New York, Raven Press, 1982, pp 29–50.

3. Fager CA: Surgical approaches to lumbar disk lesions and spondylosis. *Surg Clin North Am* 1980;60:649–663.

4. Fager CA, Freidberg SR: Analysis of failures and poor results of lumbar spine surgery. *Spine* 1980;5:87–94.

5. Fager CA: Lumbar disc disease—Surgical treatment, in Hardy RW (ed): *Lumbar Disc Disease, Seminars in Neurological Surgery*. New York, Raven Press, 1982, pp 119–145.

6. Finneson BE: Lumbar disc disease, in Finneson BE (ed): *Low Back Pain*, ed 3. Philadelphia, JB Lippincott Co, 1980, pp 287–377.

7. Freeman DG: Major vascular complications of lumbar disc surgery. *West J Surg* 1961;60:175.

8. Hardy RW: Repeat operation for lumbar disc, in Hardy RW (ed): *Lumbar Disc Disease, Seminars in Neurological Surgery*. New York, Raven Press, 1982, pp 193–1202.

9. Hudgins WR: Exposure of two interspaces for lumbar disc surgery. *J Neurosurg* 1975;42:59–60.

10. Kempe LG: *Operative Neurosurgery, Vol 2, Posterior Fossa, Spinal Cord, and Peripheral Nerve Disease*. New York, Springer-Verlag, 1970, pp 266–276.

11. Love JG: Removal of protruded intervertebral disks without laminectomy. *Proc Mayo Clin* 1939, 1940;14:800, 15:4.

12. Mixter WJ, Barr JS: Rupture of the intervertebral disc with involvement of the spinal canal. *N Engl J Med* 1934;211:210–215.

13. Shenkin HA, Haft H: Foraminotomy in the surgical treatment of herniated lumbar discs. *Surgery* 1966;60:274–279.

14. Weinstein MA, Modic MT: Computed tomography scanning of the lumbar spine, in Hardy RW (ed): *Lumbar Disc Disease, Seminars in Neurological Surgery*, New York, Raven Press, 1982, pp 51–64.

15. Weinstein PR: Lumbar stenosis, in Hardy RW (ed): *Lumbar Disc Disease, Seminars in Neurological Surgery*, New York, Raven Press, 1982, pp 257–276.

16. Wilson DH and Harbaugh R: Lumbar discectomy: A comparative study of microsurgical and standard technique, in Hardy RW (ed): *Lumbar Disc Disease, Seminars in Neurological Surgery*, New York, Raven Press, 1982.

Chapter 19

Techniques of Lumbar Posterior Decompression Procedures in the Lateral Position

Michael L.J. Apuzzo, M.D.

The major objectives in surgery of herniated lumbar discs are (1) decompression of the involved nerve root or roots and cauda equina with restitution of the normal anatomical disposition of elements of the cauda equina within the spinal and root canals and (2) maintenance of optimal biomechanical preservation of bony spinal, joint, and ligamentous elements. In accomplishing this end, minimal manipulation of neural elements is imperative, as an anatomical environment that will preclude recurrent root entrapment at the operated region is provided. Experience in the surgery of this region has indicated that patient selection is equally as important as meticulous and painstaking operative technique. This chapter will address the basic elements of operative technique as related to the lateral position for cauda equina and individual root decompression and disc excision.

The lateral position provides a physiological placement of the patient with maximum exposure of lateral elements of the main lumbar dural tube and nerve roots. At the same time, it accomplishes the provision of a postural substrate that offers maximum exposure of the intralaminar space, ligamentum flavum, and interbody spaces in the region. This is provided without the risk of increased intra-abdominal or intrathoracic pressure with secondary distention of the epidural venous complex, and, therefore, an optimum surgical field within the spinal and root canals is realized. The position is one of considerable comfort for the operating surgeon and offers the opportunity not only for assistants and nurses to view the operative procedure but also for individuals who are learning to appreciate surgical anatomy and technique.

PREOPERATIVE RADIOGRAPHIC ASSESSMENT

In preparation of the patient for surgery, certain areas of radiographic assessment are important in establishing a comprehension of the pathological alterations within the spinal and root canals. Appropriate radiographic studies will provide insights that will make the surgical endeavor safer for the patient and more rewarding for the surgeon. Computed tomography has emerged as the primary screening radiographic adjunct. This modality should be obtained based on the patient's history, neurological examination, and plain film findings. Such studies provide three-dimensional information related to root canal, spinal canal, and associated anatomy. In the event that all information coincides with the introduction of contrast media, metrizamide is not necessary; however, in the circumstance that elements of vagary exist, or issues of multiple levels of involvement are present, or findings do not absolutely relate to physical findings, myelography with the possible concurrent utilization of imaging is an important technique to establish absolute structural definition. The region of the conus medullaris should be clearly visualized.

ESSENTIALS OF POSITIONING

Following the induction of adequate general anesthesia, positioning of the patient is undertaken (Figures 19–1 and 19–2). In consideration of the lateral position the patient's painful extremity is placed superiorly. In initiating positioning, the surgeon and three assistants are the optimum number

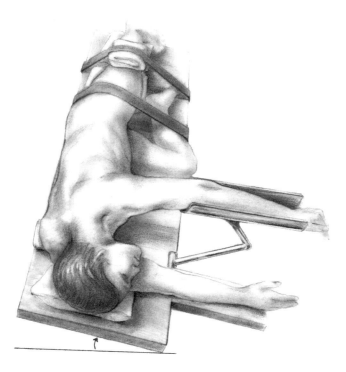

Figure 19–1 Schematic representation of lateral position. Painful extremity is superior. Operative level is at midpoint of table. Table is side-tilted away from operator to afford maximum visualization of lateral recess and to optimize lateral spinal canal visualization.

to effect this maneuver with ease. The proposed operated level is placed at the midpoint for flexion of the operating table and the patient's back is moved to the lateral table edge closest to the surgeon. The table is then fully flexed and the inferior lower extremity is flexed at the hip and knee with the knee supported by a padded kidney rest inserted at the break point.

The superior extremity is fully extended and supported medially by two pillows, one at the level of the thigh and the other at the level of the leg. At this time several bands of 3-inch cloth adhesive tape are run from one lateral runner of the operating table to the other to maintain the pelvis in a flexed position. These maneuvers accomplish the following: (1) the lumbar curve is straightened and largely reversed, (2) the ligamentum flavum at the operated level as the intralaminar space is distracted, (3) the nerve root sheaths at the superior aspect of the canal are disposed and lengthened to allow for optimum exposure and visualization of the lateral recess of the spinal canal, (4) the interbody space is distracted posteriorly and superiolaterally so that adequate evacuation and visualization within the interspace may be accomplished.

The inferior axilla is supported on an axillary roll. The upper limb is supported in a cradle. The patient's thorax is made parallel with the floor by manipulation of the reverse Trendelenburg setting of the operating table. The table is then side-tilted away from the surgeon so that the lumbar region is turned approximately 15–20° from the vertical plane.

SURGICAL TECHNIQUE

Preparation and Draping

The lumbodorsal region is appropriately prepped. Marking is then undertaken with a soft pen (Figures 19–2 and 19–3). Initially, the posterior-superior iliac spines are identified and marked. The first interspace palpable superior to a line drawn between these spines is the L5–S1 intraspinous space. This is identified and an appropriate mark for level is made. To assist with identification of the appropriate operated level a perpendicular line is drawn from the iliac crest to the midline. The relationship of this line to the L4–L5 interspace is judged

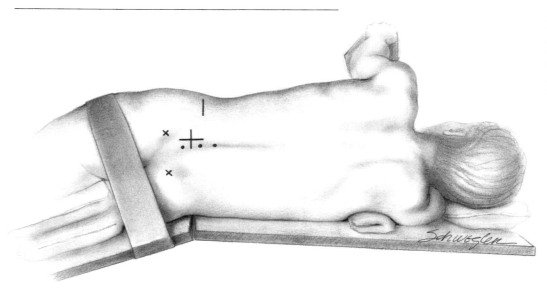

Figure 19–2 Localization of operative level in lower lumbar area of palpation of bony landmarks (Figure 19–3). Incision for single-level exploration (L) L5–S1.

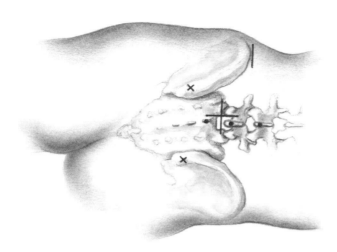

Figure 19–3 Bony landmarks for localization of level and incision. Posterior superior iliac spines (X) with first palpable interspinous space L5–S1. Iliac crest generally at L4–5 level. These guides allow for entry, but sacral identification and direct count establish absolute level of laminotomy.

according to A-P lumbosacral spine films. Rather than using x-ray identification of the proper level, it is efficacious for identification of the L4–L5 level to identify the sacrum and the L5–S1 level in all cases prior to embarking on decompression of the L4–L5 region. At higher levels x-ray identification has been used in the operating room.

For the purposes of this discussion an L5–S1 exposure for decompression of the S1 nerve root and excision of the herniated nucleus pulposus at the L5–S1 level will be described. An incision is marked 1 cm superior and lateral to the spines of L5 and S1. The length of this mark is variable (4–6 cm) according to the physique of the given patient. Infiltration is undertaken in the subperiosteal and paraspinous muscular planes at both the L5 and S1 levels with a solution of 0.5 percent xylocaine with epinephrine. Approximately 5–7 cc of this solution are used at each level. The subcutaneous tissues are then infiltrated with a similar solution in the region of the marking for the incision. A draping system that incorporates three towels, one at the superior, one at the inferior, and one at the medial surface of the field, is recommended. A Steri-drape is then placed over the three towels and marked area with a cuff fashioned on the lateral field. This will act as an anchor for the secondary laparotomy drapes that follow.

After draping, the surgeon has the option of either sitting or standing during the operative procedure. The scrub nurse is positioned to the right in the case of a right-handed surgeon and the assistant is positioned to the left. A Mayo stand is placed between the surgeon and the nurse with a secondary table at the nurse's side to augment the essential instrumentation for each portion of the procedure as it evolves. A 9 French suction apparatus is positioned on the surgeon's left and a

blunt-tipped bipolar coagulating forceps is placed on the surgeon's right for easy access.

Incision and Laminar Exposure

With incision of the cutaneous and subcutaneous spaces, the lumbodorsal fascia is identified approximately 1 cm parallel to the spines of L5 and S1. Bleeding at the cutaneous margins is controlled with Michel clips, which also prevent the displacement of the Steri-drape from the wound edge. The spines of L5 and S1 are identified by palpation and an incision is made parallel to these spines in the lumbodorsal fascia to expose the paraspinous muscular groups. The assistant introduces a hand Meyerding retractor and the surgeon, using a 20 mm Hoen periosteal elevator, develops a subperiosteal plane at the level of the spine of S1 and develops this plane inferiorly along the spine to the level of the lamina (Figure 19–4). Once the lamina is appreciated, the periosteal instrument is rotated in position and appropriately utilized so that the subperiosteal plane can be developed laterally to the level of the facet joint. The assistant introduces gauze sponges to assist the dissection of the paraspinous musculature. Attention is then turned to the L5 spine, where a similar dissection is undertaken, prior to which a Mayo scissors is employed to incise the multifidus rotator that separates the two spines in a muscular band. This dissection being completed, the gauze packings are removed, the hand Meyerding retractor is introduced laterally to the level facet joint, and palpation is undertaken. The sacrum is identified as well as the lamina of L5. Retraction of the paraspinous musculature is then maintained with a Hoen self-retaining retractor. This instrument is optimally positioned in the following fashion. Initially, the spinous component of the retractor system is placed at the midline. Secondly, the muscle retracting blade is placed over the hand Meyerding retractor and that retractor is removed. Finally, the handle of the retractor system is attached to both blades and retraction is effected. Removal of retained muscle may then be undertaken with a pituitary rongeur.

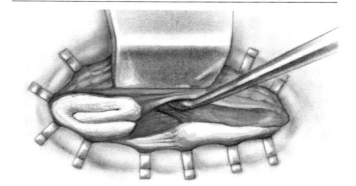

Figure 19–4 Combinations of infiltration with xylocaine epinephrine solution, meticulous identification of tissue layers and establishing of subperiosteal plane allow for rapid, virtually bloodless exposure of lamina.

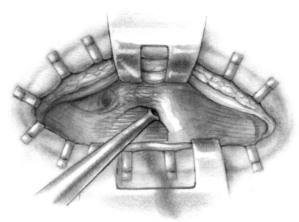

Figure 19–5 4 mm bone curette establishes sublaminar plane. A Hoen retractor system is in place. Superior and inferior lamina of level, as well as the ligamentum, is clearly identified.

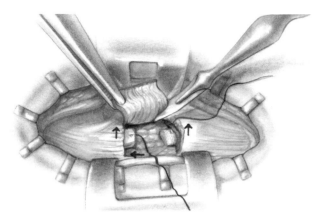

Figure 19–7 The ligamentum is excised along bony margins with protective cottonoids in the epidural space.

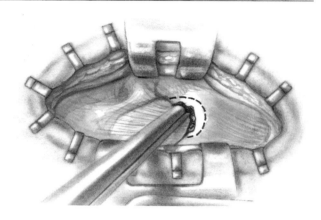

Figure 19–6 Angled bone punches are used to complete hemilaminotomy to enlarge exposure of ligamentum.

Laminotomy, Partial Facetectomy, and Foraminotomy

A 4 mm bone curette is then used under the inferior edge of the lamina of L5 to establish the plane between the leading edge of that lamina and ligamentum flavum (Figure 19–5). As has already been noted, the lateral position places the ligamentum flavum in a fully stretched position so that it is readily appreciated with a maximum visualization of the interlaminar space. Following development of the natural plane of cleavage between the ventral surface of the L5 lamina and the ligamentum flavum, a laminotomy is fashioned utilizing a Leksell rongeur. Employment of 45-degree angled bone punches of 3, 5, and 7 mm sizes with reduced depth of foot-plates to accomplish further superior and lateral extension of the laminotomy opening (Figure 19–6) are recommended. In the event that there is encroachment by a hypertrophied or a sizable facet joint, the medial aspect of this joint is appropriately trimmed either with a Leksell rongeur or a combination of bone curettes and angled bone punches.

Optimum exposure of the ligamentum flavum having been gained, this structure is then incised medially parallel to the spine with a #15 blade scalpel (Figure 19–7). A small cottonoid pledget is then introduced into the epidural space and the ligamentum flavum is excised with the #15 blade, with appropriate manipulation of the cottonoid in the epidural space to protect underlying dura during the course of this maneuver. Incision is initially made along the margin of the S1 lamina, secondarily along the margin of the L5 lamina. The ligamentum flavum is then reflected laterally and excised either with a large bone punch or by transverse incision at the region of the facet joint. The operative procedure from the stage of excision of the ligamentum flavum onward is potentially enhanced by the employment of the operating microscope setting with a 250 or 275 mm lens.

With excision of the ligamentum flavum, superior and lateral bony removal is undertaken. It is important to stress that in the course of root decompression and disc excision by this technique exposure of the lateral recess and lateral component of the spinal canal with entry into the root canal is imperative and is one of the primary surgical maneuvers in reducing unnecessary retraction on the root during decompression and evacuation of the interbody space. This bony access is acquired utilizing a combination of angled bone punches initiated superiorly and laterally, which are augmented by bone curettes. Introduction of soft cottonoids prior to the placement of bone cutting instruments is important to reduce the possibility of a dural tear or neural injury. In the event that there is considerable dorsal displacement of neural elements, it is inadvisable to introduce foot-plated instruments into the bony recess, and under these circumstances either sharp curettes or a high-speed drill should be employed to effect appropriate bony exposure. Lateral decompression may be achieved by angular undercutting of facets (Figure 19–8) employing fine-angled bone punches or curettes. This technique allows for neural decompression with maximum bone and joint preservation.

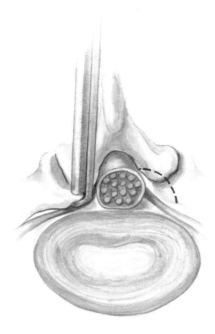

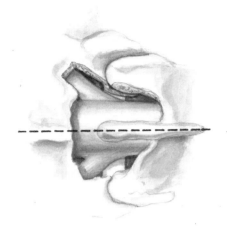

Figure 19–9 Bilateral decompression with hemilaminotomy (hemi-laminectomy) and foraminotomy (superior) is readily accomplished and is recommended in cases where a spinal stenosis or ventral mass or bilateral radiculopathy requires such action.

Figure 19–8 Undercutting of medial facet margins provides maximum decompression and visualization of lateral recess region with optimal preservation of joint.

In the event that bony spinal stenosis exists, or a large anterior mass is present, or bilateral root exploration is required, a more extensive dorsal exposure is required and easily achieved (Figure 19–9).

Root and Fragment Identification and Removal

The ultimate goal of bony exposure prior to removal of a free fragment of exploration of the interspace is complete visualization of the lateral aspect of the main dural tube, the shoulder, axilla, and a minimum of 2 cm of the appropriate nerve root. With lateral disc herniation most often there will be dorsal median displacement of the nerve root, and with the attainment of exposure of the lateral recess of the spinal canal the fragment of disc material will readily be appreciated (Figure 19–10). At this time cottonoids may be placed superior to the shoulder of the nerve root and distal and lateral on the nerve root to displace this structure slightly medially and enhance exposure of the lateral recess region. Dissection of epidural fat and/or adhesions in the region is undertaken with either a blunt-tipped or fine-tipped bipolar coagulating forceps and a #5F Frazier suction apparatus. If normal anatomical planes are obscured, it is imperative that magnification of vision be employed. For ultimate visualization, the operating microscope is far superior to the customary headlight and loupes because of the intensity of illumination provided with the microscopic light source as opposed to the standard headlight systems and because of the versatility of magnification

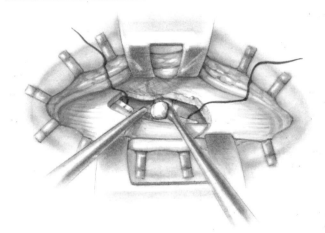

Figure 19–10 A disc fragment is identified adjacent to the interspace. Small cottonoids afford the minimal retraction that is required at the shoulder of the root.

offered. For minimization of trauma to the root, it is imperative to effect separation of adhesions particularly from the ventral surface of the root prior to extraction of a fragment from this interface. In particular, for lateral disc protrusions, a retractor is seldom necessary to mobilize the nerve root for visualization of the disc fragment and maintenance of proper exposure for interspace exploration. Therefore, with proper placement of cottonoids the fragment is further exposed and its dorsal component freed of any epidural venous complex with bipolar coagulating forceps. A cruciate incision is then made over the fibrotic tissues and a small pituitary rongeur or Rhoton forceps is utilized to gently tease the fragment from the spinal canal (Figure 19–11). With excision of the fragment, there is considerable relaxation of neural elements in the area. In the event that a fragment is not appreciated and adequate lateral bony excision and visualization have been gained, it is advisable to use angled instruments, such as an eye muscle hook or a Frazier dural guide, to explore both dorsally and ventrally along the nerve root as well as ventrally in the spinal canal in the region of the root axilla and shoulder. The fragment and/or herniation will readily be identified at this time.

Another maneuver of some value is the introduction of normal saline into the interbody space. This may be accomplished by employing a #20 spinal needle and a Luer lock syringe. A normal interspace will accept a little more than 0.5 cc of saline, whereas a degenerated interspace will readily accept saline solution without difficulty. With introduction of the saline, it is possible to identify a region of tear in the annulus by the egress of fluid and this aids in the identification of a disc fragment.

Disc Excision

With removal of the fragment and/or identification of the interspace, a generous window is fashioned through the posterior longitudinal ligament and annulus fibrosis with a #11 blade (Figure 19–12). Care must be taken to ensure that the inferior and superior edges of the window are on the inferior and superior margins of the bodies involved and that in the course of lateral extension of the window opening no injury is incurred by the superior nerve root in the area that is passing laterally in the region of the pedicle. With proper execution of this maneuver, one may then set the stage for complete visualization into the interspace. At this time, a small pituitary rongeur is introduced into the interspace and evacuation of disc material commences. It is common practice to remove only that disc material which is softened, degenerated, and lacks resistance to excision. Scoville cartilage curettes are essential for proper evacuation of the interspace and, therefore, combinations of straight, 45-degree and 90-degree curettes are used in exploration and excision of degenerated disc material (Figure 19–13).

Following the development of a dead space in the central portion of the interspace, the curettes are introduced to free degenerated material into the central portion of the dead space and then under direct vision this debris is removed. It is apparent that as more excision is undertaken, it is necessary to use the 45-degree and 90-degree curettes to bring the disc material into the central portion of the interspace for removal by the pituitary rongeur. It is obvious that care must be taken in evacuation of the interspace to avoid transgressing the anterior annulus and entering the retroperitoneal space. Provided that the dorsal opening in the annulus and posterior longitudinal ligament are adequate, the evacuation can be accomplished under direct vision, thereby reducing the possibility of such an event. Following removal of the degenerated disc material, the interspace may be inspected both by direct vision and by palpation with blunt instruments. Angled endoscopy instru-

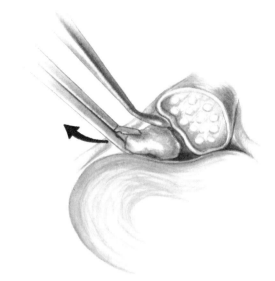

Figure 19–11 Medial-lateral fragments are easily retrieved from the lateral recess of the spinal canal with minimal manipulation and deformation of the main dural tube.

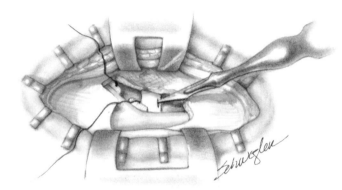

Figure 19–12 The interspace is entered with a generous window in the annulus after the free fragment has been delivered. The window should afford visualization within the central region of the nucleus.

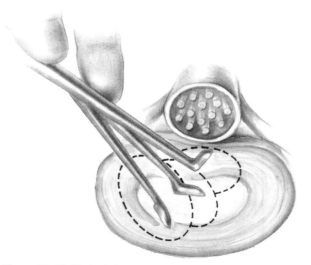

Figure 19–13 Method of technique of application of straight, 45-degree and 90-degree Scoville curettes to evacuate and free degenerated material from interspace. Index finger acts as fulcrum.

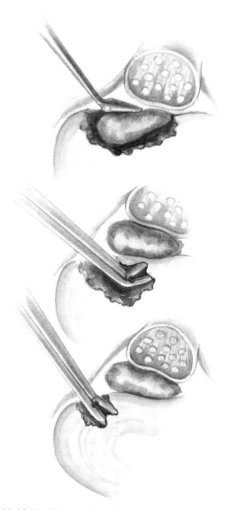

Figure 19–14 Method for excision of central or centrolateral fragment. A "void" is created in the interspace following lateral canal entry. The fragment is then dissected from the anterior dural tube and collapsed into the "void." The fragment is delivered from the "void."

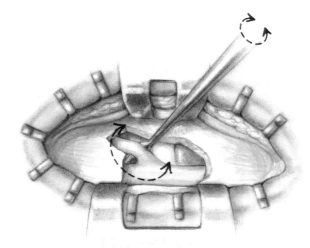

Figure 19–15 At the completion of decompression, angled instrumentation is employed to explore the root canal and ventral spinal canal to ensure the completion of absolute decompression and lack of "hidden" fragments of disc material.

completion of the procedure, a minimum of 2 to 2.5 cm of nerve root is completely visualized. Finally, exploration is undertaken with eye muscle hooks dorsally and ventrally down the root canal, followed by a Frazier dural guide dorsally and ventrally down the root canal to assure that there is no further fragment of disc material or bony encroachment or compromise in the area (Figure 19–15). Exploration is then undertaken ventrally in the spinal canal in the superior and inferior plane initially with eye muscle hooks and secondarily with the Frazier dural guide, once again to ensure freedom from encroachment of any retained disc material. Copious irrigation is then undertaken with Bacitracin, and a pledget of Bacitracin-soaked Gelfoam is placed in the foraminotomy laminotomy opening.

Closure is then accomplished in layers with meticulous hemostasis to ensure a minimal presence of blood in the muscular layer, which can be a source of irritation and postoperative spasm. Care is taken to ensure a secure closure, particularly at the level of the lumbodorsal fascia.

POSTOPERATIVE CARE

Following the procedure, the patient is allowed to stand and can walk to the bathroom to void within four hours. On the day following surgery, the patient is mobilized and ambulated both in his or her room and in the hall with assistance. This continues over the course of the next one to two days with gradually increased mobility. Mobilization is critical to reduce spasms and to increase the confidence of the patient. Complete mobilization with prolonged ambulation is encouraged to be attained within 24 to 48 hours following surgery.

ments are used to inspect the margins of removal of disc material from within the interspace.

In the event that a central fragment is present, a helpful technique (Figure 19–14) for excision involves developing a lateral window in the annulus, followed by the creation of a void within the centrolateral portion of the inner space. The fragment may then be dissected from the anterior dural tube and delivered into the inner space from which it may be excised. The interspace is then irrigated copiously with Bacitracin solution (50,000 units in 500 cc of normal saline).

Foraminotomy Completion and Final Exploration

Attention is once again turned to the root area and the displacing cottonoids are removed and the foraminotomy is completed using angled bone punches and/or curettes. At

SUMMARY

Surgery of the herniated lumbar disc is, in essence, a surgery of the nerve roots of the cauda equina. The primary objective of each procedure is to decompress a neural element and/or elements in this region and to preserve biomechanical integrity. This requires adequate bony exposure, particularly in the lateral spinal recess and region of the facet joint. A careful balance must be attained between exposure and excessive bony removal with ligamentous disruption, which would be a source of biomechanical difficulty to the patient during the early and late postoperative period. Care should be taken whenever possible to preserve the normal anatomical substrate.

The hallmark of the surgery is minimization of handling and manipulation of the involved nerve root or nerve roots by obtaining adequate lateral exposure in the spinal canal at the lateral recess region with reduction of retraction of the involved nerve roots and gentle displacement of the same by appropriate placement of cottonoids. Following removal of fragments from within the spinal canal, discectomy is accomplished with a view toward reducing the biomechanical impact of the surgery with removal of only what is estimated to be degenerated components of interspace material. This is accomplished by appropriate visualization within the interspace as well as proper employment of cartilage curettes.

Dissection under magnified visualization with intense lighting provided by the operating microscope is, at times, imperative to ensure proper handling of neural elements and optimum appreciation of dissection planes.

A critical step in the procedure is the performance of an adequate foraminotomy for decompression of the root with exploration of all ventral surfaces in the region with angled instruments. Early mobilization during the postoperative period is important to reduce spasm and functional limitation as well as to build the patient's confidence in relation to his or her own capabilities for activity.

Chapter 20

The Laminectomy Patch

John Collis Jr., M.D.

The laminectomy patch is a thin, nonadherent material that is sutured into the laminectomy opening and thus forms a barrier between the paraspinal muscles and the contents of the spinal canal. Figure 20–1 illustrates that a laminectomy patch can be used both for a tiny "laminotomy opening," as perhaps with a unilateral discectomy, as well as for larger openings. The laminectomy patch has also been used for openings that involve removal of several arches (14 or more laminae).

SURGICAL TECHNIQUE

Utilizing the laminectomy patch is rather like "replacing the ligamentum flavum," i.e., the patch is a barrier between the paraspinal muscles and the spinal canal. Using a patch that is larger than the actual laminectomy opening is important. If the patch is too small, it is difficult to suture into place, and the patch might recede into the epidural area, thereby not performing efficiently as a patch. It could conceivably irritate an underlying nerve root (in actuality, this has never occurred).

Intentionally leaving some of the soft tissue about the facet joint, sacrum, and laminae for suture attachment later makes application of the patch very simple. The edge of the ligamentum flavum can also be used to anchor sutures to the patch. Performing the procedure three or four times makes the technique easier and routine.

The suture should first be placed through the soft tissue, and then secondarily, the suture should be passed through the

patch before tying. If the suture were first passed through the patch, there might be no accessible tissue around the opening for ideal attachment.

A drill is occasionally used to form a hole in the lamina; this is necessary only with inadequate soft tissue around the laminectomy opening. Leaving Gelfoam under the patch makes suturing easier. The material used for the patch is Dura Film.*

DISCUSSION

The laminectomy patch offers the following advantages: (1) the patch, placed between the contents of the spinal canal and paraspinal muscles, seems to reduce problems following the inevitable scar tissue formed in or around nerve roots; (2) if reopening of the wound is needed, the laminectomy patch is helpful in preventing manipulative trauma to the underlying nerve root or cauda equina; it makes reopening quicker and safer; (3) the laminectomy patch can help to immediately reduce or stop epidural bleeding; it can prevent fluids from entering into the intraspinal area from the paraspinal muscle area; (4) the laminectomy patch can be used to help seal any dural opening; here the patch can be used as a reinforcement to help prevent cerebrospinal fistula; (5) the patch permits interposing Gelfoam between the nerve roots and the laminectomy patch, thereby contributing to better hemostasis and also at the same time possibly reducing the likelihood of epidural scarring; and (6) any drain left beneath the paraspinal muscles will be made more effective with the patch in place.

---

*Dura Film: Codman & Shurtleff, Inc., Randolph, Mass. 02368.

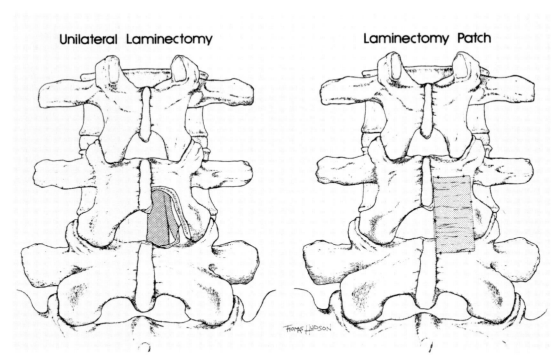

Figure 20–1 The laminectomy patch is sutured over the laminectomy defect.

From a practical point of view, there are no disadvantages to the laminectomy patch. There have been absolutely no infections, no foreign body reactions, no rejections, no seroma accumulation, no nerve root irritation. No "bleeding" complications have occurred. The laminectomy patch is not to be used with infected wounds.

SUMMARY

The laminectomy patch is an aid to spinal surgery. Its use is strongly recommended. Obviously, with experience, this becomes a quicker, as well as more efficient procedure. This technique has been found to be a consistent and practical clinical step.[1]

REFERENCE

1. Collis JS Jr and Meier G: The indications and technique for the use of a subdural patch. *Surg Gynecol Obstet* 1973;3:449–450.

Chapter 21

The Spinal Column: A Modern Tower of Babel

Charles V. Burton, M.D., FACS

Pity the poor patient with the diagnosis of "spondylosis" (*spondylos*—pertaining to a vertebrae, Gk.; -osis, condition of). If one believes that successful treatment depends upon an initial accurate diagnosis, it is evident that the patient with "spondylosis" is a low-probability candidate for rational therapy.

In actuality a nebulous diagnosis because of lack of knowledge has been a familiar pattern in medicine. American colonial medical practice was typified by diagnoses such as "noxious miasms and malicious effluvia permeating the body humours." Even in this century "dropsy" and "status thymico-lymphaticus" where often given as causes of death on autopsy reports.

Although not yet generally understood or adequately utilized, modern advanced spinal roentgenographics and imaging have now provided the clinician with the means of making specific pathologic diagnoses by correlating these data with clinical observations. The effective translation of data by medical and surgical spondylotherapists is what is presently lacking. This liability is due to two basic factors:

1. The lack of uniformly understood terminology, which has created a modern "Tower of Babel" in failure of communication between radiologist and clinician (particularly the surgeon).
2. The inherent high level of difficulty existing for radiologists and clinicians in mentally assimilating and

understanding multiplanar (mainly axial) images of the spine being produced by computed tomography (CT) and magnetic resonance imaging (MRI) scanners, particularly at the lumbosacral junction.

TERMINOLOGY

Creation of comprehensive and generally agreed-to basic informational concepts from which common terminology can be derived is critical. The following material is directed toward initiating this goal.

When Walter Dandy first accurately described the herniated disc in 1929, a focus of interest on this subject was initiated and subsequently popularized by Mixter and Barr in 1934. This recognition has proven to be a mixed blessing. While the differentiation between disc and tumor was an important step forward, it has also, quite unfortunately, focused conceptual thinking into the belief that all back pain is related to a herniated disc. The proof of this is seen in the myriad current lumbar spine CT scans in which the imager cuts through the disc spaces alone (something akin to playing cards with only half a deck). This situation reflects a general lack of understanding regarding the natural process of progressive change in the lumbar spine reflecting congenital liabilities (usually structural), acquired insults and injuries, and the superimposition of the process of aging. Because there is presently no

Note: A deep debt of appreciation is expressed by the author to his neurosurgical, orthopedic, and radiological colleagues at the Institute for Low Back Care and the Center for Diagnostic Imaging in Minneapolis, as well as our "Saskatoon Connection," for assistance in developing some of the ideas expressed in this chapter.

descriptive term, the word "spondylogression" is employed to reflect this natural progression of change.

William Kirkaldy-Willis and his associates have, in recent years, promoted the concept of "the three joint complex" and have thus provided a legitimate conceptual base to build logical thought regarding spondylogression. In Figure 21–1 a significant part of this process is depicted. With the concept of spondylogression established, the inherent understanding of clinical syndromes relating to disc, facet, and sacroiliac becomes possible. The appreciation of pathologic entities, (i.e., various forms of vertebral stenosis) also becomes possible.

THE HERNIATED DISC

Having established spondylogression as a protective conceptual mechanism, it is now safe to return to consideration of the "disc," a most important entity. At base level, it is important to point out that "disc" is a biologic term appropriate to the spine while "disk" is a technical term inappropriately applied to the medical area.

Until recently, a herniated disc was radiographically identified almost exclusively through lumbar myelography. Even when myelography was accurate, very few specifics regarding the herniation could be drawn (even with the addition of discography, which appears to have its greatest present value in the differentiation of nonherniated discogenic pain syndromes). With modern high-resolution CT and MRI imaging, it is now often possible (and will be more so in the future) to document important anatomic characteristics. In this regard, another conceptual entity is suggested—the "contained vs. noncontained" herniated disc. This is an important starting point for logical algorithmic therapeutic decisions. The concept is explored further in Figure 21–2. The posterior longitudinal ligament/disc capsule complex (PLLDC) serves as the key anatomic structure in this schema.

There are presently three basic therapeutic approaches for acute disc herniations in patients who have not had surgery. Treatment selection is determined, to a large degree, by the history, physical, and neurologic examination. In the future, selection will be more influenced by imaging information. The three approaches are as follows:

1. Conservative (noninterventional)—typified by bed rest and traction modalities of which the Gravity Lumbar Reduction Therapy Program (GLRTP) appears to provide the highest degree of physiologically effective axial traction. Clinical studies at the Institute for Low Back Care have demonstrated a 70–74 percent efficacy for GLRTP and suggest that all patients with contained disc herniations are primary candidates for initial conservative management regimens.
2. Interventional (nonsurgical)—local, epidural, and intradiscal injections of analgesics, steroids, sclerosing solu-

tions, and enzymes. In recent studies at the Institute for Low Back Care, a 70 percent good-to-excellent success rate with chymopapain for chemonucleolysis has been found. Interventional modalities appear to be most effective on patients with acute contained disc herniations who have either failed other, more conservative, therapies or who are not candidates for the latter because of other considerations.
3. Surgical—best employed for noncontained disc herniations. Statistics indicate an over 90 percent success rate in the noncontained group, with the operative procedure of choice being microsurgical discectomy. Other operative approaches and different statistics apply for chronic disc herniations and more complicated cases with concomitant additional pathology such as lateral spinal stenosis and adhesive arachnoiditis.

A more sophisticated appreciation of pathologic anatomy allows for more appropriate therapy. For example, any form of therapy, other than surgery for a noncontained sequestered disc herniation with significant neurologic deficit, represents a very low cost-effectiveness of care.

LATERAL SPINAL STENOSIS

Only within the past few years has lateral spinal stenosis (LSS) been recognized as an important clinical entity. Of particular importance to spinal surgeons has been the docu-

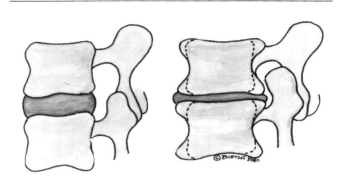

Figure 21–1 The process of spondylogression reflects a segmental phenomenon involving the three-joint complex. As acquired, insult and injury are superimposed on the segment and as weakening occurs, dynamic dysfunction results. As Kirkaldy-Willis has shown, this progresses to segmental instability. The response of the body is to absorb the deranged and degenerated disc and to promote bone hypertrophy and osteophyte formation by subperiosteal bone deposition. This healing process usually leads to a return of segmental stability. In the unusual circumstance, nerve entrapment may occur because of bony stenosis. In this example, the intervertebral disc space has markedly narrowed, the zygapophyseal joint has enlarged, and the foraminal zone has been narrowed by the anterosuperior displacement of an enlarged superior articular process from the inferior vertebrae. *Source:* Used with permission of Charles V. Burton, M.D., © 1980.

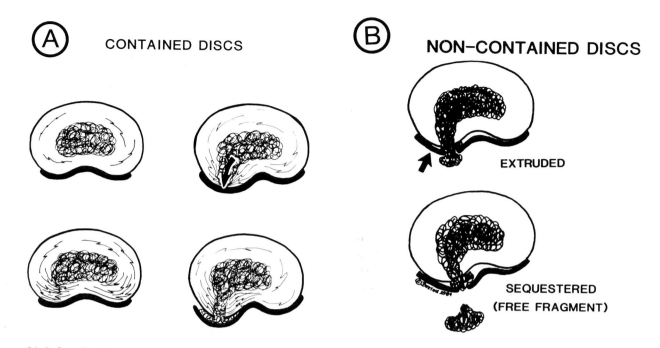

Figure 21–2 Contained and noncontained discs are compared. In (a) the progression of internal derangement and degeneration is shown. The process is initiated with annular tears that coalesce into annular fissures through which the abnormal disc material herniates. The key structure is the posterior longitudinal ligament/disc capsular complex (PLLDC), shown as a heavy black line. Even though the disc material may pass beyond the annulus (the so-called "roof disc"), as long as it does not penetrate the PLLDC, the disc herniation is "contained." In (b) discal material is now extruding through the PLLDC. At the point where continuity with the disc space is lost, the fragment is considered to be "free" and sequestered in the spinal canal. *Source:* Used with permission of Charles V. Burton, M.D., © 1984.

mentation identifying LSS as the most common reason for the "failed back surgery syndrome" because of failure to either diagnose or adequately treat LSS.

LSS represents, in actuality, a spectrum of spinal nerve compressive entities beginning with the central spinal canal and extending beyond the intervertebral foramen. Now that quality diagnostic imaging has demonstrated its capability of defining the existence and nature of LSS, it is important to create a conceptual model providing better understanding and nomenclature.

"GHOSTBUSTING"

Recently, there have been claims that myelography is more accurate in the diagnosis of LSS than lumbar CT. The Institute for Low Back Care specializes in the rehabilitation of problem low back cases referred from physicians and institutions throughout the United States. The average patient appears with a collection of diagnostic studies, which, in recent years, has also come to include a fascinating spectrum of CT scans. Based on some 15,000 lumbar CT scans the following observations may be made:

1. Lumbar CT scanning requires a particularly high level of effort and expertise to obtain satisfactory results.

2. Many of the lumbar CT scans presently being performed do not demonstrate adequate understanding of the technical processes necessary to demonstrate the pathology. Even when reviewed by expert radiologists such studies provide only a paucity of accurate information.

3. Few general radiologists at this time are expert in the interpretation of lumbar CT scans. There are, therefore, many reports of very limited value and often of a confusing or misleading nature.

4. Many radiologists are expert in performing and interpreting myelography. Their interpretations are of high value but limited by the fact that myelography is inherently limited in defining any form of lateral nerve entrapment of which LSS is the most common clinical entity.

It is clearly evident that a high-quality/high-resolution CT scan with adequate multiplanar reconstructions properly interpreted represents the most comprehensively accurate lumbar examination that can be performed at this time. The patient's interest is best served by carrying out such a study prior to being exposed to interventional therapy having significant risk. There does not appear to exist any credible evidence at this time to challenge this view.

LATERAL SPINAL STENOSIS AND COMMUNICATION

Foramen—a hole or opening, from *foro*, L., "I pierce"

A prominent "bottleneck" in the communication process between imaging radiologist and surgeon is the lack of commonly understood site-specific terminology. "Lateral recess" in California means a site within the central spinal canal but in other areas of the country it means the lateral foraminal area. This confusion is really not surprising because the definition of foramen does not even clearly identify whether it is a two-dimensional structure (opening) similar to a door or window or a three-dimensional structure (hole) similar to a canal or passage.

It can be suggested that the foramen is three-dimensional and that the course of a spinal nerve is a "spondylar passageway." This passageway begins in the central spinal canal where the preganglionic spinal nerve leaves the dural sac and continues through the intervertebral foramen (usually as the dorsal ganglionic segment) and its postganglionic spinal nerve existence into Leon Wiltse's "far out syndrome" land.

One of the most important surgical landmarks is the vertebral pedicle. The pedicle can also be selected as the base of a reference schema, designed to allow more accurate communication regarding the site of a lesion. As illustrated in Figure 21–3, the pedicle is selected as the point of reference and vertical lines are drawn at its medial and lateral borders thus creating three "zones."

Subarticular and "lateral recess" stenosis (as well as the typical dorso-lateral disc herniation) occurs within the "central zone." The "garden variety" LSS is found in the "foraminal zone" or "canal zone." It is at this location that most other forms of lateral entrapment (i.e., tumor, inflammatory, or infectious) occur. The "extraforaminal zone" represents the land of Wiltse's far out syndrome where structural anomalies, ligaments, lateral disc herniations, and tumors can occur. The L5-S1 level is most commonly involved. Of key importance to the surgeon is the appreciation of pathology involving more than one zone, which allows a surgical approach conducive to utilizing this important information.

THREE-DIMENSIONAL IMAGING

An assault on the Tower of Babel is not enough; technology must also be brought to bear on improving the safety and efficacy of lumbar diagnosis and patient treatment. For even the most astute medical observer, utilizing high-resolution imaging with adequate reconstructions requires the ability to mentally assimilate this complex information intracranially. This represents a considerable feat.

The answer to the above dilemma lies in the development of three-dimensional data display screens. An image created by Kenneth Heithoff and associates is shown in Figure 21–4. In this format, information is much more readily comprehended.

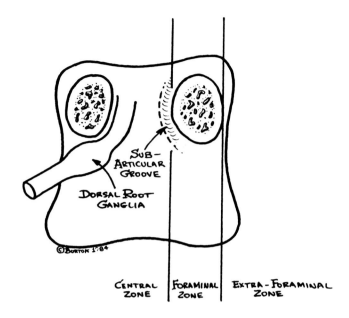

Figure 21–3 The lines at the medial and lateral borders of the pedicle define the central, foraminal ("canal"), and extraforaminal zones. On the left, an exiting spinal nerve is shown where the dorsal root ganglia is within the foraminal zone. Note the presence of a subarticular groove. The dorsal root ganglion of the S1 nerve is usually in the central zone. *Source:* Used with permission of Charles V. Burton, M.D., © 1984.

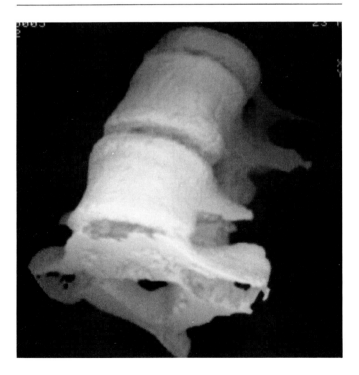

Figure 21–4 Example of three-dimensional data display. This image was created by a line drawing computer algorithm and reformatted from the basic data on a routine GE 8800 lumbar CT scan. The area of the spine shown is the same as that covered by the axial images. *Source:* Used with permission of Charles V. Burton, M.D., © 1984.

The only practical limitation to routine use of this display is the length of time that the scanning computer takes to reformat the data (about 20–30 minutes).

Although a great amount of interest is being shown in MRI lumbar imaging, it is the advent of three-dimensional data display that will have the greater value in the next decade. MRI will provide important information regarding the pathologic status of tissues such as disc and bone, but it is unlikely to replace CT for the purpose of creating accurate geographic topography guides. CT and MRI have the potential to complement rather than to compete.

SUMMARY

The Tower of Babel has represented a serious impediment to the application of new therapeutic techniques for the benefit of the patient. The recognition of the problem has opened new vistas for communication and dissemination of imaging information.

Chapter 22

On the Diagnosis and Surgical Treatment of Lumbar Subarticular and "Far Out" Lateral Spinal Stenosis

Charles V. Burton, M.D., FACS

A wise man, Ecclesiastes, writing more than 2,500 years ago, said, "Much learning is a weariness of the flesh." Certainly a great deal has already been written about the problem of low back pain. May it be of some comfort to the present reader to know that while knowledge is undoubtedly required, even more important is the ability to discern the needs of the individual patient and in what way can these be met most effectively.

—William H. Kirkaldy-Willis, M.D.[1]

The subject of spinal stenosis is certainly not "a weariness of the flesh." It actually represents an extremely important area of study for the surgeon, not only because it is a poorly understood entity but, more specifically, because it has the distinction of being the most common organic reason for the failure of lumbar spinal surgery.[2] As in aviation, where the study of crashes has contributed to greater flight safety, it has been through the study of the "Failed Back Surgery Syndrome"[3–6] that the safety and efficacy of spinal surgery has been advanced. The groundwork upon which this understanding has been built has been the exploration and definition of lateral spinal stenosis as a pathologic entity.[6–9]

In Chapter 21, "The Spinal Column: A Modern Tower of Babel," the point was made that: "Although not yet generally understood or adequately utilized, modern advanced spinal

roentgenographics and imaging have now provided the clinician with the means of making specific pathologic diagnoses by correlating this data with clinical observations. The effective translation of data by medical and surgical spondylotherapists is what is presently lacking. This liability is due to two basic factors:

1. The lack of uniformly understood terminology, which has created a modern "Tower of Babel" in failure of communication between radiologist and clinician (particularly the surgeon).
2. The inherent high level of difficulty existing for radiologists and clinicians in mentally assimilating and understanding multiplanar (mainly axial) images of the spine being produced by CT and MRI scanners, particularly at the lumbo-sacral junction."

These considerations have led to a new nomenclature concept, that of utilizing the vertebral pedicle as a reference point (Figure 22–1) thus creating central, foraminal ("canal"), and extraforaminal zones to assist in promoting more specific communication between radiologist and surgeon. The need for improved communication is clearly evidenced by the uniquely high failure rates of spinal surgery in the United States, the inordinately high cost of such failure, and the general lack of awareness regarding the subject, demonstrated by many surgeons routinely performing these operative procedures.

Note: The present level of understanding regarding the complexities of spinal stenosis reflects the dedicated efforts of many pioneers. From the standpoint of the Institute for Low Back Care in Minneapolis, our mentor has been Dr. William Kirkaldy-Willis, Professor Emeritus of the Department of Orthopedic Surgery, University of Saskatoon, Saskatchewan, Canada. We acknowledge our debt of gratitude to him and express our appreciation for his patience and consideration.

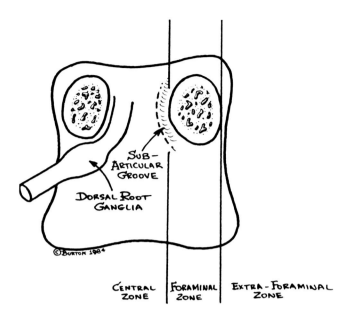

Figure 22–1 With removal of the posterior neural elements, it can be observed how the pedicle serves as a means of establishing "central," "foraminal" ("canal") and extraforaminal zones to serve as a communication guide. The relationship of an exiting spinal nerve to the pedicle as well as the position of the "subarticular groove" is shown. The location of the dorsal root ganglia to the foraminal zones varies at the different lumbar segments. *Source:* Used with permission of Charles V. Burton, M.D., © 1984.

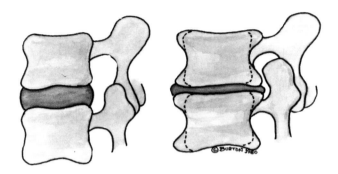

Figure 22–2 A depiction of "spondylgression," the "natural life history" of degeneration of the segmental three-joint complex based on congenital liabilities (usually structural), acquired insults and injuries, and the superimposition of the process of aging. Nature is attempting to achieve stabilization of the segment by disc absorption, subperiosteal bone deposition, enlargement of the zygapophyseal joints, and remolding of the vertebrae. Note the effect of this process on the patency of the intervertebral foramen. Lateral stenosis appears to reflect a failure of nature to achieve stabilization without neurologic compromise. *Source:* Used with permission of Charles V. Burton, M.D., © 1980.

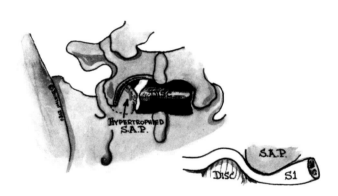

Figure 22–3 An example of subarticular stenosis in the central zone at the L5–S1 level. It can be seen that the hypertrophy of the zygapophyseal joint (compare with normal joint on right) has created decrease in volume of the subarticular area to the point where the traversing S1 nerve is being compressed. In this example, the bulging of the L5–S1 disc has produced a guillotine-like distortive force. *Source:* Used with permission of Charles V. Burton, M.D., © 1980.

Insult to a spinal nerve sufficient enough to produce clinical signs or symptoms of a debilitating nature is the basic subject of this chapter. Through an understanding of subarticular and "far out" stenosis, the surgeon will gain insight into the entire subject of spinal stenosis. Adequate diagnosis needs to be followed by adequate therapy and with the sophisticated tools available to us today, this now also includes the *prevention* of impending disease clearly identifiable at the time of diagnosis.

Another important consideration is that of iatrogenic disease; it is, at the very least, truly "bad form." The etiologic relationship between iophendylate (Pantopaque) and the production of adhesive arachnoiditis has been so well documented that its use can only be justified under the most "exceptional" of circumstances.[2–5,10,11] Epidural and perineural fibrosis represents another pathologic situation adverse to the patient when present in excessive degrees. Appropriate fat grafting has now been demonstrated to be worthy of consideration when utilized routinely in spinal surgery cases.[12]

SUBARTICULAR STENOSIS

Preganglionic spinal nerve root compression by bone in the lateral aspect of the central spinal canal is presently referred to by a number of terms including "subarticular" and "lateral recess" stenosis as well as the "superior articular facet syndrome." All of these entities involve nerve insult in the "central zone" (referred to previously) and represent an entity only recently appreciated by spinal surgeons. A major reason for this lack of appreciation is the fact that a wide laminectomy with medial facetectomy automatically relieves the problem. From the standpoint of operative approach, subarticular stenosis is among the easiest to treat, and its relief only rarely contributes to segmental instability requiring concomitant fusion.

It appears that a congenitally small or "trefoil"-shaped central canal predisposes one to subarticular stenosis. Super-

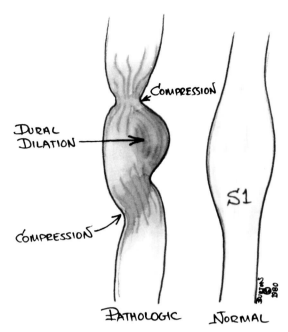

Figure 22–4 Drawing from an actual case of L5-S1 subarticular stenosis where the left S1 nerve was compressed by an overlying hypertrophied superior articular process from the S1 vertebrae. The imprint of this process can be seen on the deformed and swollen dorsal root ganglia. This has produced both areas of constriction and dilatation. Neurophysiologic research indicates that the dorsal nerve root is the most sensitive structure and when compromised becomes a prominent pain generator. This accounts for the great amount of pain and incapacitation produced without associated objective neurologic deficit. *Source:* Used with permission of Charles V. Burton, M.D., © 1980.

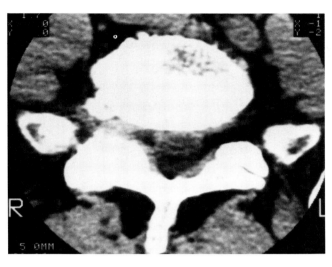

Figure 22–5 In this case of lateral entrapment, compression of the exiting L5 nerve is present in both the foraminal and extraforaminal zones. The latter is evidenced by a large osteophyte arising from the posterolateral aspect of the first sacral vertebra.

imposed upon this strata is the spectrum of degenerative disease affecting the three-joint complex.[13] This process is summarized in Figure 22–2. As hypertrophy of the zygapophyseal progresses, the traversing spinal nerve is compromised in the central zone, at the superior margin of the vertebrae and in the upper portion of the subarticular groove. This process is further enhanced by vertebral lip osteophytes and the protrusion or bulging of the associated intervertebral disc (Figure 22–3). While this is usually a chronic and progressive change, it may also be dynamic and related to body movement (particularly torque movements).

At the Institute for Low Back Care, study of this entity was initiated by a series of 20–40-year-old female patients presenting with a chief complaint of leg pain and/or numbness radiating to the feet and toes. Neurologic examination invariably showed no objective neurologic deficit and electromyography (EMG) examinations were typically unremarkable. A consistent finding was tenderness to palpation at the sciatic notch and in the popliteal fossa (bowstring sign) associated with positive straight-leg raising. Myelography and computed tomography (CT) were thought to be normal but in retrospect the diagnosis was present on CT and is now made on a routine basis. The first group of patients coming to surgery (for "exploration") were found to have rather dramatic evidence of long-standing S1 nerve compression at the L5–S1 interspace (Figure 22–4).

"FAR OUT" LATERAL SPINAL STENOSIS

A debt of gratitude is owed to Leon Wiltse for identifying and popularizing the "Far Out Syndrome."[14] In addition to compression of the L5 postganglionic spinal nerve by the alar transverse process and by transverse ligaments, we now recognize that the L5 nerve is at risk from lateral disc herniations, osteophytes, tumors, inflammatory processes, etc., at the site of the extraforaminal zone.

Recently, 235 personal cases of surgically treated lateral spinal stenosis were reviewed. In eight cases where the patients did not do well, the persistence of lateral spinal stenosis was the reason for failure. The most common reason for this failure was lack of recognition that the lateral spinal stenotic (foraminal zone) process also extended to the extraforaminal zone. Figure 22–5 represents a typical example of a "far out" osteophyte producing continued compression of the L5 nerve. It takes a bit of surgical effort to adequately address such a lesion and when both zones are involved, the surgery needs to be from the medial approach. In Figure 22–6, lateral stenosis involving both zones is identified in (a) and a postsurgical CT scan (b) demonstrates an "adequate" decompression with full-thickness autogenous fat grafting extending to the extraforaminal zone. In cases where the pathology is purely limited to the extraforaminal zone, as in the treatment of a lateral disc herniation, a paralateral surgical approach alone is adequate.

As the postganglionic spinal nerve passes lateral to the disc in the extraforaminal zone, it appears to be enveloped in tightly adherent restraining fascia (TARF), which serves as a tether when a medial-to-lateral expansion of tissue occurs. This forces compression of the spinal nerve against the patho-

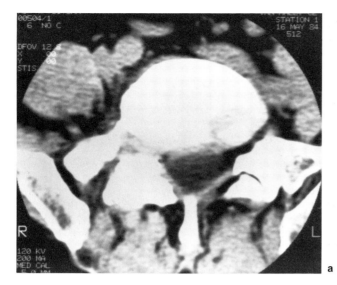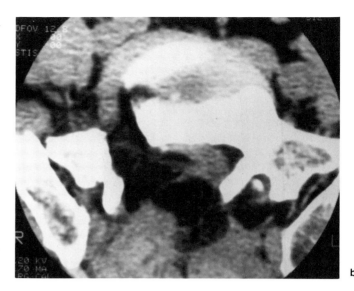

Figure 22–6 In preoperative scan (a) insult to the exiting L5 nerve by lateral stenosis is accentuated by alar-transverse process compression in the extraforaminal zone (because of a congenital transitional vertebra). At surgery (b), decompression was extended laterally to the sacral ala. Soft autogenous fat was then placed around the nerve and over the dura. The postoperative scan documents an adequate result from the radiologic standpoint.

logic process thus producing the clinical symptoms. TARF appears to be a pathologic entity particular to the extraforaminal zone and separate and distinct from the well-known dural ligaments that tether the thecal sac and spinal nerves in the central to extraforaminal zones. Using the paralateral approach, it often appears that simply releasing the TARF by surgical dissection produces significant decompression of the compromised nerve.

SURGICAL TECHNIQUE

An accurate diagnosis should suffice for appropriate treatment. In stenotic syndromes, however, this is not necessarily so. In one case, a 36-year-old male had undergone two operative procedures for the treatment of a right sciatic radiculitis. The patient's first preoperative study (and radiologist's report) identified, at the same level, a herniated disc and severe lateral spinal stenosis. The second preoperative CT scan (and radiologist's report) again identified the same lateral stenosis. The second study showed a ''bony spur'' that was removed but clinical improvement did not result. A third CT indicated that the original stenosis had never been surgically addressed and the patient is now facing a third operative procedure. This is not an unusual situation.

Given the assumption that the surgeon has the correct diagnosis and understands it, the operative procedure needs to be carried out in such a manner that a controlled microsurgical technique can be employed in a dry operative field.

Patient Positioning

Any form of positioning that avoids abdominal compression to decrease epidural vein pressure and avoids the potential complications of neck or extremity compression is acceptable.

Prophylactic Antibiotics

Based on experience, the predictions of Leonard Malis[15] in regard to substantially reducing neurosurgical infection rates by the use of intraoperative antibiotics are confirmed. Infection rates at the Institute for Low Back Care have been kept to less than 1 percent over a ten-year period by the initial use of the Malis regimen: single-dose tobramycin and vancomycin, then tobramycin alone and most recently a single operative holding room dose of one gram of monocid given intravenously (by piggyback).

Microsurgical Technique

The application of microsurgical principles requires a dry operative field. Bipolar coagulation and the use of cottonoid patties are essential. With the development of modern operating telescopes (not loupes) with coaxial fiberoptic headlights that produce magnification of up to 9× (with both depth of vision and a wide field of vision), surgeons now have at their disposal a lightweight, relatively inexpensive, and practical means of applying microsurgical principles to all spinal cases. A popular choice (Figure 22–7) is a 4×, 18'' focal distance operating telescope. If higher levels of magnification are necessary, an operating room microscope is essential.

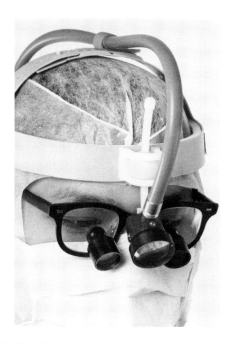

Figure 22–7 Operating telescopes (4×) being used in conjunction with a lightweight, universal movement, high-intensity fiberoptic light system. Three-dimensional movement of the lens assembly allows the surgeon to achieve true coaxial focusing of the light for working through "keyhole" or deep exposures. The telescopic lenses are mounted in the lower portion of the eyeglass to allow the operator to choose between normal field of vision and magnification/high-intensity illumination with a nod of the head. By utilizing the Gallilean principle, telescopes can be made with magnification up to 9× (with depth of field and wide field of vision) before they become too heavy and cumbersome to be worn on eyeglasses. (Photograph courtesy of Designs for Vision, N.Y.C.)

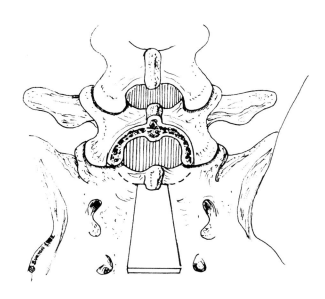

Figure 22–8 The operative approach indicated permits greatest access to intraspinal contents without significantly adding to segmental instability, if the facets are normal in size and configuration and the segment was stable to start with. Such an exposure is also "balanced" so that future remolding of vertebral structures will occur equally on both sides. In this type of approach, subarticular stenosis would be automatically alleviated by the surgeon. This inadvertent "cure" appears to be a common phenomenon. The Cloward fine-curved osteotomes are of particular value in "undercutting" the superior articular process and allowing a great deal of lateral decompression to be carried out through a medial exposure. *Source:* Used with permission of Charles V. Burton, M.D., © 1982.

Instruments

The air turbine drill and osteotomes are of particular value in spinal surgery in addition to rongeurs and curettes. Sonic powered tools, which were invented in the U.S.S.R. and advanced in the U.S., presently lack the necessary hard and sharp cutting tips.

Operative Exposure

In Figure 22–8 the operator is about to complete a bilateral inferior hemilaminotomy of L5, medial facetectomy of L5–S1 bilaterally, and bilateral superior hemilaminotomy of S1 (osteotome). This exposure would be adequate to address subarticular stenosis at any level of the spine. The surgeon must carefully inspect the preoperative CT scan to determine if the anatomy of the zygapophyseal joint allows medial facetectomy.

The surgical relief of lateral spinal stenosis can be achieved by the exposure shown but undercutting has to be carried out.

When the lesion extends to the extraforaminal zone, a subtotal or total facetectomy is required if a midline approach is desired. In a stable spinal segment, any one single element of the three-joint complex can usually be removed without creating the need for a stabilizing procedure.

Most cases of stenosis or entrapment in the extraforaminal zone (the "far out syndrome") are best approached from the paralateral incision originally described by Wiltse in 1964[16] and updated in 1968[17] and 1973.[18] Charles Ray has recently innovated a number of new paralateral operative approaches[19,20] that allow a high degree of versatility.

The greatest difficulty of the paralateral approach is finding the correct vertebral level. In this regard, preoperative marking with a dye such as lymphazurin has been of value. Under fluoroscopic control, a small amount of dye is injected percutaneously into the L5 dorsal process and into the tips of the appropriate transverse processes. Additional dye is then injected into the skin overlying these points. Roentgenographic level verification is made at surgery if the pathology is not directly encountered.

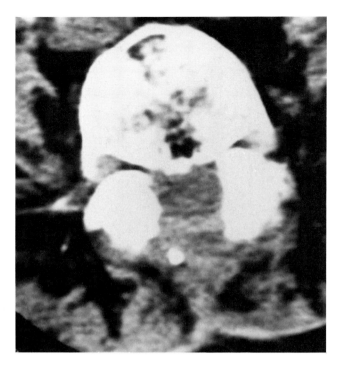

Figure 22–9 An unfortunate situation where surgery on a patient with multilevel lateral spinal stenosis producing an incapacitating "lumbar claudication syndrome" resulted in only superimposing iatrogenic epidural fibrosis on the basic problem.

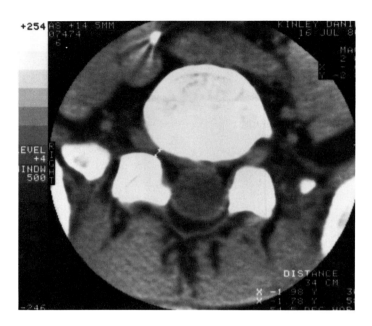

Figure 22–11 A two-year follow-up CT scan showing the residual fat from the graft, the formation of a "pseudo-ligamentum flavum" and the paucity of postsurgical epidural and perineural fibrosis. If such a patient would require reoperation, the graft can be easily separated from the dura by blunt dissection. A Cobb periosteal elevator is recommended for this.

Figure 22–10 In (a), lateral spinal stenosis is indicated on the left side produced by an enlarged facet joint. Surgical decompression has been carried out (b) and full-thickness grafts have been placed, filling any dead space and preventing the accumulation of blood. After six months to a year the graft has reduced in volume by about 30 percent and has become vascularized. At this point, the fat cannot be distinguished histologically from normal epidural fat. In most cases, a "pseudo-ligamentum flavum" (c) is formed. Note that the dural sac has reexpanded.

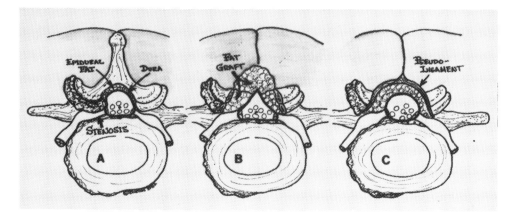

Source: Used with permission of Charles V. Burton, M.D., © 1982.

Fat Grafting

Surgeons have searched for an acceptable means of avoiding epidural and perineural fibrosis (Figure 22–9) since at least 1919 when Lexer first published on the subject.[21] In 1965, Langenskiold demonstrated that fat transplants were capable of protecting the dura from overlying scar.[22] A 1977 Institute for Low Back Care study[12] on 183 patients who underwent

full-thickness autogenous fat grafts from a separate incisional site has led to the routine use of this method on all operative cases. By being able to monitor the survival of the graft over a period of years using follow-up CT scans, it has been possible to document survival of the graft and the amount of scar tissue present. This type of grafting has now been done in over 2,000 patients.

The typical life history of a full-thickness graft is shown in Figure 22–10 and a representative follow-up CT scan in Figure

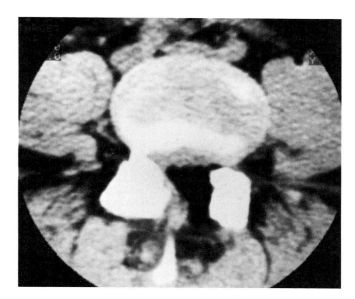

Figure 22–12 A "normal" postoperative CT scan. The full-thickness autogenous fat graft has "deflated" the dural sac. This is a routine observation and not associated with any clinical adversity other than making the radiologist quite nervous when this phenomenon is first observed.

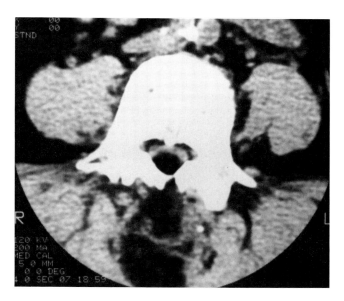

Figure 22–13 This patient developed postsurgical evidence of cauda equina dysfunction. The CT scan shows that graft not only "deflating" the dural sac but causing a concave depression in the theca. The latter appears to be the key observation. At surgery a "knuckle" of fat had passed under the superior lamina (as shown). The quality of the fat was not optimal as it was more fibrous than usual. Additional decompression and reduction in volume of the fat graft produced reversal of dysfunction. This patient was operated upon for severe central spinal stenosis in which the intrathecal nerve roots had been subjected to compression over a long period of time. During the immediate postoperative period, it is difficult to differentiate dysfunction due to a postsurgical physiologic "concussion syndrome" from other causes of dysfunction.

22–11. Until recently, the only complications encountered were at the fat graft site. In 1984, two patients with severe central spinal stenosis developed postoperatively the signs of cauda equina dysfunction. Following additional decompression and partial removal of the graft to decrease volume, both patients have experienced neurologic recoveries.

Figure 22–12 depicts a typical postoperative CT scan in which a large full-thickness graft has been employed. The flattening of the dural sac is a routine observation. A postoperative scan from a patient developing cauda equina dysfunction is shown in Figure 22–13. The graft has produced a concave depression in the dural sac. The phenomenon was present in both cases of dysfunction and appears to represent a significant finding in conjunction with the fact that, in the two cases reported, the involved intrathecal nerves had been subject to chronic compromise and were, therefore, not normally resilient.

SUMMARY

The subject of spinal stenosis is progressively becoming a better known and understood entity. Because of this, there is an ever-increasing level of medical interest, which may be the best means of improving the quality of low back care and surgical success. Subarticular and "far out" stenosis represent variations on a theme having their own special aspects and difficulties. It would appear that subarticular stenosis may often be surgically relieved inadvertently, while the "far out" form is occasionally incompletely treated even by experienced spinal surgeons.

REFERENCES

1. Kirkaldy-Willis WH: *Managing Low Back Pain.* New York, Churchill Livingstone, 1984.

2. Burton CV, Kirkaldy-Willis WH, Yong Hing K, Heithoff KB: Causes of failure of surgery on the lumbar spine. *Clin Orthop* 1981;157:191–199.

3. Burton CV: The etiology of the "failed back surgery syndrome," in Cauthen JC (ed): *Lumbar Spine Surgery.* Baltimore, Williams & Wilkins Co, 1983.

4. Burton CV: How to avoid the "failed back surgery syndrome," in Cauthen JC (ed): *Lumbar Spine Surgery.* Baltimore, Williams & Wilkins Co, 1983.

5. Burton CV: Diagnosis and treatment of lateral spinal stenosis: Implications regarding the "failed back surgery syndrome," in Genant HK (ed): *Spine Update 1984.* San Francisco, University of California Press, 1984.

6. Verbiest H: A radicular syndrome from developmental narrowing of the lumbar vertebral canal. *J Bone Joint Surg* 1954;36–B:230–237.

7. Kirkaldy-Willis WH, Mcilvor GWD: Spinal stenosis. *Clin Orthop* 1976; 115:2–144.

8. Kirkaldy-Willis WH, Wedge JH, Yong-Hing K, Reilly J: Pathology and pathogenesis of lumbar spondylosis and stenosis. *Spine* 1978;3:319–328.

9. Kirkaldy-Willis WH, Yong-Hing K: Pathology and pathogenesis of lumbar spinal stenosis, in Genant HK (ed): *Spine Update 1984*. San Francisco, University of California Press, 1984.

10. Burton CV, Wiltse LL: Editorial and symposium on lumbar arachnoiditis: Nomenclature, etiology and pathology. *Spine* 1978;3:23–92.

11. Burton CV: Lumbosacral arachnoiditis. *Spine* 1978;3:24–30.

12. Burton CV: Full-thickness autogenous fat grafts in the prevention of epidural fibrosis. *Contemp Neurosurg* 1984;5:1–6.

13. Kirkaldy-Willis WH: The three phases of the spectrum of degenerative disease, in *Managing Low Back Pain*. New York, Churchill Livingstone, 1984, pp 75–89.

14. Wiltse LL et al: Alar transverse process impingement of the L5 nerve: The far-out syndrome. *Spine* 1984;9:31–41.

15. Malis LI: Prevention of neurosurgical infection by intra-operative antibiotics. *Neurosurg* 1979;5:339–343.

16. Wiltse LL: The paraspinal sacrospinalis-splitting approach to the lumbar spine. *Clin Orthop* 1964;35:116–122.

17. Wiltse LL et al: The paraspinal sacrospinalis-splitting approach to the lumbar spine. *J Bone Joint Surg* 1968;50-A:919–926.

18. Wiltse LL: The paraspinal sacrospinalis-splitting approach to the lumbar spine. *Clin Orthop* 1973;91:48–57.

19. Ray CD: New techniques for decompression of lumbar spinal stenosis. *Neurosurg* 1982;10:587–592.

20. Ray CD: New methods for decompression in spinal stenosis. Audiocassettes CU-09, CU-10 (2 hours), from Symposium on Spinal Stenosis, American Association of Neurological Surgeons, Annual Meeting, April 1983.

21. Lexer E: Die freien transplantation en Part 1. *Neue Deutsche Chirurgie* 1919;26:264–545.

22. Langenskiold A, Kiviluoto O: Prevention of epidural scar formation after operations on the lumbar spine by means of free fat transplants: A preliminary report. *Clin Orthop* 1976;115.

Chapter 23

The Intervertebral Foramina

Leon L. Wiltse, M.D.

Recent advances in diagnosis have made it possible to recognize and often treat several conditions of the lumbar spine that were hitherto unknown. Consider the fact that spinal stenosis was relatively unknown until the late 1940s or early 1950s when Verbiest[21] published his classic work on the subject. (Elsberg and several others had written on the subject but most articles remained unclear as to the exact definition of spinal stenosis.)

Kirkaldy-Willis[11] and his associates in particular clarified the condition further. Their work specifically described the contribution of the lateral neurovascular canals to spinal nerve compression. More recently[22] it has been shown that a spinal nerve can be compressed even beyond the lateral border of the foramen, and at least at L5, clear to the anterior rim of the sacral ala. At L5, because of the peculiar arrangement of the ligaments, the L5 spinal nerve is bound to the sides of its canal and can be compressed out to the point where it passes over the rim of the sacrum and joins with other spinal nerves to form the sciatic trunk. Even certain points of the sciatic nerve and its major branches are securely fixed. For example, over the head of the fibula, the peroneal nerve is fixed as is also the tibial nerve as it passes around the medial maleolus.

This discussion will be limited to the fixation points and areas of possible compression only as far distally as the sacral ala.

ANATOMY

The segment of neural tissue inside the central and lateral canals, which is commonly called the "nerve root," is actu-ally two nerve roots—a motor and sensory—encased in a dural sleeve. This dural sleeve gradually becomes more adherent and although it varies in different people, it is not tightly adherent until it gets to the ganglion. The ganglion is principally sensory. Just beyond the ganglion the nerve fibrals become interlaced and from there on, form a true spinal nerve, sometimes called a "mixed nerve." No satisfactory name has been derived for the portion of nerve between the dura and the ganglion. The recent glossary of the American Academy of Orthopaedic Surgeons[26] calls this segment simply a "spinal nerve." Another name used by various authors for this segment of neural tissue is "preganglionic spinal nerve." The problem with this term is that on the motor side it is preganglionic, on the sensory side it is postganglionic.

In this chapter we will use the L5 nerve, and will call it simply "spinal nerve" from the time it leaves the dura until it joins other spinal nerves to become a trunk.

Immediately after leaving the foramen, the spinal nerve divides into a large anterior ramus and a small posterior ramus. Just before division, it gives off minute (two to four on each side) recurrent meningeal or sinu-vertebral branches which reenter the vertebral canal after anastomosing with a sympathetic trunk. Beyond the level of the top of the transverse process, the anterior ramus gives off a sympathetic branch (gray ramus communicans), which joins a sympathetic ganglion lying on the side of the vertebral body.

Almost immediately after leaving the dura, the intraspinal portion of the L5 spinal nerve passes between the superior articular process of S1 posteriorly and the lower one-third of the body of L5 anteriorly. Strictly speaking, this is not the

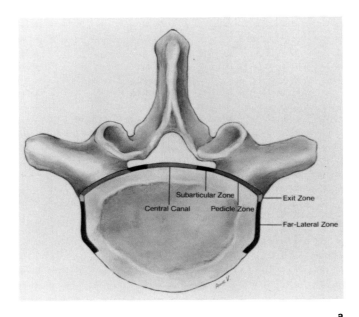

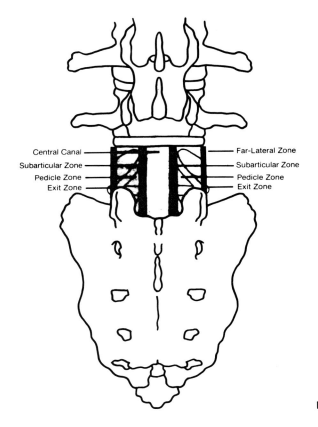

Figure 23–1 (a) Drawing of the areas where nerve compression can, and does, occur. (b) Axial drawing of areas of possible compression. The purpose of these drawings is to make it easier to communicate the area of compression.

lateral recess. The lateral recess is the space between the superior articular process of a given vertebra and the body of the same vertebra. Spinal nerves are seldom compressed at such a point unless they have been made hypersensitive by previous surgery. They can be painfully compressed only between two parts that are capable of motion, as, for example, at the point where it lies between the superior articular process of S1 and the body of L5.

The nerve can be compressed by such things as congenital narrowing, arthritic spurring, or a bulging disc, whether it is a hard fibrotic disc or a soft new rupture. Even if the patient simply leans backwards, the nerve may be compressed. This accounts for the fact that the patient with spinal stenosis so often leans forward as he or she walks.

As the nerve progresses laterally, it swings around the inferior border of the pedicle. At the point where it reaches the pedicle it enters a canal where it is encased in bone on all sides. It exits this canal through the lateral foramen. The lateral foramen has no depth; it is a window. After the nerve passes out of this window, it is in the far lateral zone.

Anteroposterior (AP) and axial figures (Figure 23–1) attempt to name the various areas or zones of the spine. The work of many other authors, but especially Casey Lee, of New

Jersey, has been drawn upon in formulating the classification that will be used in this chapter.

With the accuracy of diagnoses as to the exact location of pathology (metrizamide myelography, computed tomography scan, magnetic resonance imaging), it becomes more important than ever that exact terminology be used.

MOTION OF THE SPINAL NERVES WITH BODY MOVEMENTS

The L5 spinal nerve is securely attached at several points and virtually no gliding or slipping motion occurs. The motion that does occur, which is seen so frequently at surgery, is due to flexion and extension between vertebral segments. This gives the impression of a gliding motion but actually it is a tightening and slackening of the nerve. A fair amount of stretch of the nerve is also available. The nerve roots inside the dura have plenty of slack. If this slack above was not available, the intradural roots might be overstretched and perhaps even paralyzed by certain things. Since the nerve is securely fixed at the foramen, if it was not free proximally, a very hard jerk on one or both legs might damage the roots severely.

When performing interbody fusions, many surgeons put strong spreaders between the vertebral bodies and spread them as much as 1.8 cm. Because the nerve is fixed distally, most of the increase in length has to be taken up by pulling the nerve down from the more cephalic direction. Those who have done interbody fusions have noted that nerve trouble from over-stretching virtually never occurs, and relief is often immediate and complete.

Spencer[18] has postulated that the relief that is so often obtained after chemonucleolysis is the result of the disc space narrowing as the bulging disc becomes soft, thus giving slack to the nerve and taking away some tension. This is certainly an attractive idea with regard to that portion of the nerve far out laterally, where the nerve is bound at points on either side of the disc. It does not, however, explain why removing a bulging disc, which is inside the bony canal, gives such prompt relief since the nerve roots at this level already have plenty of slack.

COMPRESSION OF A SPINAL NERVE IN THE ENTRANCE ZONE

For the nerve to be painfully compressed in this area there has to be motion plus one of the following:

1. A bulging disc. This can be a soft disc but more often it is a hard disc.
2. Osteoarthritic build-up around the vertebral body margins or on the articular processes. Often several areas show osteoarthritic build-up.
3. Marked narrowing of the disc space.
4. An expanding tumor.

If the patient has had previous surgery, the nerves may become supersensitive. Very little motion is required to produce pain. Often, merely tugging on the nerve with body movements is enough to produce pain.

Decompression obviously involves the enlarging of the nerve channel. Sometimes complete removal of the pars and portions of the articular processes to channel the nerve is necessary. Wray[24] has stated that there are cases where an uncovertebral process lying anterior to the nerve can produce pain, and relief can only be obtained by getting in front of the nerve and cutting this process off. However, Rouschning has stated that what appears on the CT scan to be a hook or process is actually a ridge.[17]

The ganglion, because it is an enlarged area in the nerve, may be more easily compressed by a bulging disc in the bony pedicle zone. Decompression is still the treatment of choice. If the ganglion has been damaged by previous surgery, it may cause pain, and decompression may not be effective. Actual removal of the ganglion has been used occasionally for this situation.

One of the problems in decompressing the ganglion is that it is so far laterally that satisfactory decompression involves sacrificing all of the posterior support on that side. In other words, the pars and the articular processes must be removed. Fusion at that level may be indicated and will be discussed later in this chapter.[25]

Ganglionitis,[7] of S1 in particular, has been reported to cause trouble. Again, decompression seems to be an excellent method of treatment.

Surgical decompression of the lateral neurovascular canal is rather simple if one sacrifices the articular processes and exposes the nerve all the way to a point beyond the foramen. However, the posterior stability should be saved if possible.

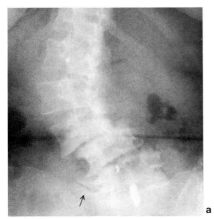 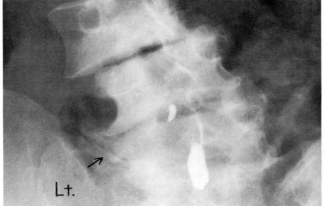 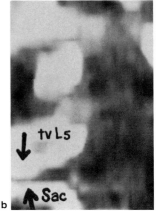

Figure 23–2 (a) Typical standing anterior posterior roentgenogram showing the left transverse process impinging upon the sacral ala. The patient's symptoms, plus neurological and EMG findings, indicated L5 spinal nerve involvement. *Source:* Reprinted with permission from *Spine* (1984;9:32), Copyright © 1984, JB Lippincott Company. (b) Ferguson AP view of the same patient. *Source:* Reprinted from *Multiplanar CT of the Spine* (p 385) by SLG Rothman and WV Glenn Jr, Aspen Publishers Inc, © 1985. (c) Coronal view of a CT scan of the same patient as shown in Figures 23–1a and 23–1b. Note that the part labeled TV L5 (transverse process of L5) lies against the part labeled Sac (sacral ala). *Source:* Reprinted with permission from *Spine* (1984;9:32), Copyright © 1984, JB Lippincott Company.

The computed tomography (CT) scan, and recently magnetic resonance imaging (MRI), are our main diagnostic tools in determining the degree of compression in this area. Even the metrizamide myelogram does not extend laterally far enough. All other available diagnostic aids should, of course, be used. Electromyography (EMG) and nerve conduction studies are valuable. Selective nerve blocks can be especially valuable in localizing the involved spinal nerve.

The paraspinal approach is generally the best for this area[6] (Figure 23–2) unless both laminae have to be decompressed. In this case a midline approach is probably necessary. Removing the medial swing of the articular processes is easy and safe, but if the lateral canal is still blocked beyond that, the problem is much more difficult. Channelling the canal and still saving stability can be done only to a limited extent. Through the paraspinal approach, one can reach both the entrance zone and the exit zone and still save the stability.

Hazlet and Kinnard[10] have stated that if one articular process is removed at a single level, clinical instability will not result. This statement is probably true, provided the development of instability is not already in progress as, for instance, in even slight degrees of degenerative spondylolisthesis.

A one-level unilateral fusion on the opposite side is usually done if a total decompression is necessary on one side. If the disc space is narrow, a unilateral fusion will usually result in solid arthrodesis. If the disc space is wide and succulent, an anterior interbody fusion can be added in a week to ten days if there is concern for the development of instability.

THE FAR OUT SYNDROME: SPINAL NERVE COMPRESSION LATERAL TO THE FORAMEN

Impingement of a spinal nerve anywhere out to the point where it exits from the lateral border of the intervertebral foramen has been well described and is generally accepted;[5,16] however, nerve compression farther laterally is less well known. Failure to recognize the fact that the nerve can be compressed even farther laterally than the point where it exits from the intervertebral foramen accounts for a fair number of failures of lumbar spine surgery. Because of the far lateral position of the compression, the phrase ''far out syndrome'' has been suggested.[2,22]

In the following pages, far lateral compression of the L5 spinal nerve will be the principal one described since it is the nerve most commonly affected. However, except for the sacral nerves, virtually any other spinal nerve can be similarly compressed. The following causes of far lateral compression are described in sequence:

1. Alar transverse process bony impingement
2. Ligamentous compression beyond the foramen
3. Compression by a bulging or ruptured disc lateral to the foramen

ALAR TRANSVERSE PROCESS BONY IMPINGEMENT

In these cases the lateral mass, and the base of the transverse process, and occasionally the entire transverse process, impinge on the ala. This syndrome has been noted in two types of patients: (1) elderly individuals with degenerative lumbar scoliosis and (2) a somewhat younger population with isthmic spondylolisthesis and at least 20 percent slip.

Description of the Two Types of Bony Compression

Type I (and probably the most common) is the elderly individual with degenerative lumbar scoliosis or asymmetric disc degeneration at L5, causing tilting of the fifth lumbar vertebra. These patients usually have a primary lumbar curve that causes the transverse process of L5 to dip downwards toward the sacral ala (Figure 23–3). Also, because of rotation, the same transverse process moves posteriorly and hits the ala.

Occasionally, there may be compression at the concavity of the major curve but it is more commonly seen in the concavity of the compensatory lumbosacral curve down at the L5 level.

While the most common place for the far out syndrome to occur is between the transverse process of L5 and the ala of the sacrum, it can occur higher in the lumbar spine and occasionally it is noted that the two pedicles and transverse processes are tightly jammed together (Figure 23–2) at higher levels where there is sharp angulation. The pathology is basically the same as that seen with scoliosis at L5–S1.

Type II includes a somewhat younger population group with isthmic spondylolisthesis[23] and at least 20 percent slip who also develop the same syndrome as Type I. While 20 percent slip is the smallest degree of olisthesis, 30 percent is more

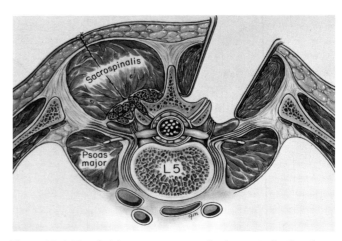

Figure 23–3 Two Gelpi retractors seem to be the most effective. If one need only reach the transverse process and ala, it is not necessary to expose the lamina as far medially as in the drawing. *Source:* Reprinted with permission from *Journal of Bone and Joint Surgery* (1968;50A: 920–923), Copyright © 1968, Journal of Bone and Joint Surgery Inc.

common. In the 30 percent slip group, it can occur bilaterally but is usually unilateral because the forward slip is often slightly asymmetric.

Many people with isthmic spondylolisthesis have somewhat enlarged transverse processes but not nearly to the point of being considered transitional vertebrae. The radicular pain in spondylolisthesis patients has traditionally been explained on the basis of fibrous tissue compression of L5 or bony compression of S1. Also, stretching the S1 signal nerves with progressive slip has been incriminated in cases of high-grade olisthesis.

As the vertebral body slips forward, the transverse processes move in an anterior, as well as a caudal direction, allowing the transverse processes to settle down against the sacrum. We have seen this type of nerve compression in cases of spondylolisthesis at the fourth level also, and there is no reason why it could not occur at higher levels.

In screening patients for the presence of this syndrome, the Ferguson view (20 degrees caudocephalic anteroposterior x-ray) is the most helpful. When this view is compared with the routine AP view, one can easily see how much better the Ferguson view delineates this condition than does the standard AP. Myelography usually is done in these patients and, in the degenerative type (Type I), it characteristically shows at least some central canal stenosis. A CT or MRI scan is required to show alar transverse process impingement. It is important, however, to alert the radiologist doing the scanning to use a "wide window" for inclusion of the area clear to the tip of the transverse process of L5 and also the sacral ala.

Sciatica in Type II patients is usually one-sided. The symptoms and physical signs are those of the sciatica type of spinal stenosis.

On myelography, the spondylolisthesis cases (Type II) will show a certain amount of canal compromise at the level of olisthesis, but again computerized axial tomography or MRI scanning is by far the procedure of choice to demonstrate far lateral compression.

Technique of Decompression

Type I Degenerative Scoliosis

The patient is placed in the kneeling position. Either a midline or a paraspinal approach can be used. The paraspinal approach is usually preferable since it makes removal of part of the pedicle and transverse process much easier. Often there is so much central stenosis that both laminae must be removed in the lower levels. In these cases, a midline approach is necessary.

The spinal nerve must be traced out laterally and all overlying bone removed. Usually, the caudal third of the pedicle must be removed along with at least the lower half of the transverse process (Figure 23–4). It may be simpler to remove the entire transverse process, and it is doubtful if saving the

cephalic half is of any value, unless fusion is contemplated. The cephalic border of the ala can be removed if this seems easier. This removal has the advantage of totally detaching the sickle ligament, thus eliminating any chance of constriction by this ligament (Figure 23–5). A fusion is usually not attempted on the decompressed side. Unless the disc at L5 is very narrow and osteoarthritic, a one-level unilateral fusion is done on the other side (Figure 23–6). Advanced age and poor general health may preclude fusion, however. If possible, the unilateral total decompression is limited to one level. Even then, further slip is a real danger.

Type II Spondylolisthesis

In the case of spondylolisthesis, the paraspinal approach is used if possible (Figure 23–7). Only a unilateral decompression is done, unless the pain is severe in both legs. The pain is, however, usually largely unilateral. It is not absolutely necessary to remove the entire lamina of L5. The L5 nerve can simply be channeled out through the defective pars and the lower portion of the pedicle removed along with the base of the transverse process (or the entire transverse process). Some of the cephalic border of the ala can be removed if it seems to be impinging.

The use of pedicle screw devices may make it possible to lift L5 off of the nerves and thus make extensive decompression unnecessary.[13]

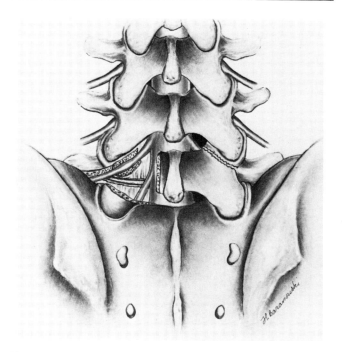

Figure 23–4 In order to get the L5 spinal nerve decompressed, it is necessary to take off at least the lower half of the pedicle and some of the transverse process. *Source:* Reprinted with permission from *Spine* (1984;9:35), Copyright © 1984, JB Lippincott Company.

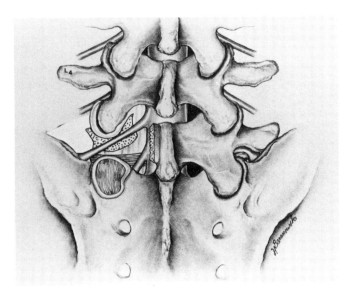

Figure 23–5 Sometimes, in order to get the L5 nerve unequivocally decompressed, it is necessary to totally remove the transverse process. *Source:* Reprinted with permission from *Spine* (1984;9:35), Copyright © 1984, JB Lippincott Company.

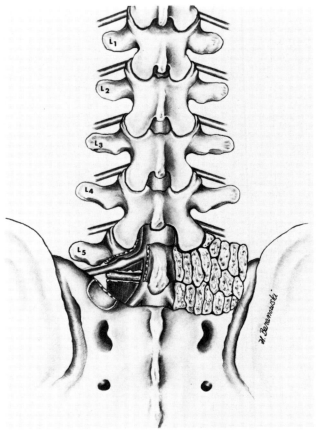

If it is necessary to decompress both sides, a fusion should not be done at the same time unless internal fixation is used, which jacks the vertebrae apart. The device may keep the graft from migrating medially. Cloward[3] recommends his operation in this situation.[19]

Figure 23–6 Type of unilateral fusion done. *Source:* Reprinted with permission from *Spine* (1984;9:39), Copyright © 1984, JB Lippincott Company.

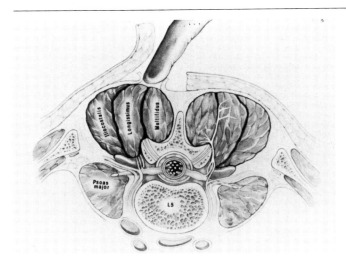
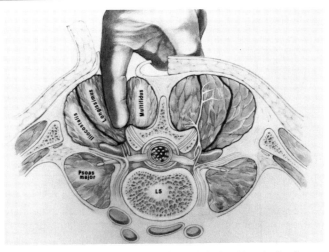

Figure 23–7 (a) This shows the paraspinal approach. A midline skin incision is used. The skin is pulled over. The fascia is incised longitudinally one and a half finger breadths lateral to the midline at the level where the articular processes of L4 and L5 articulate. The multifidus and longissimus separate well. The finger can be plunged between the muscles down to the L4–5 facets. *Source:* Presented in an exhibit by LL Wiltse and D Spencer at a meeting of the International Society for the Study of the Lumbar Spine, Cambridge, England, April 1983. (b) The finger can be plunged between the multifidus and longissimus at the level of the apophysis of L4 and L5. The multifidus swings laterally at the L5 level and attaches to the ligament. It can be cut away from the ligament almost bloodlessly. *Source:* Presented in an exhibit by LL Wiltse and D Spencer at a meeting of the International Society for the Study of the Lumbar Spine, Cambridge, England, April 1983.

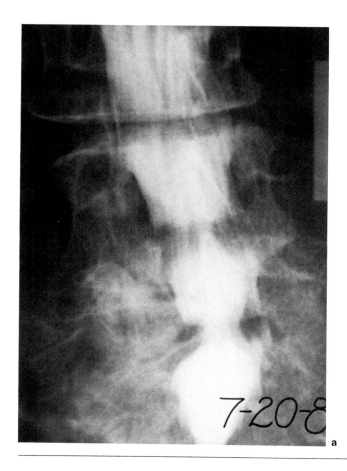

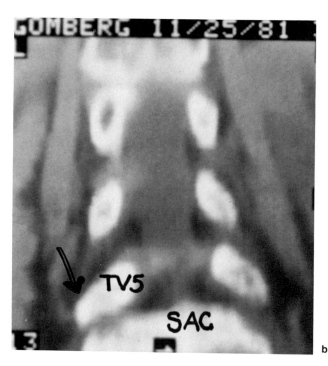

Figure 23–8 (a) AP myelogram of a 69-year-old woman with very severe leg pain. (b) Coronal CT scan shows marked impingement of TV 5 (transverse process of L5) on Sac (sacral ala) on the left. *Source:* Reprinted with permission from *Spine* (1984;9:38), Copyright © 1984, JB Lippincott Company.

Typical Cases

Case 1

The following case is representative of Type I, degenerative scoliosis. The case involves a 69-year-old Caucasian woman who had low back pain and severe left leg pain with numbness in the L5 distribution for two years. Prior to surgery she was unable to walk because of back and especially leg pain. Roentgenograms showed that she had degenerative scoliosis and a narrowed disc space that was asymmetrically narrowed. The transverse process of L5 on the painful side was lying against the ala of the sacrum (Figures 23–7a and 23–7b).

Myelography demonstrated the typical central spinal canal stenosis in the lower lumbar canal, which is so frequently seen in these cases. The CT scan uncovered the pathology. In both sagittal and coronal views, the transverse process on the painful side was down against the ala of the sacrum (Figure 23–8).

The patient underwent surgical decompression of the painful L5 level with removal of the lower half of the left pedicle and the entire left transverse process. A unilateral fusion on the right was done. In her case, it was believed that because of the marked narrowing of the fifth interspace, no further stabilization beyond the unilateral fusion would be necessary. She is currently approximately four years postoperation and is doing well, and her unilateral fusion is solid.

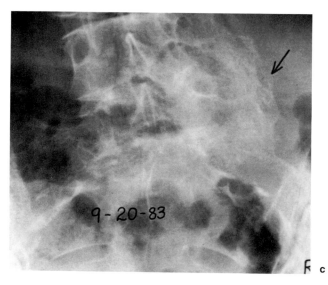

Figure 23–8 (c) AP x-ray, two years postoperation, shows that the lower half of the pedicle and transverse process has been removed on the left. A unilateral fusion has been done on the right from L5 to S1. Because of the narrowing of the L5 disc space, an interbody fusion was not added. The patient obtained a solid fusion. The same type of unilateral fusion alone on this patient shown in Figure 23–5. *Source:* Reprinted with permission from *Spine* (1984;9:38), Copyright © 1984, JB Lippincott Company.

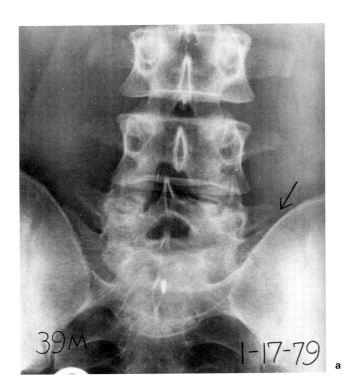

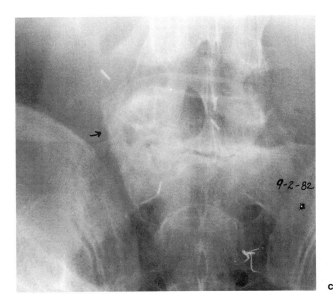

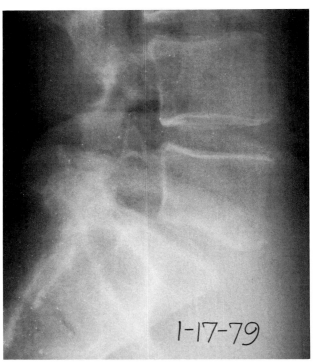

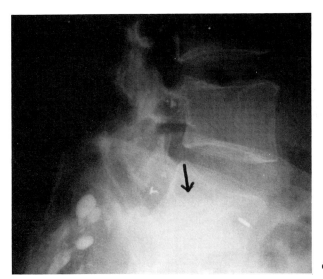

Figure 23–9 (c) AP x-ray 21 months postoperation. Note a total decompression was done on the right and a one-level fusion on the left. (d) A lateral view 21 months postoperation shows an interbody fusion at L5–S1 using fibula. *Source:* Reprinted with permission from *Spine* (1984;9:40), Copyright © 1984, JB Lippincott Company.

Case 2

A 39-year-old man with isthmic spondylolisthesis and 20 percent slip presented with low back and right leg pain. Two years previously he had undergone a right-sided laminectomy at L5 but without relief. On examination there was decreased sensation in the L5 nerve distribution, and sciatic tension tests were markedly positive on the right side. The CT scan showed approximation of the pedicle, the base of the transverse process, and even the tip of the transverse process to the ala of the sacrum (Figure 23–9).

Figure 23–9 (a) AP x-ray of a 39-year-old man with isthmic spondylolisthesis. Note close proximity of the right lateral mass and transverse process of L5 to the ala. At surgery the nerve was seen to be compressed all the way out to the lateral third of the shaft of the transverse process. (b) Lateral view preoperatively. *Source:* Reprinted with permission from *Spine* (1984;9:40), Copyright © 1984, JB Lippincott Company.

At surgery a complete decompression was done on the right side with removal of the lower half of the pedicle and, because of the marked compression of the nerve, the entire transverse process. A contralateral one-level posterolateral fusion was done at the same time. Because his L5 disc was fairly wide, failure of arthrodesis with only a one-sided fusion posteriorly was a concern, so an interbody fusion was done approximately ten days after the posterior operation. He was allowed to be mobile immediately (Figures 23–5 and 23–6).

The question might be asked, just how common is this syndrome? In the middle-aged adult with more than 20 to 30 percent slip in isthmic spondylolisthesis, the condition is extremely common and probably accounts for many of the failures of the Gill operation. For many years, Gill et al[27] advocated complete removal of the loose element along with any fibrocartilaginous mass, extra ossicles of bone, and even the proximal stumps of the pars bilaterally. If one goes further and removes the caudal half of the pedicles and a portion of the transverse processes, instability will be quite severe and further significant olisthesis is very likely to occur. In many of these cases, there is some lateral tilt of L5 and one transverse process is closer to the ala of the sacrum than the other; thus the decompression can be unilateral. The pain is also usually unilateral, or at least tolerable, in the less painful leg. If a total decompression can be done on one side only (the painful side), then the other side can be fused. If a unilateral fusion is contemplated, it is advantageous to use a paraspinal approach.

An important question is, will a unilateral L5 to sacrum fusion produce arthrodesis in a high percentage of cases when the graft is only at one corner of the tripod? If there is marked narrowing of the fifth disc space, it probably will. If the fifth disc space is quite normal, it may not. The number of unilateral fusions is as yet too small to have reliable statistics. As a result, if in doubt, an interbody fusion can be added.

Theoretically, the Cloward operation should be ideal in this particular situation if the pseudoarthrosis rate it not too high. If an anterior abdominal approach is used with fibular struts, the strut grafts must be stood on end and the vertebral bodies jacked apart severely. Perhaps by using fibular struts and jacking the vertebrae apart severely, posterior decompression may not be necessary. One thing to remember is not to do a Gill operation posteriorly and fibular struts anteriorly. These struts will tip over and olisthesis will increase.

In the older patient, with the Type I far out syndrome (degenerative scoliosis) with very marked narrowing of the fifth interspace and severe osteophytic overgrowth, it is likely that a unilateral total decompression without fusion can be done without danger of serious instability. If a unilateral paraspinal approach can be used for decompressing at the one painful level, the instability should be relatively little. Because a one-level fusion adds relatively little to the procedure, a unilateral fusion can be done. With the development of methods of jacking the vertebrae apart with pedicle screws and posterior rods, it may very well be that, in the future, the lateral masses can be lifted off the nerves and fused without decompression.[19]

Figure 23–10 shows a case where the far out compression was on the left side, but above a transitional vertebra. The case demonstrates that far lateral compression can also occur at the L4–5 level above a transitional vertebra.

LIGAMENTOUS COMPRESSION BEYOND THE FORAMEN

Clinical compression of the spinal nerves, especially L5, can be produced by ligaments. MacNab[14] has stated that in spondylolisthesis, the corpora transverse ligament can sharply compress the L5 spinal nerve, much like a guillotine does. As the L5 vertebra slips forward, this ligament descends on the nerve, compressing it between itself and the sacral ala.

There is a ligament attaching the spinal nerve to the farthest lateral expansion of the posterior longitudinal ligament at the level of the disc.[9] Also, there is a ligament caudal to the nerve,[18] that attaches the spinal nerve to the caudal pedicle.[20] There are also multiple small fibrils attaching the nerve to the side of the vertebral body.

The spinal nerve at the exit zone of the foramen, located at the distal border of the ganglion, is securely attached[8] by fibrous bands between it and the periosteum and the capsule.[1] The transforaminal ligaments also have attachments to the nerve as it exits. Also, in a few specimens attachments to the superior pedicle were found.

After it exits from the intervertebral foramen, the nerve passes through a tunnel formed by the intertransverse ligament posteriorly and the lumbosacral ligament (the sickle ligament) anteriorly (Figure 23–11a). The nerve must also pass through a V-shaped opening, formed by the sickle ligament and the sacral ala (Figure 23–11b). The sickle ligament was first implicated by Danforth and Wilson[5] in 1925 and more recently by Lombardi.[12] Large lateral osteophytes from the sides of the bodies of L5 or S1 or a large lateral disc herniation can constrict the nerve in the lumbosacral tunnel.

The lumbosacral ligament (sickle ligament) is most often in the form of an inverted "V." It consists of two fascial bands, arising from the transverse process of L5, one going to the body of S1 and a lateral band to the sacral ala. The sickle ligament attaches to the inferior border of the transverse process of L5 and extends medially and caudally anterior to the L5 spinal nerve to attach to the bodies of L5 and S1 and the sacral ala. At the point where the L5 spinal nerve passes out between the limbs of the "V," the ligament is attached to the nerve by fibrous bands both front and back[12] (Figures 23–12a,b). Thus, in effect, this segment of spinal nerve is tethered at both ends by fairly strong bands and in its middle by fibrils, so that any mass under the tethered segment can put tension on the nerve.

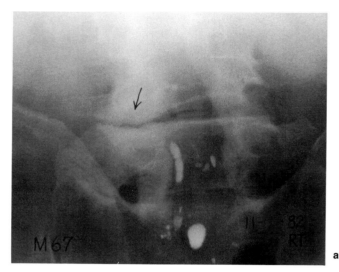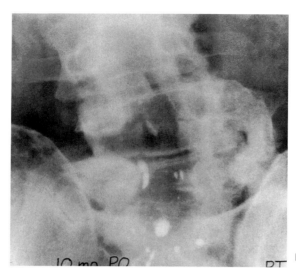

Figure 23–10 (a) Note severe lateral impingement on the left between the lateral mass and transverse process of L4 and a transitional L5. Two midline decompressions had been done in two years. (b) A total decompression on the left and a unilateral fusion on the right was done. The patient obtained a solid fusion and complete relief of pain.

To completely free the L5 nerve, one must surgically snip the attaching ligaments all the way from the foramen to a point past the rim of the sacral ala.

The S1 spinal nerve is securely tethered at the point where it passes out of the anterior S1 foramen. Before that point, it is only lightly attached, and after that point it is attached to the front of the sacrum of a few small fibrils.

The L4 spinal nerve has most of the same tethering ligaments as does L5 but does not have anything resembling a sickle ligament.

In spondylolisthesis, the transverse process of L5 slides anteriorly and caudally. Since L5 is anchored to the ala and will not move, either traction or compression can cause symptoms.

In the case of scoliosis with tilt of the L5 vertebra on S1 with large osteophytes at the vertebral margins, the tethering of the L5 nerve holds it and thus allows it to be pinched between the lateral mass, the transverse process, and the ala of the sacrum.

FAR LATERAL (EXTRAFORAMINAL) DISC PROTRUSION AS A CASE OF SPINAL NERVE COMPRESSION

Before the advent of CT or MRI scanning,[4] it was not possible (short of anatomical dissection) to visualize a spinal nerve lateral to the point where water-soluble contrast ceased to flow into the dural sheaths that cover the spinal nerves. However, since CT is being used extensively, not only are disc ruptures in the vertebral foramina seen (Figure 23–13) but also the far lateral disc. If a large extrusion of the disc material occurs at the point where the nerve crosses the disc space, the spinal nerve can be compromised either by compression or by traction (Figure 23–14). As stated before, the L5 nerve is securely tethered both at the level of the foramen and also

where it passes over the rim of the ala between the limbs of the lumbosacral (sickle) ligament. Thus, there is a 2.5 to 3 cm segment of the L5 spinal nerve that is securely bound at each end, and to some extent, bound by small fibrils at its middle. An extrusion at the point where the spinal nerve crosses the lateral side of the disc can cause symptoms characteristic of a typical ruptured disc in the central canal.

Although there is no absolute proof, exuberant osteophytes or a hard, bulging annulus may also cause symptoms of compression.

Table 23–1 lists the areas shown in Figure 23–1 (a and b) where a disc can rupture. A large rupture at L5, as far laterally as 90 degrees, can cause trouble, and there has been a report on two in the literature, that large ruptures, even in front, have caused pain.

POSSIBLE SYMPATHETIC DISTURBANCE BY A FAR LATERAL DISC

As more and more patients with a far lateral disc are seen, it may be concluded that there could be an occasional disc that presses upon the sympathetic chain since a few patients seem to have causalgic type pain. This has not been proven. Sympathetic blocks have been used with limited success. They are difficult at L5.

Table 23–1 Areas of Nerve Compression

I. CENTRAL CANAL
   A. Mid Central
   B. Lateral Central
II. LATERAL NEUROVASCULAR CANAL
   A. Entrance Zone
   B. Pedicle Zone
   C. Exit Zone
III. FAR LATERAL ZONE (out to 90 degrees)

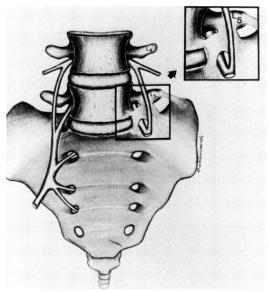

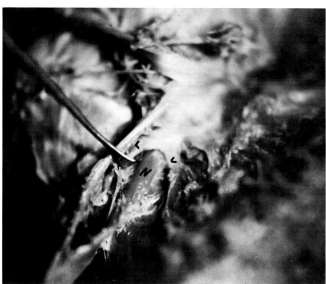

Figure 23–11 (a) Drawing of sickle ligament. (b) Photograph of sickle ligament. The two limbs of the V-shaped ligament are labeled L. The L5 nerve is labeled N. *Source:* Presented by JS Lombardi at a meeting of the International Society for the Study of the Lumbar Spine, Montreal, Canada, June 1984.

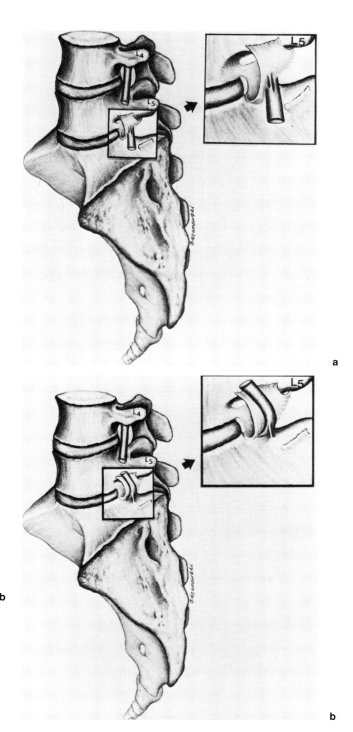

Figure 23–12 Ligamentous attachments of the L5 nerve in the lateral foramina.

SURGERY FOR FAR LATERAL DISC DISEASE

A paraspinal approach is ordinarily used to reach the posterolateral areas of the disc. In most cases, it is not necessary to expose the laminae (Figure 23–15). The outer facets of the articular processes, the posterior surfaces of the transverse processes, and the cephalic 2 cm of the posterior surface of the sacral ala should be denuded of soft tissue (Figure 23–16).

If the transverse process of L5 is in the way, the lower half of it is removed. The intertransverse muscle and ligament are carefully removed (Figure 23–17). A half circle of bone,

about 1 cm deep, is removed from the cephalic border of the ala (Figure 23–18a). This detaches both the intertransverse ligament and the sickle ligament. If the surgeon wishes, the muscle medial to the facet can be pulled and the lamina decompressed without sacrificing the pars (Figure 23–18b).

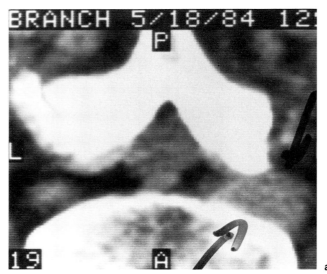

a

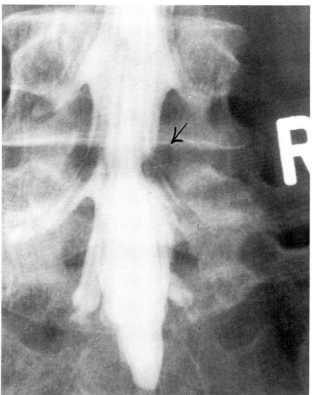

b

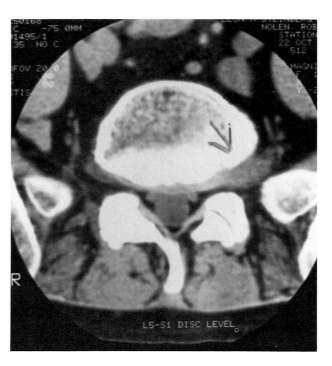

Figure 23–14 Large extruded disc far laterally under the L5 spinal nerve as it crosses the disc space. This disc was removed through a paraspinal approach. The intertransverse ligament was removed and a half circle of the ala was also removed. The nerve was very tightly bound down. The patient was relieved of pain.

Figure 23–13 (a) Lateral disc part outside and part inside the foramen. A classical right midline discectomy relieved patient's pain. The fact that midline discectomy relieved the pain indicates that the nuclear material was pulled medially. (b) Note defect on myelogram in spite of the fact that most of the nuclear material is outside the bony foramen.

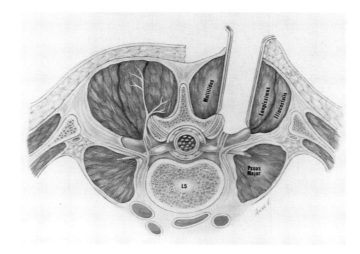

Figure 23–15 Paraspinal approach to the lateral disc. It is not always necessary to expose the lamina.

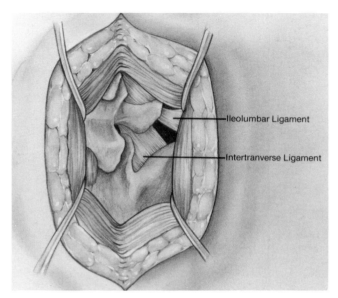

Figure 23–16 The ala, the transverse process, and the lateral border of the articular processes are denuded.

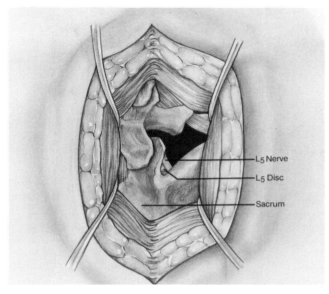

Figure 23–17 The intertransverse muscle and ligament are removed at the L5 level. The intertransverse ligament is thick and strong.

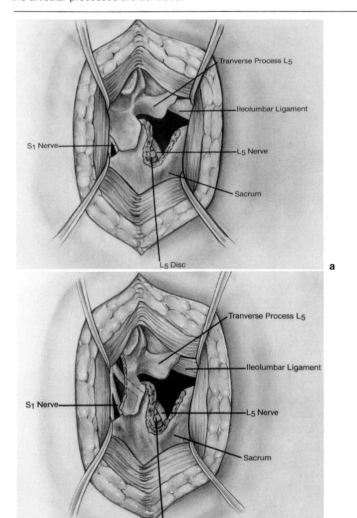

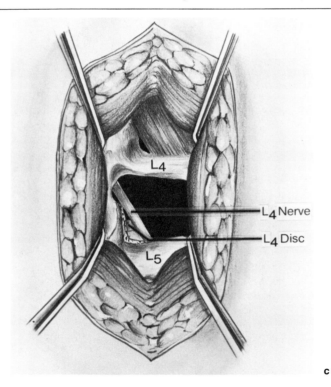

Figure 23–18 (a) A half circle of bone, about 1 cm deep, is removed from the ala. (b) If the surgeon wishes, the muscle can be pulled medially and the area of the subarticular zone decompressed. (c) This drawing shows the final stage of the approach to a far lateral disc at the L4 level instead of the L5.

Only bipolar cautery should be used in this area. Surgicell can be used to plug holes where bleeding occurs if cautery does not work well. A headlight is necessary and magnification is valuable. The L5 nerve will be found to be very tightly tied down and often difficult to move in any direction. A bulging disc is often located exactly under the nerve so the use of an angulated pituitary rongeur may be necessary. Freeing the nerve from a large exuberant osteoarthritic mass underlying it is all that is necessary in some cases.

Figure 23–18c shows the final stage of the approach to a far lateral disc at the L4 level rather than L5 level.

If the surgeon prefers, a midline approach can be used, as seen in Figure 23–19. This approach is not only very effective but also is more familiar to most surgeons.

The wound is closed routinely. Postoperative care is the same as for a classical discectomy.

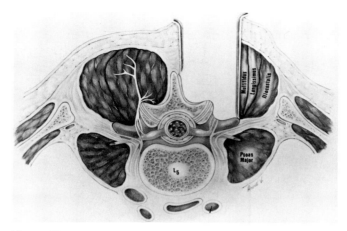

Figure 23–19 A midline approach, as shown here, can be made if preferred.

REFERENCES

1. Brieg A: *Adverse Mechanical Tension in the Central Nervous System.* New York, John Wiley and Sons, 1978, p 159.

2. Burton C: Personal communication, November 1981.

3. Cloward RB: Personal Communication 1981.

4. Dandy W: Concealed ruptured intervertebral discs. *JAMA* 1941; 821–823.

5. Danforth MD, Wilson PD: The anatomy of the lumbosacral region in relation to sciatic pain. *J Bone Joint Surg* 1925;7:109–160.

6. Enslin TB: Debridement and fusion of the lumbosacral area through an iliolumbar approach. *Orthop Clin North Am* 1975;6–1:291–297.

7. Fredrickson B: First sacral root ganglion. Read before the annual meeting of International Society for the Study of the Lumbar Spine, Montreal, Canada, June 1984.

8. Galub B, Silverman B: Transforaminal ligaments of the lumbar spine. *J Bone Joint Surg* 1969;51A–5:947–956.

9. Godard M, Reid J: Movements induced by straight leg raising in the lumbosacral roots, nerves and plexies and the intra pelvic section of the sciatic nerve. *J Neurol Neurosurg Psychiatry* 1965;28–12:12–18.

10. Hazlet JW, Kinnard P: Lumbar apophyseal process excision and spinal stability. *Spine* 1982;7:171–176.

11. Kirkaldy-Willis WH, McIvor G: Editorial comment. *Clin Orthop* 1976;115:2–3.

12. Lombardi JS, et al: The lumbosacral ligament. Read before the annual meeting of the International Society for the Study of the Lumbar Spine, Montreal, Canada, June 1984.

13. Louis R: Personal communication, 1972.

14. MacNab I: The corpora transverse ligament. *Backache.* Baltimore, Williams & Williams Co, 1977, p 55.

15. MacNab I: The negative disc exploration. *J Bone Joint Surg* 1971;53A:891–893.

16. Putti V: Pathogenesis of sciatic pain. *Lancet* 1927;2:53–60.

17. Rouschning W: Personal communication, June 1984.

18. Spencer D, et al: Anatomy and significance of fixation of the lumbosacral nerve roots in sciatica. *Spine* 1983;8–6:672–679.

19. Steffee A: A new method of using pedicle screws and plates for fixation of the lumbar spine. Read before the meeting of the North American Lumbar Spine Association, Vail, Colo., June 1984.

20. Sunderland S: Meningeal neural relations in the intervertebral foramen. *J Neurol Neurosurg Psychiatry* 1974;40:752–763.

21. Verbiest H: A radicular syndrome from developmental narrowing of the lumbar vertebral canal. *J Bone Joint Surg* 1954;36B:230.

22. Wiltse LL, et al: Alar transverse process impingement of the L5 spinal nerve: Far out syndrome. *Spine* 1984;9–1:31–41.

23. Wiltse LL, et al: Classification of spondylolysis and spondylolisthesis. *Clin Orthop* 1976;117:23–29.

24. Wray C: Causes of nerve root compression. Read before the meeting of the North American Lumbar Spine Association, Vail, Colo., June 1984.

25. Yuan H: Personal communication (1984).

26. American Academy of Orthopedic Surgeons: *Glossary of Spinal Terminology.* Chicago, American Academy of Orthopedic Surgeons, 1985.

27. Gill GG, Manning JC, White HL: Surgical treatment of spondylolisthesis without spine fusion. *J Bone Joint Surg* 1955;37A:493–518.

Chapter 24

The Paralateral Approach to Decompressions for Lateral Stenosis and Far Lateral Lesions of the Lumbar Spine

Charles D. Ray, M.D., FACS

Approaches used in surgery have always been an important element of the surgical art. Preferred approaches must address the characteristics of the overlying skin and intervening structures such as muscle, bone, fat, organs, and nerve tissue, as well as the lesion. Other considerations include the potential of injury to important nearby structures, problems in healing or recovery, and discomfort to the patient. To this important list of factors one must also add the simplicity or complexity afforded the surgeon and his or her team. Foremost is the need for the procedure to be appropriate to the target lesion, that is, how well the approach permits one to address the pathology.

Since the reports of Dandy in 1926 and Mixter and Barr in 1934, nearly all lumbar spinal surgery has utilized a midline approach. This has been largely due to current knowledge of pathoanatomy which was primarily derived from available methods of diagnosis. Plain x-radiographs of the lumbar spine have value for many lesions but lack detail regarding the status of neural foraminae and the nerve structures traversing them. The contrast myelogram yields progressively less detail as the structures progress laterally, since the dural sleeves stop at the ganglia and much pathology may lie distally.

In recent years, tomographic techniques and a fresh interest in the gross anatomy of lateral lumbar structures have shown that a significant percentage of symptomatic lesions lay further lateral than was previously known. High-resolution computed tomography (CT) proved to be the most important technique to show the presence and extent of such lesions. Further, the CT scan has helped the surgeon to plan particularly appropriate operative approaches to these lesions.

Watkins described a paraspinal approach for posterolateral fusion of the lumbar and lumbosacral spine.[15,16] Variations of this operation have been widely used for nearly 30 years; although of late, they have apparently been used with less frequency. This paraspinal approach was not intended to afford an access for lateral decompression; if decompression was ever performed via this approach during fusion, it was incidental to the purpose of the procedure.

Wiltse et al[18] and others have described variations of the Watkins technique.[17] The approach of Wiltse et al is to split the sacrospinalis muscle longitudinally; although, when bone was to be taken, their approach was essentially the same as that of Watkins. Wiltse et al felt that the slightly more medial approach permitted the inclusion of laminae as well as facets and transverse processes in the fusion. After reviewing the technique presented here with Wiltse, Watkins felt that it was the most lateral yet attempted, especially for purposes of

Note: The author wishes to express his appreciation for the suggestions and encouragement shown by: his associates at the Institute for Low Back Care, Minneapolis, Drs. Charles Burton, Alexander Lifson, and Richard Salib; Prof. William Kirkaldy-Willis, Department of Orthopaedics, University Hospital, Saskatchewan, Canada; and especially for the outstanding work using high-resolution CT scanning contributed by Dr. Kenneth Heithoff, Center for Diagnostic Imaging, Minneapolis. Although the first case operated by the author using this concept was done in 1979, the initial patient for whom the procedure was specifically applied as a result of CT scan findings was operated on in March 1982. Kevin Gracie aided in photography and the making of video recordings of the cases. Christie Marlene Ray assisted in the surgical photographs; Gerald Kolb and David Pickop made the CT scan prints. The author rendered the sketches from which final art work was realized by Bob Doig.

decompression rather than fusion (personal communication, November 1983). The method given here, referred to as the paralateral approach since it is quite lateral but parallel to the spinal axis, avoids longitudinal splitting of the paraspinous muscle. The targets lie more anterolateral to the surfaces used in fusions. Further, by not splitting the muscle, there seems to be less overall bleeding and less postoperative discomfort.

It has become clear that the paralateral approach may be utilized to deal with a number of laterally placed lesions. In contrast with a midline approach for the same laterally placed lesions, the posterior structures (e.g., dorsal spinous processes, laminae and zygapophyseal joints, associated ligaments and muscles) are more completely preserved. Such preservation should help to maintain stability and thus, hopefully, obviate, in many cases, a need for subsequent fusion. The paralateral approach traverses the intramuscular fascial planes (between spinal erectors and quadratus lumborum, for example), and therefore, there is no need for a large, relaxing incision. Retractors are small and the force of retraction is low, in contrast with midline approaches to the same laterally placed lesions. As a consequence to the smaller, gentler approach, patients generally have much less postoperative pain and muscular soreness than with equivalent midline approaches.[9]

The approach used presently is made feasible and important only through the advent of high-resolution CT scanning of the lumbar spine. A number of clinically important lesions have been found with greater frequency than previously suspected.[1-7] Those that are particularly appropriate for this approach are laterally placed lesions in cases where there is no significant pathology in the central canal. Bilateral paralateral approaches are technically more complex than when exploring a second side through a midline incision. However, multi-level, single-sided paralateral approaches are quite reasonable. Since lateral stenoses are often bilateral, or since the second side may be quite suspect, the choice between paralateral and midline approaches may hinge on the certainty of the diagnosis, anticipated technical challenge, experience of the surgeon, and expectation for long-term stability of the decompressed segment. These anatomical considerations are guided by careful study of the plain films, transaxial CT scans, and parasagittal reformatted images.[5,8,12,13]

In most cases, parasagittal reformatted CT images have proven essential in clarifying the anatomy. Sequential, parallel transaxial scans of 5 mm or less, often made with a 2 mm or 3 mm overlap of the slices, are usually required, especially at the L5–S1 level. Reformatting then provides high detail of the foraminae and exiting nerves.[1,3,5,7] A few full-trunk (total body) scan slices are also helpful for the study of muscle masses, fat deposits, fascial planes, major vessels, and configuration of the iliac crests and lumbosacral and sacroiliac junctions. These latter structures also bear upon the selection and detailed planning of the surgical approach to be utilized.

Clearly, the anatomical path between the skin incision and the target must be studied in advance.

In most male patients, the iliac crest lies higher than in females, as shown in Figure 24–1. In patients having a high intercristal (IC) line, the L5 transverse process is often large and lies quite close to the superior aspect of the sacral ala. This may reduce the L5–S1 "window of access" to a narrow slot. Further, in such cases, the iliolumbar and iliotransverse ligaments are usually quite well developed. All of these structural details may influence the decision to use the paralateral approach, the exact route to be taken, and the complexity of the dissection when one reaches the target. The full-body cross-section CT may indicate the need to resect a portion of the iliac crest in order to gain a straight line access to the lesion.

TECHNICAL CONSIDERATIONS

This paralateral approach presents a very different dimension in surgery of the lumbar spine. The principal consideration is that the approach must be appropriate and there must be no significant reason for exploration or decompression in the central canal, even though a direct view of the central posterior dura is possible to a limited extent during the dissection from a

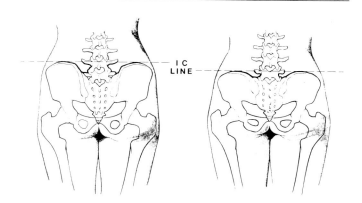

Figure 24–1 Intercristal (IC) line between the iliac crests shown in two types of pelves, typically male and female. The IC line on the left figure passes through the upper body of L4. Since the transverse processes and other anatomic structures of L5 are in close proximity to the sacral alae and ilium, this situation provides considerable lateral ligamentous support and stability of L5, especially the L5–S1 disc space. In the figure on the right, the IC line passes through the L5 body. The L5–S1 disc and facets are considerably more vulnerable to rotary and translational forces. In the lefthand case, disc and facet degenerations are far more likely to occur at L4–5, whereas on the right, they occur more frequently at L5–S1. The paralateral approach to L5–S1 is more difficult in the left case but this space is less likely to be subject to trauma, including spondylolysis with spondylolisthesis, lateral stenosis, or lateral disc rupture. Therefore, both the bad and good news of the IC line location, from a paralateral approach point of view, is that this anatomic contributor to the location of pathologic change also provides for an easier approach to its surgical solution. *Source:* © Charles D Ray Ltd, 1985.

far lateral aspect. Location and extent of the exposure should be well planned in advance.

Paralateral exposures usually require small incisions, a few centimeters long. The dissections to the target are largely simple digital divisions of muscle fibers with gentle retraction. However, in the depths of this small wound, dissection at the target can be technically difficult. Procedures at L5–S1 vertebral level and especially those with spondylolisthesis are particularly challenging at first because of the relative strangeness of the lateral anatomy, the limited exposure, and the deep dissection. With experience, however, the procedure becomes more ''logical'' and the exposure to lateral anatomy is a very rewarding experience to the operator and the assisting team.

The surgeon might well spend time in the anatomical laboratory prior to beginning this approach in order to adequately expose the course of the L5 nerve as it descends into the presacral space, or to expose and decompress lumbar roots as they wind around the medial aspect of the pedicle at the upper aspect of the foramen. The high-resolution CT scans must be at hand during the surgical procedure and will be a constant reference source. One must practice three-dimensional mental image reconstruction as one extrapolates from the scans to the patient.

The operating microscope is used with a 250 mm working distance objective, 6 to 10 power magnification, and wide-angle 12.5 power eyepieces. Ordinary bone-cutting instruments must be quite sharp and longer and smaller than those

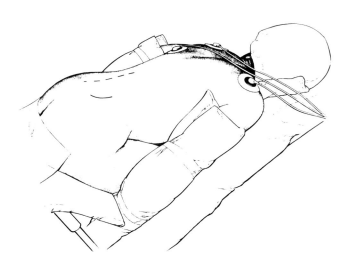

Figure 24–2 Positioning of patient on a modified kneeling seat frame. The axial line of lumbar spines is marked with a dashed line. The location of an L4–5 paralateral incision is shown as a short, solid line. Incisions for an L5–S1 approach have a medial curve ("hockey stick") extension at the inferior end, following along the iliac crest. Very muscular patients are perhaps easier to approach paralaterally if placed on a standard laminectomy frame. This is related to the tightening of paraspinous muscle as the patient's thighs and lumbar spine are flexed. *Source:* © Charles D Ray Ltd, 1985.

ordinarily used in midline decompressions. The amount of tissue resection required is generally only enough to facilitate visualization of the deep target. The only bone and ligament removed is appropriate to the decompression. With the exception of sometimes cutting out a segment of the iliac crest for visualization, no bone of significance is usually removed until the lesion itself is reached. This is distinctly different from the midline approach to a laterally placed lesion, where the majority of bone removal is for visualization of both the lesion and the involved nerve structures. The bone is important in the maintenance of stability.

It is essential to identify the correct level at decompression; this is much more difficult than with midline approaches. Since the incision and surgical exposure are quite small and the dissection is often deep, it is easy to become lost and disoriented near the target area. Although it is clearly preferable to mark both the skin and the underlying inferior edge of the transverse process at the vertebral level to be decompressed, useful marking is seldom achieved. Of the substances used for injection-marking, a relatively good one is Lymphazurin® (1% isosulfan blue dye for lymphography, Hirsch Industries, Inc., Richmond, VA 23219). About 0.7 mL are injected deeply and 0.1 mL into the immediately overlying skin.

The dye must be injected not more than a few hours before surgery or it may disappear from the depth, although it will still be present in the skin. Unfortunately, any injected marker is not easily found in the deep tissues since one must be right upon it in order to see it and in the region of paraspinal structures, every available surface is covered with muscle. It is nonetheless quite useful to have the skin marked directly dorsal either to the tip of the transverse process or the spinous process at the level to be approached. The plain films and digital exploration are used for further orientation.

Wiltse et al have reported the use of a small wire drilled into the transverse process and cut off flush with the skin.[18] A Kopans spring hook localizer (as used to mark breast lesions), inserted under fluoroscopic control, has been tried, but such markers are both tedious to use and to find in the depths. When arriving at the target level, the wire should be easily located and then pulled out. None of the above marking techniques is very reliable. On the other hand, with experience and a good set of plain spine films on hand, the structures (especially the transverse processes at the L5–S1 and L4–L5 levels) can usually be identified by the exploring finger prior to inserting the retractor. If all else fails, the location must be checked with a lateral x-ray film at the operating table.

SURGICAL TECHNIQUE

Most patients are positioned on the operating table in a modified knee-chest (tuck) or seated position (Figure 24–2). For very muscular patients, however, this 90 degree thigh flexion may so tighten the posterior paraspinous muscles as to make lateral wound retraction difficult. In such cases, placing the patient on a standard laminectomy frame may be preferred. Many patients are operated upon under local anesthesia. This technique, as stressed by the late R. Eustace Semmes, requires a gentler handling of the nerve tissues, allows the patient to help in localizing the symptomatic level or lesion, and promotes more rapid recovery (patients eat, have normal bowel and bladder function, and are ready to go home at least one or two days earlier than those having equivalent procedures under general anesthesia).[14] The surgeon must, however, be quite familiar with the use of local anesthesia or it will probably fail.

A surgical assistant is usually not needed. The surgical microscope is usually preferred but it is relatively inflexible. A fiber-optic headlight, together with optical magnification, allows for a quicker surgical procedure. If the microscope is indeed used, one may find it preferrable to elevate the table rather high and to stand, rather than to operate while seated.

An incision of approximately 5 or 6 cm in length is made just at the gentle folding edge of the paraspinous muscle mass (sacrospinalis group), about 10 to 12 cm lateral to and parallel with the lumbar midline. The incision is centered just inferior to the skin marking. Since fat grafts are important in prevention of postoperative fibrosis around nerve and dura,[2] a small fat graft of about 10 to 20 ml volume is obtained when cutting through the subcutaneous tissues. Just below the fat layers, the lumbodorsal fascia is cleared of tissue with a sharp, rounded elevator and then cut along the lateral fold with the cautery cutting tip. Two fingers are inserted to palpate straight medially, dissecting beneath the spinal erector muscle mass, to the tip of the transverse processes. Gentle division of muscle and fascia suffices.

At the L4–L5 or L5–S1 levels, the inferior half of the incision curves medialward to follow the iliac crest ("hockey stick" incision). Muscles are detached from the iliac crest leaving some fascia attached to facilitate reapproximation at the time of closure.

As the vertebral body is approached, one must first find the dye marker or otherwise identify the lateral bony anatomy. A medium Cobb elevator clears muscles from over (posterior to) the transverse processes and the facet capsule and the long, flat blade of a standard (or preferably two-tooth, modified) Taylor retractor[10] is carefully inserted above the lamina and hooked over the facet joint (Figure 24–3). The standard, one-toothed Taylor is somewhat unstable. A long loop of gauze passed over the opposite side to the operating table and hooked to a 1- or 2-kg weight holds the modified Taylor in place. A cerebellar retractor may be opened near the skin margins for improved visualization; one blade of it is placed beneath the Taylor. Large, flat blades of a Scoville retractor may also be inserted and opened (Figure 24–4). Stable exposure is essential. Ideally, only a small amount of muscle needs to be resected from around the deep bony structures if the retractor is wide enough and positioned well.

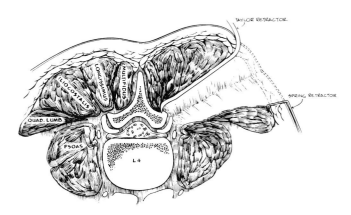

Figure 24–3 Cross-section through L4 just below the level of the pedicles (through the neural portion of the foramina). The paraspinous muscles have been retracted with a modified Taylor retractor, the distal handle of which is tied with a long gauze strip over the edge of the operating table to a 1 kg weight. A small hooked spring retractor pulled downward by an attached rubber band opens the lower wound for improved visualization. In some cases, a Scoville retractor with deep, straight blades may give better visualization. A weighted speculum does not work as well. By pulling further downward on the lower aspect of the exposed quadratus lumborum and other tissues, one may achieve a direct lateral exposure sufficient to visualize the more medial portion of the posterior disc annulus. Note that the distance to the lateral target via the paralateral approach is only slightly greater than via a midline approach. *Source:* © Charles D Ray Ltd, 1985.

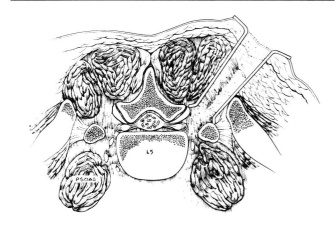

Figure 24–4 Cross-section through L5 just below the level of the pedicles (through the neural portion of the foramina). The paraspinous muscles have been retracted with a modified Scoville retractor. If a portion of the posterior iliac crest is resected (and portions of the sacral ala, if needed), the approach may be directed quite far laterally to follow the dashed line. *Source:* © Charles D Ray Ltd, 1985.

Figure 24–5 diagrams the usual anatomy encountered during the procedure. Figure 24–6 is a retouched photograph of a videotape still-frame on the paralateral approach; the view is almost identical to that shown in Figure 24–5.

At the L4 and higher levels, the surgeon follows along the inferior edge of the transverse process, with a small, sharp osteotome and a medium (Scoville) curette, and detaches the intertransverse ligament, muscle, and other fibers from the bone by scraping. Tiny arteries receive bipolar coagulation. The lateral aspect of the vertebral body between the transverse processes (guideposts for the procedure) adjacent to the target is quickly reached. Dissection and resection are continued along the junction of transverse process and vertebral body, then along the body itself, the facet capsule, and the superior edge of the next transverse process below.

Sometimes the most helpful structure that leads to the root is the neurovascular bundle of the posterior primary division. This cluster of small, sometimes tortuous arteries bleeds with conviction and is usually the only such structure in the neighborhood to do so (Figures 24–5, 24–6, 24–7, 24–9, and 24–11). The segmental artery arising from the aorta passes around the vertebral body, swings laterally, and a branch passes over the ganglion. It then participates in the medusa ("distribution point") neurovascular bundle of the posterior primary division and also serves as a primary arterial supply to the ganglion. This arterial branch and its subsequent branches

should be preserved, if at all possible. If the medusa is cut, the accompanying small arteries may be a nuisance. One millimeter arteries (and larger) do not occlude as well by bipolar coagulation as do smaller ones. These vessels should not be cauterized too closely to the ganglion, even with the bipolar coagulator, because the patient may develop a transient (perhaps permanent) dysesthesia from the burn.

A very small metal hemostatic clip (Ligaclip) may be used to occlude the artery without causing much artifact on subsequent CT scans. In Figure 24–6, the location (at the letter M) indicates where the clip is placed on the medusa. An absorbable polymer ligature clip works well for this application and is radiotransparent (Absolok ligating clip, stock number AC 100, made of violet polydioxanone by Ethicon, Inc., Somerville, NJ). This latter clip requires a longer stalk of structures to be clipped, however, than does a Ligaclip. The use of bipolar coagulation is essential.

Paralateral dissections are tedious but not difficult. In general, as the more medial aspect of a pedicle or facet is approached considerable caution must be exercised not to injure the tightly adjacent root sleeve or dura. Parts of the lamina or superior facet making up the posterior roof of the

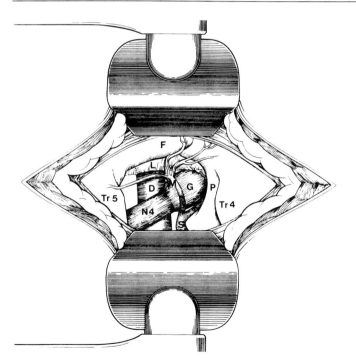

Figure 24–5 Paralateral approach at the right L4–5 level (or higher). Normal anatomy at the target is diagrammed. Indicated are: (D) disc margin, (F) superior facet of L5, (G) ganglion L4, (L) lateral reflection of the ligamentum flavum most prominent in the ligamentous (inferior) portion of the neural foramen, (M) medusa-like neurovascular posterior primary bundle showing muscular and articular (facet) branches, (N4) L4 nerve, (P) pedicle of L4, (S) segmental artery, (Tr4) transverse process of L4, and (Tr5) transverse process of L5. Blades of the Scoville retractor are shown. *Source:* © Charles D Ray Ltd, 1985.

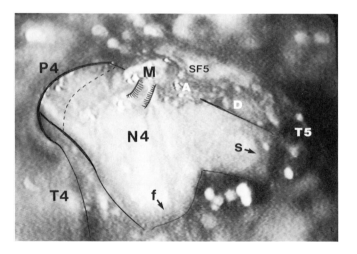

Figure 24–6 Retouched still-frame from a videotape made by the author illustrating the paralateral technique for decompression of lateral stenosis, left L4 segment. The up-down stenosis was present between the left L4 pedicle and a disc bar arising at L4–5 (plus a lateral bulging of the annulus). CT scans of an identical, but right-sided, case are shown in Figure 24–7. Shown here are: (N4) left L4 ganglion, (M) posterior primary neurovascular stalk or medusa, (P4) partially resected inferior L4 pedicle (original margin of pedicle contributing to the stenosis indicated by the dashed line across the root), (T4) partially resected inferior aspect of the left L4 transverse process, (A) small mass of Avitene hemostatic agent, (D) lateral margin of the disc where the portion lying ventral to these nerve structures has been driven inward by impaction to complete the decompression, (SF5) superior facet of L5, (T5) superior margin of the transverse process of left L5, (f and s) descending L4 nerve contributions to the femoral and sciatic. *Source:* © Charles D Ray Ltd, 1985.

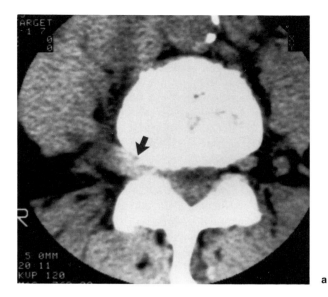

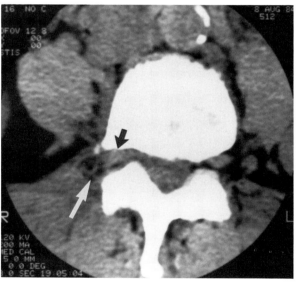

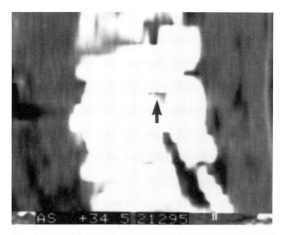

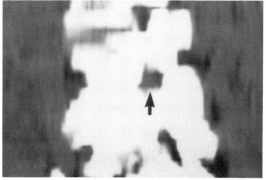

Figure 24–7 Up-down stenosis on the right of the L4–5 level. An identical, but left-sided, case is shown in the video still-frame illustration, Figure 24–6. (a) The L4 nerve is entrapped and displaced laterally by a combination of a disc bar and annulus at the L4–5 disc margins, compressing the ganglion cephalad against the inferior margin of the L4 pedicle. The fact that this is indeed an up-down stenosis is not clear in this transaxial image. This was the preoperative condition. (b) Parasagittal reconstruction showing the up-down stenosis. (c) Postoperative scan showing the decompression (black arrow) and a small fat graft (white arrow). The direction of the approach is also indicated by the white arrow. (d) Parasagittal image showing the excellent decompression achieved. *Source:* © Charles D Ray Ltd, 1985.

Figure 24–8 Preoperative scan showing a large, far laterally herniated disc on the right at the L3–4 level. This paralateral case was performed under local anesthesia with the patient observing the procedure in a video monitor screen. No bone, portion of the facet joint, or posterior ligamentous structure was removed. The incision measured 28 mm in length. Patient was discharged, symptom free, on the third postoperative day. *Source:* © Charles D Ray Ltd, 1985.

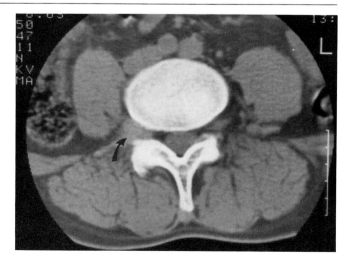

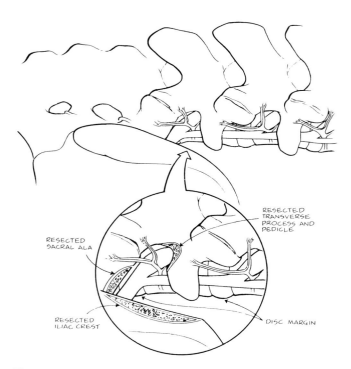

Figure 24–9 Paralateral approach to the right L5 nerve and L5–S1 structures. Portions of the L5 transverse process, inferior pedicle, sacral ala, and iliac crest have been resected to provide adequate exposure. At each level, the segmental artery, arising from the aorta or iliac artery, divides just anterior to the ganglion. One branch passes medialward below the pedicle. Another branch crosses laterally over the ganglion to join in with the emerging posterior primary nerve complex to form a medusa-like neurovascular bundle (see text). *Source:* © Charles D Ray Ltd, 1985.

40 minutes. None of the facet, or other structures, was disturbed. This technique has proved to be far superior to a midline approach for these lesions.[4]

The fact that the anatomy of the lumbosacral segment is quite different from higher lumbar segments is well appreciated. From the paralateral aspect, the L5–S1 segment dictates special considerations (Figure 24–9). For example, in order to achieve good decompression throughout the foraminal canal, it is often necessary to resect part of the inferior aspect of the L5 pedicle or its transverse process, superior portions of the sacral ala, and sometimes a segment of the iliac crest.

One must "pick up" the nerve near the foramen and follow it laterally as it curves toward the retropelvic space. Many lesions are located quite far from (ventral to) the foramen and one must remove a significant notch of bone from the medial sacral ala. Exact plans must be made in advance and the scan details followed closely if an adequate decompression is to be achieved.

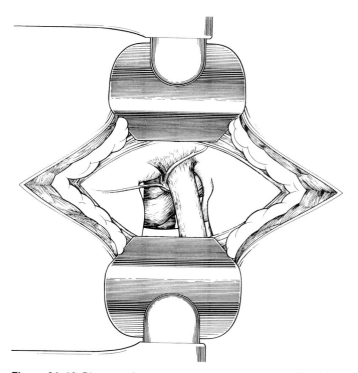

Figure 24–10 Diagram of a case during decompression at the right L5–S1 level showing a well-developed iliolumbar ligament (see also Figure 24–11). In this situation, the root and ganglion are trapped between a lateral disc bar or spur and the rather hypertrophic ligament. Several well-formed varieties of this and the various iliotransverse ligaments are commonly seen at the L5–S1 space. They may also be found at the L4–5 level if the intercristal line is quite high (see Figure 24–1). Note the inferior displacement of the posterior primary neurovascular medusa bundle around the ligament. Since the root and ganglion may swell somewhat after the decompression, a wider margin of the disc bar may be taken and parts of it may be compressed medialward with special, flat impactors or "drift" punches. *Source:* © Charles D Ray Ltd, 1985.

foramen, or discal osteophytes anterior to the root, may be removed with small osteotomes, as small as 3 mm wide. Sometimes, it is best to hollow out portions of the bony structures with an air turbine and then with long-handled, miniature curettes to collapse the remaining shell of cortical bone away from the neural tissues. One must be careful not to cause a thermal injury to the root by the high-speed burr as it thins the hard cortical bone of the medial pedicle. In general, all instruments must be long since the target is often 15 cm or more deep to the skin incision.

Figure 24–7 shows the pre- and postoperative CT scan images of a case having a decompression for up-down stenosis at the L4–5 level. The adequacy of the decompression, yet complete preservation of the dorsal supporting structures, is well demonstrated. This patient has had a complete remission of his lateral entrapment syndrome.

In Figure 24–8 one sees a typical, far laterally herniated disc, causing marked debilitation and pain. This proved to be a large free fragment lying ventromedial to and elevating the L3 ganglion and nerve. The paralateral decompression was performed under local anesthesia with a procedure time of

An iliolumbar (iliotransverse or lumbosacral) ligament or complex of ligaments is normally found at L5–S1, postero-laterally overlying the ganglion or nerve. Often the lum-bosacral ligament has a remarkable resemblance to the nerve itself although it crosses the nerve in a more transverse direc-tion as it courses from the inferior rim of the transverse process or pars interarticularis and facet capsule on its way to the iliac crest (Figures 24–10, 24–11). The ligaments are simply cut and their attachments curetted away. This may be done using the cautery knife, being careful not to bring heat too close to the nerve. A patient who is awake will report when the surgeon is getting close to the irritable nerve or ganglion at the correct level.

The bony decompression begins by resecting along the inferior aspect of the L5 pedicle. On reaching the ganglion, the anatomy will become clearer. The inferior pedicle may be burred away, undercut with the burr and collapsed away, or cut with a small osteotome.

After resection, the remnants of the pedicle can be impacted away from the ganglion using special drift punches.[8] This leaves a smooth surface presented to the nerve. Once the nerve is free cephalad, it can be retracted in that direction in order to reach and deal with the disc bar or spur that is so often found caudad and medial to the ganglion. Usually the surgeon pre-fers to impact the bar or spur rather than to burr it away since the latter technique leaves a ragged margin having loose rem-nants of annulus.

Loose portions of the annulus may best be resected using the cautery knife, placed, of course, at a safe distance away from the nerve structure. With some very prominent osteophytes, a small sharp osteotome may be used to cut a triangular wedge in the apparent sides of the osteophyte's attachment to the ver-tebral body, beneath (medial to) the root and ganglion. This compressive piece is then dissected free. More frequently, however, it is better to impact the offending, cut osteophyte into the underlying bone using the drift punches. See Fig-ures 24–9, 24–12, and 24–13.

Far lateral discs at any level may be slightly more difficult to remove than central ones since the nerve is often swollen and tightly adherent to the disc material. However, once having freed the ganglion or nerve from the adherent disc material, it is easier to empty out the disc space of remaining degenerated material. This is so because one can reach further across the oval-shaped disc space through a hole placed in the long-axis hole (laterally placed) of the space than one can through the short-axis (posterior) hole. Laterally extruded fragments, however, may sometimes virtually pop out of the lateral inter-muscular septae. The majority of laterally herniated discs occur at L3–4; next more frequently they are found at L4–5.[4]

Where there is an overgrowth of a lateral fusion causing stenosis,[2,12] the new bone is trimmed away appropriate to the decompression. Rather than locating the nerve first in the upperpart of the foramen, as with the usual stenotic case, the nerve may have to be located as it passes beneath the trans-

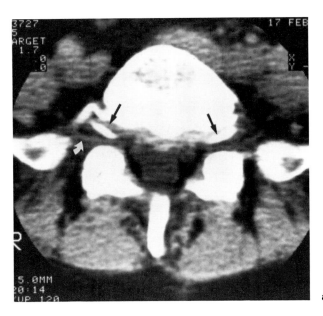

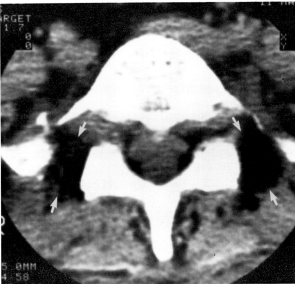

Figure 24–11 CT scans of a patient having bilateral disc spurs, lateral stenosis, and entrapment of emerging roots (L5) beneath tight iliolum-ber ligaments (see Figure 24–10). (a) Preoperative scan at L5 showing bilateral stenosis and spurs (black arrows). The iliolumbar ligament is best seen on the right (white arrow). (b) Postoperative scan, same level, showing wide bilateral paralateral decompression of spurs, re-section of medial portions of the sacral alae, and fat grafts (between white arrows) placed over the decompressed L5 nerves. *Source:* © Charles D Ray Ltd, 1985.

verse process or ala. The nerve is then followed cephalad and medialward as the offending, overlying, new fusion bone is removed (see Figures 24–14 and 24–15). Again, details shown on the CT scan films must be followed closely as the de-compression progresses.

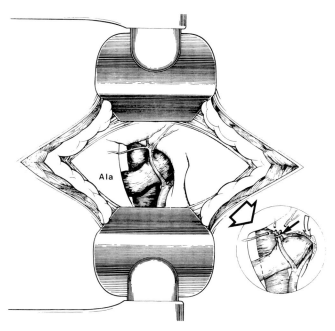

Figure 24–12 Diagram of case for a paralateral approach, right L5–S1 level (also see Figure 24–13). A spondylolisthesis with lateral hypertrophy of the L5 pedicle and the S1 superior facet, along with collapse of the L5–S1 disc space, is present. The ganglion has been compressed from above, downward between the pedicle of L5 and the superior disc rim of S1. The nerve is displaced laterally over the lateral disc bar. The insert shows the narrowed proximal L5 root after the pedicle and part of the transverse process have been resected (open arrow). The ganglion has rounded up after having been released from compression. The distal root is no longer displaced laterally by the disc bar (dashed line). A small hemostatic metal clip has been used to occlude the cut neurovascular medusa bundle (arrow). Smaller distal neurovascular bundles have been coagulated. The sacral ala was partly resected but this is not shown in the diagram (see also Figure 24–9). *Source:* © Charles D Ray Ltd, 1985.

It is essential that each entrapped root, ganglion, or nerve be very well decompressed and a good layer (5 mm or so) of fat placed around it, even if this requires removal or impaction of some apparently uninvolved adjacent bone. Thus, at the conclusion of the decompression, portions of the fat graft are placed around the root, ganglion, or nerve to separate it from bone, scar tissue, and injured muscle.[2] When a free fat graft is used, as many intact fat globules as possible should be utilized since cut ones will soon atrophy.

Before closure of the wound, an epidural microcatheter for postoperative administration of morphine is placed in the epidural space through a stiff, plastic feeding tube, extending cephalad for 10 to 15 cm. The free external end of the microcatheter is then brought out the nearby flank through a standard 18-gauge epidural needle. A Milipore injection filter is attached to the end of the catheter and 4.0 mg of morphine sulfate in 4.0 ml solution without preservative is given.[11]

Sutures reapproximate the fascia but not muscle. A running subcuticular skin closure is used with an absorbable suture.

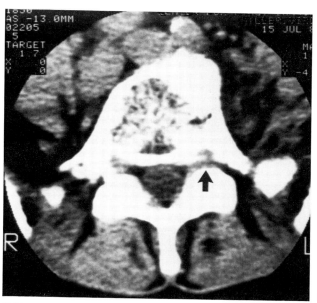
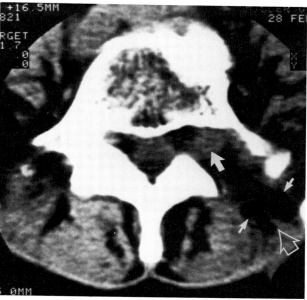

Figure 24–13 CT scans showing marked unilateral stenosis and L5 root compression (also see Figure 24–12). (a) Preoperative scan through the L5–S1 space showing the area of maximum stenosis, entrapping the ganglion. (b) Postoperative scan, fifth day. Resections of superior facet of S1, a part of the inferior facet of L5, and portions of L5 transverse process and inferior pedicle via paralateral approach. Not seen in these scans are the portions of the sacral alae and posterior iliac crests resected during the approach. The free L5 nerves (large arrow), fat graft (between the small arrows), and direction of the approach (large, open arrow) are shown. The superior facet of S1 was largely preserved caudad to this CT level. *Source:* © Charles D Ray Ltd, 1985.

Closed drainage is generally used for 48 hours to manage any delayed oozing of blood that may occur from the fat donor area, cut muscle bundles, or bone surfaces.

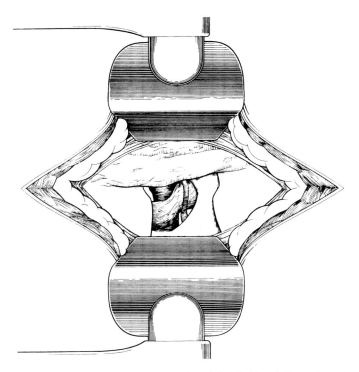

Figure 24–14 Paralateral approach at right L3–4 level. Present are: a laterally bulging disc, a collapsed space with a tight root-pedicle relationship, and an overgrowth of a lateral fusion contributing to a lateral stenosis. Bony portions to be resected are: transverse process and pedicle, disc bar, and lateral fusion mass. The paralateral approach here permitted retaining the fusion and other posterior and lateral structures. At closure, bone margins and neural structures were separated from each other by portions of the fat graft (also see Figure 24–15). *Source:* © Charles D Ray Ltd, 1985.

POSTOPERATIVE CONSIDERATIONS

As mentioned above, patients generally recover rapidly and ambulate within a few hours after the procedure. There should be little wound pain. Most patients are sent for warm-pool therapeutic aquatic exercises on the second or third postoperative day. Morphine (2 mg) without preservative is administered daily for two to three days, as needed, via the epidural catheter.[11]

If disproportionate discomfort is seen in the early postoperative period, a course of Decadron in a substantial (4 mg q.i.d.) descending dose over a period of seven to ten days can be helpful. In spite of the usually rapid immediate recovery, some patients have a rather slow long-term recovery. Repeat CT scan has often shown some persistence of nerve swelling in these cases. It should be remembered that, regardless of the surgical approach used, patients with preoperative loss of sensation or some true motor weakness do not recover normal function as well or as quickly after decompressions. Patients having such loss are warned that the postoperative recovery may well extend into several months.

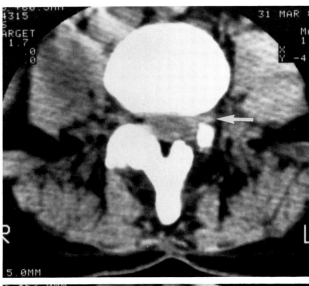
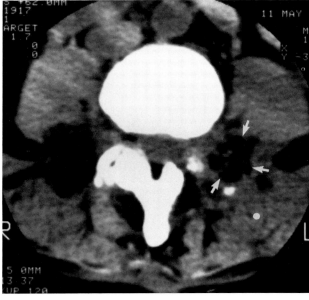

Figure 24–15 CT scans in a case of two-level paralateral decompression. Only one level is shown (also see Figure 24–14). (a) Preoperative scan at L3, the level immediately above an L4–S1 posterolateral fusion. A lateral stenosis (arrow) is seen beneath the remaining portion of the inferior facet and pedicle of L3. (b) Fourth-day postoperative scan, same level. The stenosis has been resected. A fat graft (between white arrows) has been placed to cover the exposed neural tissues. Some swelling within the muscle along the approach path is present (around the white dot). *Source:* © Charles D Ray Ltd, 1985.

FURTHER COMMENT ON CT SCANNING

In Figures 24–7, 24–8, 24–11, 24–13, 24–15, transaxial and parasagittal reformatted CT scan images are shown for a few typical cases. CT reformatted images are often indispensable in establishing a clear anatomical diagnosis and localization of stenosis. Such reconstructions can be performed only on parallel scans that have been made contiguously. That is, interrupting the continuity of adjacent scans and tilting the CT scanner gantry unit in order to parallel each disc space prohibits the use of recent computer software necessary for off-axis or parasagittal reconstructions. Further, there is rarely anything of radiologic interest inside the disc space; therefore, it is virtually senseless to make slices paralleling the disc end plates at the expense of slices that aid in the study of stenosis.[1,3,5,7]

SUMMARY

The paralateral approach in selected cases of lumbar nerve, ganglion, or root compression from lateral stenosis, spondylo-

listhesis with lateral entrapment, and laterally ruptured discs or disc spurs is a new surgical concept. Although similar in certain technical aspects to lateral approaches for lumbar intertransverse process fusions, the intent of the approaches and surgical procedures used differs considerably. The paralateral approach, while perhaps more difficult technically than equivalent midline approaches, is anatomically more appropriate. Decompression without destabilization can be achieved in selected cases.

The approach takes its appropriate place among other techniques used by lumbar spine surgeons only when accurate anatomic diagnoses have been made through the use of good, high-resolution CT scans that are correctly interpreted in light of the clinical findings.

REFERENCES

1. Burton CV, Heithoff KB, Kirkaldy-Willis W, Ray CD: Computed tomographic scanning and the lumbar spine. Part II: Clinical considerations. *Spine* 1979;4:356–363.

2. Burton CV, Kirkaldy-Willis WH, Yong-Hing K, Heithoff KB: Causes of failure of surgery on the lumbar spine. *Clin Orthop* 1981;157:191–199.

3. Glenn WV, Rhodes ML, Altschuler EM, Wiltse LL, Kostanek C, Kuo YM: Multiplanar display computerized body tomography applications in the lumbar spine. *Spine* 1979;4:282–352.

4. Godersky JC, Erickson DL, Seljeskog EL: Extreme lateral disc herniation: Diagnosis by computed tomographic scanning. *Neurosurgery* 1984; 14:549–552.

5. Heithoff KB, Ray CD: Principles of the computed tomographic assessment of lateral spinal stenosis, in Genant HK (ed): *Spine Update 1984*. University of California at San Francisco, 1984, Chap 19, pp 191–233.

6. Kirkaldy-Willis WH, Wedge JH, Yong-Hing K, Reilly J: Pathology and pathogenesis of lumbar spondylosis and stenosis. *Spine* 1978;3: 319–328.

7. Lifson A, Heithoff KB, Burton CV, Ray CD: High-resolution computed tomography scan of lumbosacral spine, in *Contrast Media in Computed Tomography. Excerpta Medica*. International Congress Series 561:183–187.

8. Ray CD: New techniques for decompression of lumbar spinal stenosis. *Neurosurgery* 1982;10:587–592.

9. Ray CD: The paralateral approach to lumbar decompressions. Poster session, abstract 21–W, *Proceedings of annual meeting American Association of Neurological Surgeons*, Washington DC, 1983, p 191.

10. Ray CD: Two new retractors for lumbar spinal surgery: Technical note, 1985, unpublished.

11. Ray CD, Bagley R: Indwelling epidural morphine for control of post lumbar surgery pain. *Neurosurgery* 1983;13:388–393.

12. Ray CD, Heithoff KB: Techniques for decompression of lumbar spinal stenosis "guided" by high-resolution CT scans. *Mod Neurosurg* 1982;1: 31–36.

13. Ray CD, Heithoff KB, Stauffer A: Lumbar lateral spinal stenosis: Classification and etiology, 1985, unpublished.

14. Semmes RE: *Ruptures of the Lumbar Intervertebral Disc: Their Mechanism, Diagnosis and Treatment*. Springfield, Ill, Charles C Thomas Publisher, 1964.

15. Watkins MB: Posterolateral fusion of the lumbar and lumbosacral spine. *J Bone Joint Surg* 1953;35A:1014–1018.

16. Watkins MB: Posterolateral fusion of pseudarthrosis and posterior element defects of the lumbosacral spine. *Clin Orthop* 1964;35:80–85.

17. Watkins RG: Bilateral paraspinous lumbosacral approach, in *Surgical Approaches to the Spine*. New York, Springer-Verlag, Chap 28, pp 176–182.

18. Wiltse LL, Bateman JG, Hutchinson RH, Nelson WE: The paraspinal sacrospinalis-splitting approach to the lumbar spine. *J Bone Joint Surg* 1968;50A:919–926.

Chapter 25

Disc Herniation in Children

Joseph F. Hahn, M.D.

Disc problems in children are not common. There is no large series in the literature. The incidence of disc disease in children less than 18 is between 0.9 and 3.2 percent.

In June 1981, the Cleveland Clinic Foundation reviewed a series of children presenting with a chief complaint of back pain.[7] Although it was thought to be an infrequent complaint, approximately 350 children presented with this complaint during a four-year period. These cases were further broken down into those requiring follow-up or those requiring only one visit. The patients needing follow-up were selected out because of continuing complaints. There were 165 patients in the latter category, or 47 percent.

This follow-up group was further subdivided to those with nonsurgical lesions and those with surgical lesions. Nonsurgical lesions included spondylolisthesis, Scheuermann's disease, scoliosis, fractures, and disc space infections. Surgical lesions included herniated discs, fusions for trauma, diastematomyelia, and tumors. The number of patients with disc problems in this group requiring surgery was eight, or approximately 2.2 percent, which correlated very closely with those reports already in the literature of disc disease in youngsters.

Of interest in this series is the finding that the most common presenting complaint requiring follow-up in the form of therapy is spondylolisthesis. This was true approximately 25 percent of the time. Spina bifida occulta was noted in 32 patients or 9.1 percent of the time. This again falls within the expected range. Youngsters in our series with spondylolisthesis presented most often with the L5–S1 level affected. There was nothing unique about their presentation, and they presented with back and leg pain that was unilateral or bilateral. Scheuer-

mann's disease again presents in the young adolescent age group but can be distinguished by changes on x-ray involving the narrowing of the disc space, irregularity of the vertebral body end plates, and wedging on the vertebral bodies themselves. Disc space infection was found in only two patients (0.5%) in this age group.

Most children who are seen for disc disease at the Cleveland Clinic present to the Sports Medicine clinic and are seen immediately. Most children with disc protrusions do not complain of back pain but of mechanical tension signs. They relate problems such as an inability to touch their toes or to flex or bend the spine. Because of the presentation without back pain, these patients are often diagnosed as having chronic strains of their hamstrings or quadriceps. They are tried on various forms of therapy prior to eventually being treated for their disc problem. In evaluating the patients seen in Sports Medicine, it is the consensus that most of these individuals respond to conservative therapy (well over 50 percent).

An earlier paper from the Cleveland Clinic reported a series of disc protrusions in the young.[10] The research was done in 1972 and included young adults. Of the series of 69 patients, 43 were less than 19 years of age. In reviewing the ten years since this report, that is, to 1982, there were 10 additional cases in the age group less than 19 years of age. In the original paper, as well as the next 11 cases, the average duration of symptoms was unchanged. It was not uncommon to see children who had had problems for 8–10 months before attention was turned to the disc as a causative factor. The majority of children had symptoms for anywhere from 4–14 months. Trauma did not appear to be a causative factor unless one considers athletic activity as a form of trauma. More often than not, no initiating cause could be determined and the children reported a gradual onset of difficulty.

The presentation of children with disc problems has been well worked out. Two typical cases will be described.

Case 1

The patient was a 15-year-old male who presented for evaluation of pain in the back of the left knee. The pain was reportedly gradual in onset and had been present for seven months. There were no complaints of numbness, tingling, or paresthesias. The pain was increased by sitting, moving about, or walking. There was no complaint of back or hip pain. The patient had an arthrogram, which was negative; an ultrasound of the left knee, which was normal; a computed tomography (CT) scan of the back, which was felt to be equivocal; and a myelogram, which showed an L5 disc protrusion. He had mechanical signs and was unable to touch his toes. His physical examination showed remarkable back spasm on flexion and positive bilateral straight-leg raising. The back spasm was worse on the left than on the right. The remainder of his neurological examination was normal.

Figure 25–1 shows scoliosis of the spine. Figure 25–2 demonstrates the equivocal CT scan at L5 disc level. The myelogram showing the obvious disc protrusion is seen in Figure 25–3. The patient underwent a partial hemilaminectomy with removal of a large disc protrusion. At one year following surgery, he has resumed all activities and is presently on the varsity basketball team.

This case is not unusual for disc problems in young patients. The duration of symptoms, namely seven months, is usual. The lack of neurologic signs and preponderance of mechanical signs is quite common.

Case 2

The patient was a 13-year-old male who presented for evaluation of low back and left lower extremity pain. Approximately four months prior to this evaluation, he was lifting some heavy logs while chopping wood with his father. About two weeks following this, he developed left lower extremity pain and was put on conservative therapy including 16 days of bedrest. He did have some relief of the pain but stated that every time he tried to become active, the pain recurred. He described the pain as intermittent and sharp and that it was brought on by changes in position. His neurological examination was normal. He had a positive straight-leg raising test on the left at approximately 30°. In trying forward flexion he was unable to bend more than 10°. There was thought to be a mild weakness of his left psoas but this was possibly secondary to pain. A CT scan demonstrated a large protruded disc at the L5 interspace. Figure 25–4 illustrates the CT scan.

Once the diagnosis of disc protrusion is considered at the Cleveland Clinic, the patient has a lumbar CT scan. If the test

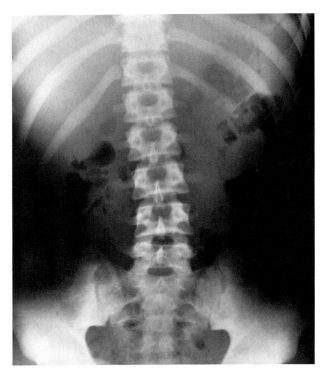

Figure 25–1 Plain x-ray of lumbar spine showing slight scoliosis (Case 1).

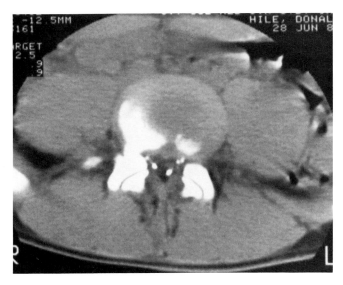

Figure 25–2 Lumbar CT scan at level of L5. Disc protrusion is not evident (Case 1).

is unequivocal, myelography is not done. If the CT scan is *not* revealing, the next step is myelography. At present a study with magnetic resonance scans is being performed to see if myelography can be circumvented. Discograms are no longer done.

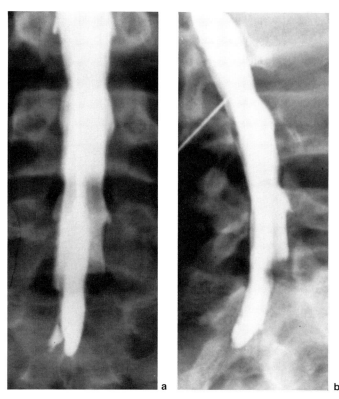

Figure 25–3 (a) A-P myelogram showing cut-off nerve root at L5–S1 (Case 1). (b) Oblique myelogram confirming disc protrusion (Case 1).

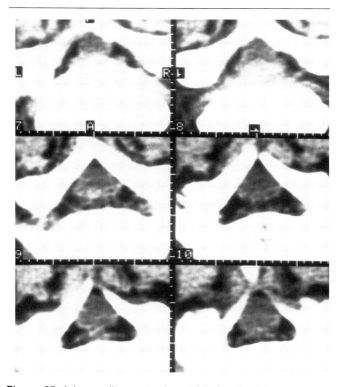

Figure 25–4 Large disc protrusion at L5 disc level best seen on sequence No 8 (Case 2).

SURGICAL TECHNIQUE

A standard operative approach in dealing with young children with disc disease is used. Although the spine may not be fully developed, a standard partial hemilaminectomy is done in each case. The amount of bone removed from the lamina is usually less than ½ cm in diameter. The ligamentum flavum is incised and removed with a Kerrison punch to expose the compressed nerve root so that it can be retracted medially. In young people, this is usually not difficult because there is virtually no facet hypertrophy. Every attempt is made to leave the facet intact and to not enter the facet joint itself.

A Kerrison punch can be used with an angled head to undercut the medial facet and gain access if the fragment has migrated up along the nerve root cephalad. The disc in young people is usually not normal. However, it does not appear to be more fibrocartilaginous because of its age. Children with all varieties of protrusion to frank herniation have been encountered. In those individuals where the disc is simply bulging, it again has been degenerative, even in young teenagers.

Once the disc is removed, the nerve root is covered with a free fat graft and the muscles, fascia, subcutaneous tissue, and skin are closed in the usual fashion.

Results indicate that surgery for disc disease in this age group is excellent. As was mentioned earlier, the individuals are carefully selected. No individual is operated on without positive radiologic findings. For this reason the clinic's success rate has been above 90 percent. Success has been measured in the return of individuals to normal as well as the return of individuals to all their premorbid activities. Well over 90 percent of the children are in this category. Although there has been a great deal of concern about future back problems for the patients, this has not been the case. There seems to be no incidence of back pain or recurrent disc problems in any of the children involved in the clinic's series.

A question has been raised about the feasibility of using intradiscal chemonucleolysis on children. This type of therapy has not been used in anyone below the age of 14 at the clinic. In reviewing the literature, no cases below the age of 20 have been encountered. Watts has suggested that at present, chymopapain should not be used in children.[11]

In order to get some idea of trends that exist in dealing with young patients with back problems, a review of several series was compiled.[1–12] Including the clinic's 53 patients, a total of 454 patients were reviewed. Several interesting trends were apparent from this review.

There did not appear to be any significant difference between the number of males versus females. There has been some thought in the past that perhaps disc problems are more common in young males because they were generally more active in sports. This has not been confirmed. In fact, it appears that there really is an equality between the sexes. There were several instances where the numbers did equal one another but, on the whole, there were more males than females. However, it was not statistically significant.

As was alluded to earlier, it was thought that trauma played an important role in the onset of disc problems in young people. In fact, the range was from a low of 6 percent in the paper by Kamel and Rosman[8] to 100 percent in the paper by Chotigavanich and Techakumpuch.[1] On the whole, however, the incidence of trauma related to sports or falls seems to be significant approximately 30–35 percent of the time.

The duration of symptoms ranged anywhere from two months to five years. It was not unusual for young patients to have complaints of back and leg pain for many months before the appropriate diagnosis was made. There are probably several reasons for this lack of appropriate diagnosis; namely, lack of familiarity with the problem, hesitancy to attribute back pain to a herniated disc in a young patient, and reluctance to do invasive studies on younger people. In the clinic's series, the patients were often referred for further evaluation once the diagnosis was made. It was not unusual for patients to have complaints for many months; the average time was in the range of eight months.

The difference between disc disease in youngsters versus disc disease in adults has been the subject of much discussion. In analyzing the series, the overwhelming complaint was back pain as well as leg pain. There were very few instances where back pain was the only complaint. In almost every case, it was a combination of back and leg pain or leg pain alone. In every series, this complaint was present over 90 percent of the time. In fact, if the patient's complaint is back pain alone, it is very unlikely to be due to a herniated disc.

The overwhelming finding was that of positive mechanical signs in young patients with herniated discs. Again, the findings of positive straight-leg raising tests, Laseague's maneuver, inability to touch the toes, or restriction of forward bending were present over 90 percent of the time. In fact, it was quite unusual to find a series that did not have these findings.

Neurologic signs, which include changes in sensation, muscle weakness, and/or changes in reflexes, were much less frequent. A positive neurological sign was found in the neighborhood of 50 percent. Not all children had changes in all three and it was not unusual to have a young patient with sensory changes only. However, it was quite striking that the mechanical signs were virtually always present, whereas neurologic signs were present less than half the time.

The surgeries that were undertaken on these children were of all forms. There was no one type of surgery that was done to make a clear-cut indication as to what is "best." However, the need for fusion did not appear to be borne out and, in fact, most of these young patients did not have fusions. The types of surgeries ranged from partial hemilaminectomies to total laminectomies. Some researchers concluded that it was important to do a total laminectomy in the younger patient because removal of the disc might be more important. However, others did not think this was the case.

Myelography was the radiographic test used most often. In this series the test had to be positive for inclusion of the patient in the study. At the Cleveland Clinic, discography was done in 43 patients, therefore, some had had myelography and some discography. In any event, to be included in the series of 454 patients, it was required that a positive radiographic test be completed.

In reviewing the literature and the clinic's series, it is apparent that young patients with disc problems have a high incidence of other anomalies. These range from spina bifida to block vertebrae to spondylolisthesis. The incidence is in the range of approximately 30 percent, which is certainly higher than the general population.

The results of surgery can be classified as excellent. In every series, excellent results were found to be greater than 90 percent, regardless of the type of the surgery undertaken and regardless if fusion was present or not. This correlates well with the results of disc surgery in adults. The incidence of recurrence in one series was thought to be in the range of 5–6 percent, which again correlates well with adults.

In reviewing the clinic's series, nothing was found that is out of the ordinary. Trauma was found to be an associated factor in approximately 40–50 percent of the cases. The overwhelming finding was positive straight-leg raising tests in all patients (53 patients) and an inability to forward flex in approximately 90 percent of the patients. Eighty-one percent of the patients had a gait disturbance and walked with a noticeable limp. In contrast, there was certainly less than 50 percent having neurologic findings. Eighteen percent had loss of reflexes and only 25 percent had a sensory loss. Approximately 20 percent had a weakness of an appropriately innervated muscle. Of those who had myelograms, all were positive. The surgery was certainly not unusual and at the present time minimal surgery is being performed as described previously. The results at the present time reveal that 96 percent of those who had been followed for more than two·years had an excellent result.

There are several points that stand out:

1. It is unusual for a patient below the age of 19 to complain of back pain.
2. If a young patient complains of leg pain and/or back pain and leg pain, a herniated disc should be high in the differential diagnosis.
3. Positive straight-leg raising test and an inability to flex the spine are present in an overwhelming number of patients, usually in the 90 percent range.
4. Absence of neurologic signs does not rule against a herniated disc in a young patient.
5. There is approximately a 30 percent incidence of bony abnormalities in youngsters with herniated discs.
6. The patients tolerate surgery extremely well and there is little need for fusion.

7. The results in long-term follow-up are excellent, in the neighborhood of 95 percent.

8. The recurrence rate appears to be no greater than for the adult population.

REFERENCES

1. Chotigavanich C, Techakumpuch S: Herniation of the lumbar disc in children and adolescents. *J Med Assoc Thai* 1983;66:367–375.

2. Clarke NMP, Cleak DK: Intervertebral lumbar disc prolapse in children and adolescents. *J Pediatr Orthop* 1983;3:202–206.

3. DeOrio JK, Bianco AJ: Lumbar disc excision in children and adolescents. *J Bone Joint Surg* 1982;64A:991–996.

4. Epstein JA, Epstein NE, Marc J, Rosenthal AD, Lavine LS: Lumbar intervertebral disc herniation in teenage children: Recognition and management of associated anomalies. *Spine* 1984;9:427–432.

5. Fisher RG, Saunders RL: Lumbar disc protrusion in children. *J Neurosurg* 1981;54:480–483.

6. Grobler LJ, Simmons EH, Barrington TW: Intervertebral disc herniation in the adolescent. *Spine* 1979;4:267–278.

7. Hahn JF, Mason L: Low back pain in children, in Hardy R (ed): *Lumbar Disc Disease.* New York, Raven Press, 1982, pp 217–228.

8. Kamel M, Rosman M: Disc protrusion in the growing child. *Clin Orthop* 1984;185:46–52.

9. Kurihara A, Kataoka O: Lumbar disc herniation in children and adolescents. *Spine* 1980;5:443–451.

10. Nelson CL, Janecki CJ, Gildenberg PL, Sava G: Disc protrusions in the young. *Clin Orthop* 1972;88:142–150.

11. Watts C: Use of chymopapain in children, editorial. *J Neurosurg* 1985;59:1108.

12. Zamani MH, MacEwen GD: Herniation of the lumbar disc in children and adolescents. *J Pediatr Orthop* 1982;2:528–533.

Chapter 26

Postlaminectomy Syndrome

John O'Brien, M.D.

The purpose of this chapter is to review the problem of persistent pain that follows posterior surgery of the lumbar spine performed for symptoms of back and leg pain. The most common causes of failed back surgery (loosely termed, postlaminectomy syndrome) are reviewed and the mechanism of persistent pain discussed in some depth. Finally, a surgical procedure, "the simultaneous combined anterior and posterior fusion" is outlined from experience over the past five years in more than 150 patients.[18]

THE PROBLEM

Failed back surgery is one of the most daunting challenges in all of clinical medicine.[16] After the laminectomy has been performed, and the pain recurs after three months or so, when no obvious cause can be found, the physician suspects a psychogenic component and refers the disabled patient to a psychiatrist. The sequence of events is all too common, as in the following example:

The patient has an accident at work and over the next few weeks there is gradual onset of back and leg pain. There is initial suspicion because the patient did not report the injury to the doctor at the work site (so-called delayed onset back pain).

The pains persist in spite of some conservative care, and investigations are performed: A myelogram is "suspicious," a computed tomography (CT) scan is "equivocal," and peripheral neurology is not really "specific." In spite of lack of hard evidence, a laminectomy is performed and it is negative (Figures 26–1 and 26–2).

This typical case history raises several points that are very important in the correct handling of patients with acute low back and leg pain.

1. Sciatica as a diagnosis
2. Pain referred to a limb
3. Discogenic pain
4. Delayed onset low back pain

Sciatica as a Diagnosis

Sciatica is defined as "neuralgic pain along the course of the sciatic nerve." It is dependent upon inflammation or injury to the nerve or its roots and is most commonly the result of a herniated disc of the lower lumbar or upper sacral spine.[8]

Many workers, however, have shown that pain in the leg may be referred from a localized lesion of the back or hips. Kellgren, in a classic paper titled "Sciatica," described how he could abolish the leg pain in the majority of sufferers by infiltration of the tender zones in the back with local anesthesia. Those not relieved by this simple technique had "true" sciatica, that is, compression of a nerve root.[12]

Pain Referred to a Limb

The phenomenon described as "pain referred to a limb" has been a source of confusion for centuries (see the above definition of sciatica). The simple fact is that any tissue deep within the motion segment, when injured or irritated, may produce pain referred to a limb.[17] (See Figure 26–3).

Figures 26–1 and 26–2 Discography demonstrating an abnormal disc.

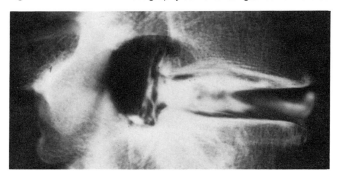

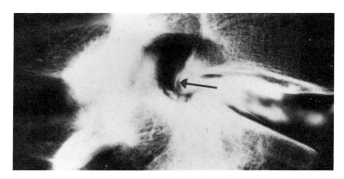

In flexion (top) the motion segment has a wide intervertebral foramen and flattening of the posterior annular fibers. In extension (bottom) the same motion segment shows marked narrowing of the intervertebral foramen. An annular bulge is now apparent in the intervertebral foramen and would account for a filling defect on myelography (arrow).

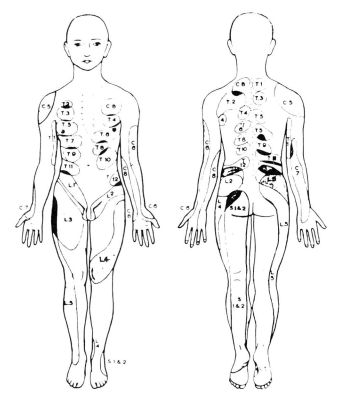

Figure 26–3 Homunculi to illustrate the patterns of deep pain produced by the injection of the corresponding interspinous ligaments. Note the large anterior component of the thoracic pain patterns and the extensive distal referral into the leg from the lower lumbar segments.

Of the deep tissues within the segment, the facet joints and the disc are the most likely pain sources. The disc is especially so because it has a rich sensory nerve supply in the outer half of the annulus fibrosus.[20] The best analogy to this referred pain is diaphragmatic irritation producing deep pain felt in the corresponding shoulder joint.

Discogenic Pain

The recent important discovery of nerve fibers in the outer part of the disc clarified the cause of pain referred to a limb in the presence of a negative myelogram, once a cause of misunderstanding and of a high incidence rate of negative laminectomy (Figure 26–4).

The painful disc can be accurately investigated only by the use of discography, in spite of strong and long-standing opposition to the study.[10]

Delayed Onset Back Pain

The phenomenon referred to as "delayed onset back pain" has not been a commonly recognized syndrome since the

thirties.[11] The name describes itself; the accident may be forgotten or obscured by associated injuries or fractures. The onset may be gradual over weeks or months and this has important medico-legal implications. It is vital that the sufferer not be abandoned as a malingerer because he or she did not see the factory doctor at the time of the lifting accident.

FAILED LAMINECTOMY

The period of pain relief enjoyed by the patient before recurrence of symptoms is felt to be important in understanding the mechanism of failure of the back operation.

In a referral center it is not uncommon to hear that the patient awoke from the anesthetic with severe leg pain, a sure indication of surgery at the wrong level or of significant trauma to the nerve root during exploration. The latter carries a guarded prognosis even with reconstructive surgery.

The common occurrence of pain three months after surgery is likely to be the result of the so-called "neurectomy effect." The adjacent tissues have been denervated by the exposure and are renervated with recurrence of symptoms about three

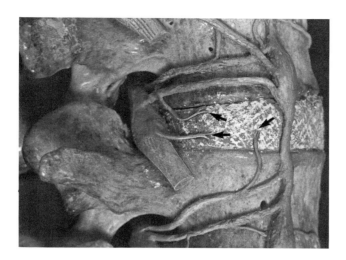

Figure 26–4 A model demonstrating the nerve supply of the lumbar intervertebral disc. The small nerve fibers (arrows) provide a rich sensory nerve supply for the outer half of the annulus fibrosus.

months later. This would also explain a discogenic pain source (as opposed to a nerve root compression/sciatica complex). In this situation again there has been enough denervation of the structures (plus enforced bed rest) to provide three months of relief from symptoms.

A third common presentation is recurrence twelve months to two years after surgery. The patient may return to work and with minimal lifting or bending, all of the symptoms recur. This may be related to an inherently unstable segment produced by the back surgery. Such a phenomenon should be regarded as an unsatisfactory result if the aim of surgery was to provide a pain-free stable spine for most if not all of the patient's life.

Late failures five years later after surgery do occur, their regularity depending on the detail of the follow-up. The world literature indicates that between 40 and 50 percent of laminectomy patients are disabled with pain of some severity, many actually unable to hold employment.[13]

THE SEQUELAE TO CONVENTIONAL DISC REMOVAL

There is no doubt that posterior lumbar disc removal is ideal and often successful when the indications for its use are correct. There exists only a minimal surgical trauma and no marked arthritic changes in the spine. This is particularly so in the younger patient with a large disc fragment compressing a nerve root. Conventional disc surgery in the teenage population, however, has not been altogether successful and in fact a follow-up of over 20 patients more than 10 years after surgery confirmed that almost half, by the time they had reached their late twenties, were significantly disabled and unable to be employed.[3]

DIAGNOSIS

The diagnosis of postlaminectomy syndrome is self-evident. Symptoms of back and leg pain have recurred after spinal surgery, which may have initially appeared successful. It is crucial that if the wrong level has been operated on, and this is a common problem, it should be corrected with revision surgery.

THE MECHANICS OF POSTLAMINECTOMY SYNDROME

There are many different causes of pain to account for failure of surgery performed for low back and leg pain.

Inadequate Preoperative Work-up

Inadequate preoperative workup is commonly seen, including the failure to provide the patient with sufficient conservative treatment before surgery. It is essential to identify the anatomical source of the pain before embarking on surgery. This is the reason "exploration" is to be discouraged.

The scientific basis of successful low back surgery rests totally on defining the anatomical source of pain. The wrong level of surgery is said to be one of the most common errors; failing to find a disc and exploring up and down the spine renders more segments unstable and increases the likelihood of postsurgery disability.

Incorrect Interpretation of Radiological Data

While CT scans provide sophisticated details of the disc and vertebrae it must be kept in mind that they do not point to the anatomical pain source and can, therefore, be misleading. This is particularly true when there is questionable clinical information and doubtful signs.

The same can be said for myelography. Shapiro[19] pointed out many years ago that there is a *one-third* incidence of false-positive myelograms in the general (nonback pain) population. Perhaps nuclear magnetic resonance (NMR) will shed further light on the subject, but similarly, it will not identify the elusive pain source.

Indications for Surgery in the Postlaminectomy Syndrome

The indication to reconstruct the spine after failed back surgery is made to a large extent on the degree of disability suffered by the patient. Back pain disability has been difficult to assess objectively and the development of a disability index scored by the patient has proved a very valuable method of assessment.[5]

It is obvious that if the patient is coping with day-to-day activities in spite of the pain, if the pain is controlled by moderate pain medication, there is not significant loss of mobility, and life is tolerable, then surgery should not be considered.

The Low Back Cripple

At the other end of the spectrum is the patient who has continual back pain with referred pain to the limb(s), who is virtually housebound and spending much of the day in bed, obviously unemployed, addicted to narcotics and alcohol, separated from his or her family, and potentially suicidal. It is this patient group, more common than previously recognized, that can benefit from reconstructive surgery: a simultaneous combined anterior and posterior fusion.

Simultaneous Combined Anterior and Posterior Fusion—Historical Perspectives

The anterior and posterior fusion for the postlaminectomy syndrome has been evolving for several years. It was John Cobb in 1952 who stated that "scoliosis is the most serious and it is the most difficult problem in orthopedics."

Experience in Hong Kong in the sixties demonstrated that the anterior correction of scoliosis by the late Alan Dwyer[4] and the distraction rod of Paul Harrington[9] when used separately were not adequate for the most difficult scoliosis after polio-

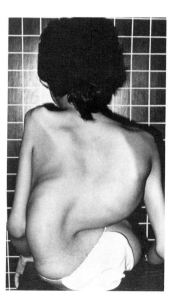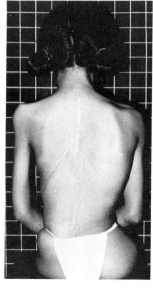

Figures 26–5a and 26–5b Photographs of the posterior view of a patient with severe paralytic scoliosis before and after surgery. The surgery performed was a combined staged anterior Dwyer and posterior Harrington rod. Note the dramatic correction of the scoliosis and pelvic obliquity with these techniques, which were developed in Hong Kong in the early seventies.

myelitis. Nevertheless, when used in combination they provided an effective, in fact dramatic, solution to a previously unsolved problem.[14]

Over the 1970s and 1980s, an effective method of combined anterior and posterior surgery for correction of the most severe spinal deformities (Figures 26–5a and 26–5b)[15] has been developed based on the Hong Kong experience. Failed back surgery, however, has remained an unsolved problem. A common attitude is that if symptoms recur or persist after laminectomy, then psychological counseling is called for.

It seemed rational in the early eighties that if combined anterior and posterior surgery could solve the most difficult paralytic scoliosis with pelvic obliquity, then perhaps it was worthy of a trial in the postlaminectomy syndrome group. This concept has a sound anatomical basis because the motion segment is a three-joint complex, namely two facet joints and the intervertebral disc. To guarantee blocking all movement within the segment, stiffening the whole complex is required, that is, arthrodesis of both front and back of the segment(s) involved.

THE SIMULTANEOUS COMBINED ANTERIOR AND POSTERIOR FUSION

Early Developments

For many years anterior fusion of the previous laminectomized levels was the treatment of choice (and for single-level lesions it is still practiced). The aim of the surgery was to rehabilitate the patient with maximum speed. However, if pseudarthroses was encountered (not uncommon when the corresponding neural arch is missing), the delay in rehabilitation was often significant.

The Combined-Staged Operation

The next step was to combine the fusions, staging them by an interval of two weeks. The only objections to this system is the added stay in the hospital, as well as the added metabolic disturbance resulting from two surgical procedures, two anesthetics, osteoporosis, and delay in rehabilitation.

THE SIMULTANEOUS COMBINED ANTERIOR AND POSTERIOR FUSION (SCAPF)

In the first group of patients posterior fusion was done first, then the patient was turned during the anesthetic and the interbody fusion was then performed.

The biggest objection to this approach was that the instrumentation of the posterior segments flattened the lumbar lordosis leading to secondary flattening of the thoracic kyphosis and subsequent spinal pain above the fusion.

By a series of tried and tested steps, the simultaneous combined anterior and posterior fusion has evolved. It is simple in its concept but does require studied techniques in both anterior and posterior surgery.

The principles of the simultaneous operation are as follows:

1. All movement in the affected segment(s) is blocked by the combined fusion thus eliminating friction of the nerve root emerging at that segment.
2. The disc(s) containing nerve fibers in the outer half of the annulus[20] is totally excised and replaced with bone graft with maximal distraction of the segment, thus correcting any height loss (and correcting any deformity). This also restores the lordosis of the lumbar spine and opens the reduced intervertebral foramina.
3. Nerve root decompression is achieved by distraction of the motion segment and correction of the deformity with opening of the lateral canals and the intervertebral foramina. The nerve roots are *not* directly decompressed.
4. Further immobilization of the posterior structures is obtained by rod instrumentation of the remaining neural arches and the use of a massive bilateral bone graft. The patients are often 3–4 cm taller after the procedure.

Preoperative Planning

Detailed studies before surgery should include discography (to define the anatomical pain source) as well as tomography. CT scans and other investigations have not been used routinely.

Planning the Extent of the Fusion

The surgeon is guided by the results of the discography and by the extent of the previous back surgery performed. The instrumentation used in all cases obviously needs to extend from one intact neural arch to another; usually this involves L4 and L5 segments.

THE SURGICAL PROCEDURE

The Anterior Lumbar Fusion

A left-sided extraperitoneal approach is used, which can be either the muscle cutting incision using diathermy or the more recent alternative approach to the lumbar spine described by Fraser.[6] A good deal of time has been spent on the research and development of special instruments to distract the disc space and to keep it distracted while all the soft tissue is removed.

The lumbosacral joint is approached usually between the bifurcation of the vessels, and the L4 segment is approached medial to the vessels. The presacral nerve is easily identified crossing the midline of the L5 disc and coursing from left to right across the disc. Damage to this nerve will produce retrograde ejaculation, but it should be emphasized that it is clearly seen and palpated and easily retracted with Steinman pins driven into the vertebral bodies. Care with the vessels and the viscera is implied if one is performing anterior spinal surgery.

It is common in this group of severely disabled patients to find a significant inflammatory response in the prevertebral tissues[16] and outer annular fibers. This inflammatory reaction can produce matting and adhesions tacking down the vessels onto the disc, which may be very friable and easy to tear. In this context the iliolumbar vein is very vulnerable because it is often anomalous; it may require ligation and division to approach the L4 segment and it may be thick, short, very thin-walled and easily avulsed, possibly producing a calamitous bleed. Handling of tissues, it must be stressed again, is of the utmost importance in this form of surgery and the techniques need to be taught and not be assumed.

The Instruments

The instruments, which have been designed by Middleton, are constantly being updated and provide easy and safe complete removal of the disc (Figures 26–6 and 26–7).*

1. The *vertebral spreader* is powerful and when the annulus has been subtotally removed, distraction with the spreader will restore the anatomical disc height. After the spreader has been used and the space increased, this space is then maintained by *spacers*, which are modifications of an early undescribed design by the late Homer Pheasant. They maintain the disc space widely open so that safe and careful dissection of all the soft tissue down to raw bleeding subchondral bone may be performed.
2. The *curettes* are of several types, including a long-handled sharp pear-shaped curette, which takes the complete end plate out. The recesses can be cleared of soft tissue with the beaked commonly available curettes or a long-handled variation of those designed by Middleton (Figure 26–7).

The Approach

One space is done at a time; traditionally the lowest space is done first. X-ray control to identify the level is usually unnecessary because the lumbosacral promontory is easily felt. Before surgery it is essential to decide whether the lowest segment is an easily accessible joint or whether it may be technically difficult. If it is deeply set and obliquely placed within the pelvis, it may present technical difficulties and in fact be hazardous. For this reason, it is sometimes advisable to perform a transperitoneal approach (though this is not commonly needed).

*These are available from J.K. Middleton "Surgical Instruments," 132 Gathurst Lane, Gathurst, Nr. Wigan, Lancashire, U.K.

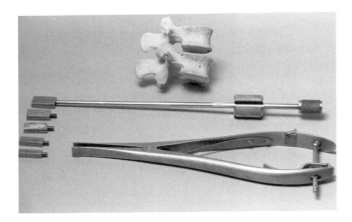

Figure 26–6 A powerful self-locking spreader together with a series of interbody spacers that maintain the height of the disc space so that careful and complete removal of the disc can be completed with safety. This design is a modification of a similar set of instruments shown to the author by the late Dr. Homer Pheasant. Instruments currently being developed, updated, and manufactured by J.K. Middleton.

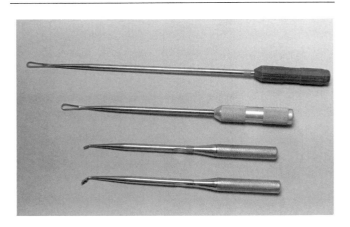

Figure 26–7 The curettes of the beak-nosed and pear-shaped variety permit complete and careful removal of all disc tissue and cartilagenous end plate. Instruments currently being developed, updated, and manufactured by J.K. Middleton.

The Bone Graft

Bone is removed from the patient's left iliac crest through a separate incision with preservation of the crest itself. A window technique, popularized by Freebody,[7] is employed because it has been found that removal of the crest is not only cosmetically disfiguring but can produce significant long-term physical impairments.

It is important to remove as much bone as possible but at the same time to avoid fracture to part of the hemipelvis. This practice can be disabling and in one patient required reconstruction with plate and screws, which all points to the one

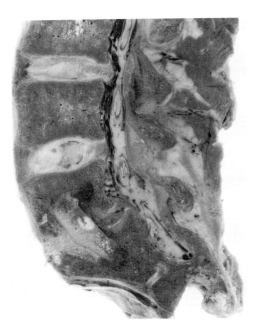

Figure 26–8 A sagittal section of the lumbar spine in which an anterior lumbosacral fusion was performed by the Freebody technique. The patient died 30 days after surgery with pulmonary embolism. The specimen is fascinating because it shows that disc tissue has been left in the posterior part of the lumbosacral disc space and it has actually invaded the posterior part of the graft, which is at right angles to the space itself.

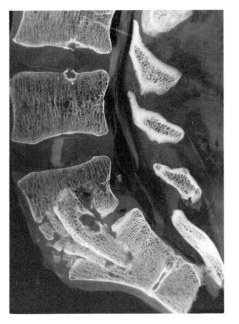

Figure 26–9 A lateral x-ray of the specimen. Compare closely with Figure 26–8. Note the erosion in the posterior part of the iliac crest graft due to invasion by the remnants of disc tissue in the posterior part of the space. This important specimen demonstrates that it is absolutely essential to clean the space entirely of disc tissue.

Figures 26–10, 26–11, and 26–12 A series of three photographs to demonstrate the basic technique involved with removal of the disc and the use of the special instruments designed for this purpose.

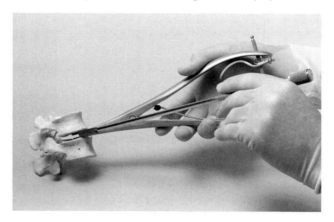

(a) The interbody space is spread widely and one of the spacers of appropriate height is put into the segment to keep the space open for radical dissection and removal of the disc.

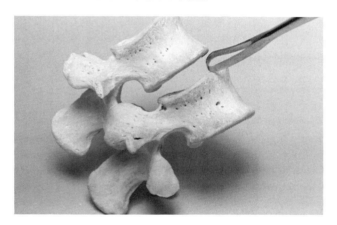

(b) The pear-shaped curette is shown cleaning the cartilagenous end plate.

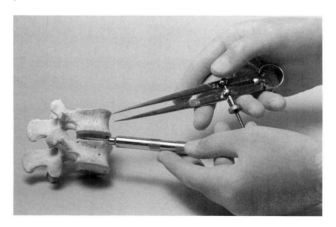

(c) Measurement of the height and depth of the cleaned disc space is important so that precisely shaped bone grafts can be cut to replace the removed disc.

recurring problem in this type of reconstructive surgery: obtaining enough good-quality bone, particularly when multiple levels need to be grafted from the front and back. The use of blocks of bone cut precisely according to the height and depth of the cleared disc space is the preferred method. One-third of the bone in the anterior grafting is usually prepared by the Cloward technique.[1] This ensures that adequate volume of bone is available to completely pack the disc space with maximal distraction. Complete removal of the disc, including end plates, is essential, leaving only part of the posterior annulus. Remnants of disc left in place are likely to produce an unacceptably high level of graft nonunion (Figures 26–8 and 26–9).

When the lowest level has been excised and grafted, the four Steinman pins are removed and dissection is then carried out to expose the L4 disc on the left side of the vessels. Care must be taken to ensure that the iliolumbar vein is not damaged during retraction of the iliac artery and vein to the right side.

Replacement of Disc with Bone (Figures 26–10, 26–11, and 26–12)

The same technical procedure is repeated exactly at this level. This level is usually easier because it is in direct line with the eye of the surgeon, rather than obliquely placed, as is the lumbosacral disc. It is important, if there is a significant component of leg pain, to be careful with dissection of the posterior annulus because the most common pathological finding with anterior lumbar fusion is a hole in the posterior annular fibers through which disc tissue is "squelched out" with time and compression during walking. It is, therefore, common to remove large fragments of disc tissue that are stuck through the annulur fibers into the spinal canal. It is usual to place at least three (and sometimes four) grafts side by side in each motion segment that has been fully distracted by the instruments demonstrated (Figures 26–6 and 26–7).

The Closure

The wound is adequately irrigated with Betadine solution and closed in anatomical layers. The iliac crest wound is carefully reconstructed to avoid a Trendelenburg lurch and a suction drain is placed into the hip wound but not into the retroperitoneal space.

The Turning of the Patient

Teamwork is of the essence for this operation because the complete cooperation of the theater nursing staff, the anesthetist, and the surgical assistants is required. The patient is usually catheterized before surgery and full cooperation of the team is needed to turn the patient into the face-down position from the left oblique position. This requires major readjustment of the bean bag, which is used for virtually every spinal operation. Care must be taken to avoid any compression of the abdominal viscera thus eliminating unnecessary extradural venous bleeding during the reopening of the laminectomy wound.

The Posterior Instrumentation and Fusion

The previous laminectomy wound is usually reopened; the length of the incision depends entirely on the length of the instrumentation. Diathermy dissection is performed when possible to reduce the blood loss. The best retractors for the erector spinae muscle mass are of the Keon Cohen design popularized by Crock.[2] Wide lateral dissection is performed out to the tips of the transverse processes and if part or all of a lamina(e) is missing, then careful dissection is required to avoid injury to the cauda equina. Once the soft-tissue dissection has been completed, a decision can be made regarding the implants to be used. If three segments or more are to be instrumented, then double Harrington rods from the ala of the sacrum to the first intact neural arch are preferred for mechanical reasons. If, however, only two segments are required to be instrumented the Knodt rods are inserted from the neural arch of the sacrum to the neural arch of L4. They are easily applied and quickly inserted and distracted until they just begin to bend.

The Bone Graft for the Posterior Fusion

The bone graft is taken through the same incision from the posterior lateral part of the iliac crest, again preserving the upper part of the crest itself. This autograft is mixed with femoral head allograft, which is usually readily available from hip joint replacement surgery.

The lateral gutters are extensively decorticated and the bone graft is packed into these gutters, being careful not to leave bone fragments proximal to the highest fused motion segment. This is done to prevent the bone graft from growing proximal and rubbing on the next mobile motion segment, "the so-called impingement syndrome."

Wound Closure

The wound is irrigated with a concentrated iodine solution and debridement is performed to rid the wound of dead and dying muscle tissue. To minimize this dead tissue, the retractors are altered occasionally throughout the posterior procedure. Important points in technique include:

1. wound drainage if required, but not necessarily routine
2. muscle closure without excessive tension, which will only produce ischemic muscle and add to the scarring already present
3. careful closure of the thoracolumbar fascia, the relevance of which has been recently stressed by Tesh and coworkers
4. metal clips to the skin.

Postoperative Care

As is to be expected, patients who have endured two major surgical procedures require relatively large volumes of pain medication, ideally delivered by the infusion technique, so that blood levels are maintained at a constant level. Morphine or one of its derivatives is ideal, at least for the first 48 hours. During this period of time, the patient may be nursed flat in bed and rolled onto the right side; they usually resist rolling onto the left side, which involves pressure over the left iliac crest donor site wound. Nasogastric tubes are not routine unless a transperitoneal anterior approach has been employed. This is not common, but in the meantime, fluids by mouth are avoided until bowel sounds have reappeared. It is customary to expect their absence for 24 to 48 hours.

Drains need regular checking; when they have ceased to be purposeful, they may be removed, usually 48 hours after surgery. There is therefore no specific nursing detail required in the immediate postoperative phase, other than turning the patient, controlling the pain with medication, and regulating fluids. Catheterization will usually have been employed, particularly in the older and multi-operated patient, who invariably will have difficulty with voiding in the early postoperative period. However, it should be stated that because of the biomechanical fixation of the fusion technique, the stability is so ensured that patients are able to stand with support 24 hours after surgery if they have not been catheterized and if they wish to pass urine.

Customarily these patients are kept for a minimum of 12 to 18 hours in the intensive care or recovery ward until the basic signs have stabilized and settled. X-rays are not routinely done during this period unless there is concern relating to a respiratory complication, unusual spinal pain, unexpected leg pain, etc.

By the third day, the patients have usually settled and the bowel sounds have reappeared, by which time they will have started some fluids and now can commence on a light diet. They rarely need very much in the first instance and it will take a couple of days before their appetites reappear. Ideally, the first light food by mouth is hot tea with dry toast. This gives the upper alimentary tract a firm substance to maneuver and encourages the rapid return of normal peristalsis.

There is no reason why these patients cannot be encouraged to sit and take a few steps by the third day.

After the simultaneous double operation the patients are usually happy to be discharged from the hospital 10–14 days after surgery. It must be emphasized that it is the speed of rehabilitation and the relief from pain that have been the most gratifying aspects of this surgical procedure (Figures 26–13 and 26–14).

Complications

Complications are few and usually of a minor nature, although, naturally, deep vein thrombosis is an ever-present

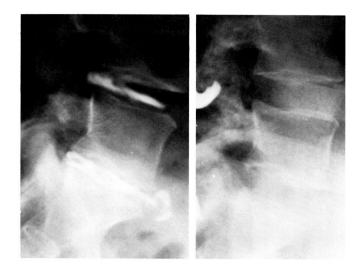

Figures 26–13 and 26–14 X-rays before and after the simultaneous combined anterior and posterior fusion. Note that discography is essential to identify the anatomical pain sources before the operation itself can be planned. Strong distraction is required so that maximum bone graft can be used. Many of these patients are 4–5 cm taller, a feature that should be explained before surgery!

threat. Patients have generally had early bone healing. Occasionally, resorption of some of the lateral bone graft has been noted on radiographs taken at six months.

An interesting but fortunately small group of patients have developed severe postoperative psychoses previously described by Crock.[2] Whether this is due to drug reaction or to the resorption of toxic metabolites from the circulation adjacent to the disc is not at all clear. These patients can pose a particular problem because they are often quite paranoid and capable of injuring themselves.

THE RESULTS OF THE SCAPF OPERATION

The SCAPF operation evolved over the past five years and publication has been deliberately delayed to be sure that the results of such a major and new approach to an old problem are worthwhile. The available evidence suggests that if the patients are under 40 and have not had multiple repeat laminectomies and myelograms with intractable nerve root scarring and leg pain, one can anticipate an excellent result. The excellent good result in over 150 patients followed very closely for the past several years indicates that there is invariably a significant improvement and the majority of patients can return to activities that previously they could not contemplate for many years before surgery.

CONCLUSIONS

The postlaminectomy syndrome is a complex and very disabling problem that is one of the major challenges in the whole of clinical medicine. It is recognized that the current approach to the problem of back and leg pain is that when the evidence is present of disc lesion, "a laminectomy is performed." If symptoms are not relieved or they recur after laminectomy, then the current fashion is to abandon all thoughts of further surgery and to concentrate on a psychological approach with pain medicines, etc.

The new surgical approach that has been presented is an entirely opposite approach. If it can be demonstrated that the patient is seriously and genuinely disabled from previous back surgery, then a simultaneous combined anterior and posterior fusion is performed using the technique briefly outlined above. This is a new approach to an old problem and it does not necessarily mean that it is not the correct one. Experience over five years with a significant number of patients indicates that if the nerve roots are not surgically decompressed and the motion segments affected are merely distracted and fused from the front and back, there is an excellent chance that the patient can be rehabilitated, a challenge that has not been previously addressed.

REFERENCES

1. Cloward RB: Gas-sterilized cadaver bone grafts for spinal fusion operations—A simplified bone bank. *Spine* 1980;5:4–10.

2. Crock HV: *Practice of Spinal Surgery.* New York, Springer-Verlag, 1983.

3. Curtin J, O'Brien JP, Park WM: Natural history of the surgically treated herniated lumbar intervertebral disc in the adolescent. *J Bone Joint Surg* 1977;59B:506.

4. Dwyer AF, Shafer MF: Anterior approach to scoliosis: The results of treatment in fifty-one cases. *J Bone Joint Surg* 1974;56B:218–224.

5. Fairbank JCT, Davies JB, Couper J, O'Brien JP: The Oswestry disability low back pain questionnaire. *Physiotherapy* 1980;66:271–273.

6. Fraser RD: A wide muscle-splitting approach to the lumbosacral spine. *J Bone Joint Surg* 1982;64B:44–46.

7. Freebody D, Bendall R, Taylor RD: Anterior transperitoneal lumbar fusion. *J Bone Joint Surg* 1971;53B:617–627.

8. *Gould Medical Dictionary,* ed 3. New York, McGraw-Hill, 1972.

9. Harrington PR: Treatment of scoliosis. *J Bone Joint Surg* 1962;44A:591.

10. Holt EP: The question of lumbar discography. *J Bone Joint Surg* 1968;50A:720–726.

11. Jones Sir R, Lovett RW: *Orthopaedic Surgery,* ed 2. New York, Oxford University Press, 1933, chap 31, p 670.

12. Kellgren JH: Sciatica. *Lancet* 1941;1:561–564.

13. O'Brien JP, Evans G: A review of laminectomies: A correlation of disability with abnormal spinal movement. *J Bone Joint Surg* 1978;60B:439.

14. O'Brien JP, Yau ACMC: Anterior & posterior correction and fusion for paralytic scoliosis. *Clin Orthop* 1972;86:151–153.

15. O'Brien JP, Dwyer AP, Hodgson AR: Paralytic pelvic obliquity. *J Bone Joint Surg* 1975;57A:626–631.

16. O'Brien JP: The role of fusion for chronic low back pain. *Orthop Clin North Am* 1983;14:639–647.

17. O'Brien JP: Mechanisms of spinal pain, in Wall, Melzack (ed): *Textbook of Pain,* London, Churchill Livingstone, 1983.

18. O'Brien JP, Dawson MHO, Heard CW, Momberger G, Speck G: Simultaneous combined anterior and posterior fusion. *Clin Orthop* 1986;203:191–195.

19. Shapiro R: *Myelography.* Chicago, Year Book Medical Publishers, 1962.

20. Yoshizawa H, O'Brien JP, Smith WT, Trumper M: The neuropathology of intervertebral discs removed for low back pain. *J Pathol* 1980;132:95–104.

Chapter 27

Lateral Recess, Lateral Canal, and Foraminal Stenosis

William H. Kirkaldy-Willis, M.D., and Ken Yong-Hing, M.D.

DEFINITION

The nerve canal extends from the place where the spinal nerve leaves the dural sac to the foramen. The foramen is the door by which the nerve exits from the spinal canal and as a door, it has no thickness. The lateral part of the nerve canal begins opposite the medial border of the superior articular process and passes obliquely outward and downward to the foramen. It is in this lateral part of the nerve canal that lateral stenosis, and its result, lateral spinal nerve entrapment, develops.[4,9]

ETIOLOGY

Developmental changes sometimes, but rarely, result in one or more narrow lateral canals. Narrowing of a canal may be one of the sequelae of a vertebral fracture. Most commonly, lateral stenosis is the result of advancing degeneration that, of course, involves other parts of the vertebrae as well as the lateral canal. The sequelae of chemonucleolysis are loss of disc height, subluxation of articular processes, and the development of lateral stenosis. Lateral stenosis may follow an operation for a disc herniation, particularly when the operative field was obscured because of inadequate hemostasis or when the tissues have not been handled with adequate care.[8,10,13,25]

PATHOGENESIS AND PATHOLOGY

The pathological changes that are the result of degeneration are similar, though not identical, to the changes that follow a poorly executed operation. For brevity and simplicity, only the changes that occur during the degenerative process will be discussed here. These changes are of two kinds. The first is continuing loss of disc height with subluxation of the posterior joint. As the upper vertebra moves slightly backward on the lower vertebra, the superior facet (process) slides upward and forward on the inferior facet of the same posterior joint. This markedly narrows the foramen, and of more importance, the lateral canal medial to it.

The second kind of change is the result of the attempt by the tissues to repair the process occurring in the disc and posterior joints. This reparative process results in the formation of new bone both around the circumference of the vertebral bodies on either side of the disc and on the surfaces of the articular facets. The facets enlarge. It is the posterior joint subluxation, together with the facet enlargement by osteophytes, that produces lateral stenosis. The bulging annulus fibrosus of a narrow degenerate disc further reduces the size of the lateral canal and entraps the nerve.[10,13] Each spinal segment is a disc, two facets, a traversing spinal nerve, and an exiting spinal nerve (which is the more cephalad nerve). For example, at the L4-5 segment, there is the L4 disc, the superior facet of 5 and the inferior facet of 4, the exiting L4 nerve, and the traversing L5 nerve. The L5 nerve becomes the exiting nerve at the L5–S1 segment.

There are two main sites at which a nerve can be entrapped. The first traversing nerve can be entrapped medially, between an enlarged superior articular process and the back of the same vertebral body in what is called the subarticular recess. Second, the exiting nerve can be entrapped more laterally between the pedicle, the anterior aspect of the superior process, and the back of the disc and vertebral body (Figure 27–1). Two more sites of entrapment have recently been described. Ray has described the site far laterally, in the region of the foramen, where the nerve is entrapped by the foraminal ligament. Wiltse has described entrapment between the transverse process of L5 and the ala of the sacrum, the "far out syndrome."

The sites of nerve entrapment can be explained more simply by specific examples. At the L4–5 level the traversing nerve may be entrapped in the subarticular recess formed by the L5 superior facet and the back of the body of L5.[12] At the same intervertebral level, the exiting nerve may be entrapped at the L4 pedicle between the front of the L5 superior facet and the disc and L4 level. Thus, two spinal nerves may be entrapped at any one intervertebral level. In this example, the L4 and L5 spinal nerves are entrapped at the L4–5 intervertebral level (Figure 27–2).

Conversely, any one spinal nerve may be entrapped in different ways at two intervertebral levels. For example, the traversing L5 spinal nerve may be entrapped at the L4–5 intervertebral level in the subarticular recess between the L5 superior articular facet and the L5 vertebral body. At one intervertebral lower level, L5–S1, the same now-exiting L5 spinal nerve, may be entrapped between the S1 superior articular facet and the L5 pedicle and vertebral body.

It is worth emphasizing, because of its great consequence, that two nerves may be entrapped at one intervertebral level. Conversely one spinal nerve may be entrapped at two intervertebral levels. This must be kept constantly in mind during investigation and surgical decompression for lateral stenosis.[10,21] Moreover, if the lesions described by Ray and Wiltse are not just rarities, then the spinal nerve may be entrapped at two intervertebral levels. At one of these two levels—the intervertebral level at which the nerve exits from the spinal canal—the nerve may be entrapped at three sites. It may be entrapped by the tip of the articular facet, by the foraminal ligament, and by the transverse process.

Three phases of degeneration are recognized:[25] (1) the early phase of dysfunction, (2) the middle phase of instability, and (3) the final phase of restabilization. During the middle phase of instability, one vertebra moves abnormally backward and forward and rotates on another. Because of the abnormal movement, lateral stenosis in this phase is intermittent and is termed dynamic and recurrent. During the final phase of restabilization, movement of one vertebra on an adjacent one is greatly reduced or absent. In this phase any lateral stenosis is fixed or static. Recognition of these two types is of vital importance in planning treatment,[7,14] as will be discussed later.

SYMPTOMS AND SIGNS

Sometimes the patient complains of low back pain. More commonly he or she complains of buttock and trochanteric and posterior thigh pain that radiates to the knee. The pain may pass below the knee down the lateral calf or posterior calf to the ankle. Occasionally, the pain extends to foot and toes. In the presence of instability, the pain may be exacerbated by rotational movements of the trunk.

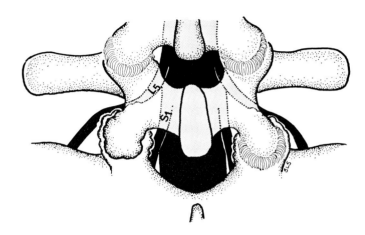

Figure 27–1 Two pairs of nerves may be entrapped at any one level, ie, the L5 and the S1 nerves at L5–S1. *Source:* Reprinted with permission from *Orthopedic Clinics of North America* (1983;14:3), Copyright © 1983, WB Saunders Company.

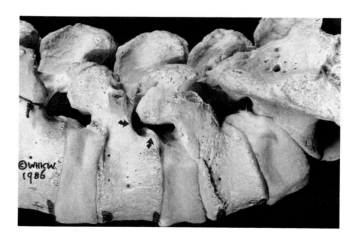

Figure 27–2 Skeleton of the lumbar spine. The L4 nerve may be entrapped between the pedicle of L4 and the tip of the superior articular process of L5 (arrow on left): the L5 nerve may be entrapped at the same L4–5 level between the part of the superior articular process of L5 and the osteophyte growing backwards from the posterior aspect of the body of L4 (arrow on right). *Source:* Copyright © William H. Kirkaldy-Willis, 1986.

Movements of the lumbar spine are not greatly restricted. Straight-leg raising is usually slightly diminished. Frequently, neurological findings are normal. There may be some change in sensation over the L4, L5, or S1 dermatome. Diminution of the ankle reflex and reduction in muscle power are rare findings. The Lasègue test is rarely positive. The Bowstring test (tenderness over the posterior tibial or lateral popliteal nerve at knee joint level) and sciatic notch tenderness are often positive.[4]

As will be discussed later, these symptoms and signs do not differ greatly from those of a facet, sacroiliac, or muscle syndrome. They do no more than suggest the diagnosis of lateral spinal stenosis.[11]

In the presence of instability, forced extension of the lumbar spine or forced rotation of the trunk on the pelvis may exacerbate the patient's pain.[15]

RADIOGRAPHIC FINDINGS

Next, it is convenient to determine whether there is any instability by use of dynamic radiographs. AP views in left and right lateral bending may demonstrate malalignment of the spinous processes or translation of one vertebra on the next. Lateral views in flexion and in extension may show that the upper vertebral body moves backward into retrospondylolisthesis on the lower body and that this is more marked in extension. A shift of 2 mm or more is significant. These findings enable the physician to determine whether the lateral stenosis, if present, is dynamic (in the phase of instability) or if it is static (in the phase of restabilization).[14,15]

CT scan images enable the physician to confirm the presence of, and assess the degree of, lateral stenosis.[16,21]

1. In the most medial type of lateral stenosis, the subarticular recess between the body and disc and the superior facet of the same vertebra is narrow (for example, the recess between the superior facet of S1 and the body of the sacrum and L5–S1 disc (see Figure 27–3).
2. More laterally, between the medial and lateral margins of the pedicle, and at a higher level, the upper exiting nerve may be entrapped in a narrow part of the canal between the anterior aspect of the superior facet and the back of the body and disc above it. This narrowing, seen on a CT slice just below the pedicle, is between the front of the superior facet and the back of the vertebral body (Figure 27–4).

OTHER INVESTIGATIONS

A selective nerve block is useful in determining which spinal nerve is entrapped. For example, when the L5 nerve is approached at the L5–S1 foramen, the patient's pain may be

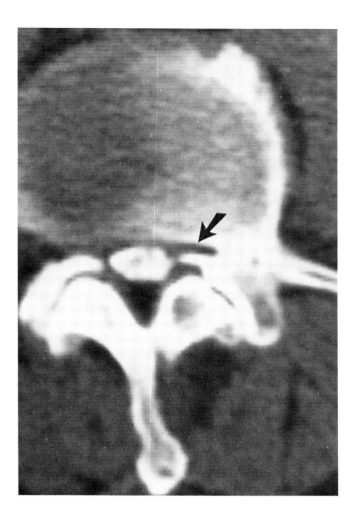

Figure 27–3 CT image. Entrapment of the L4 nerve (left of arrow) at the same L4–5 level as in Figure 4 between the back of the body of L4 and the superior articular process of L5. *Source:* Reprinted from *Managing Low Back Pain* by WH Kirkaldy-Willis (Ed) with permission of Churchill Livingstone Inc, © 1983.

reproduced as the tip of the needle touches the nerve, or as contrast is introduced into the fibrous nerve sheath. If the pain is abolished on injection of local anesthetic, the diagnosis is more certain. Correlation of this test with CT findings enables the physician to tell both which nerve is entrapped and the likely site of entrapment.[24]

Electromyographic studies demonstrate the presence or absence of a radiculopathy that is too subtle to detect by clinical tests. These studies provide useful confirmatory evidence.

Discography is also sometimes helpful. An abnormal contrast outline may be useful in confirming the level of instability. Injection of saline may reproduce the patient's pain and identify the painful disc.[23]

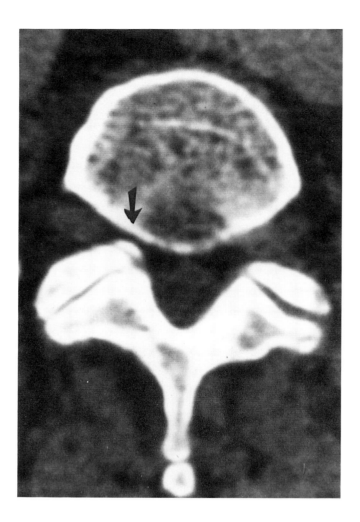

Figure 27–4 CT image. Entrapment of the L5 nerve medially (right of arrow) between the back of the body of L5 and the part of the superior articular process of L5 in the subarticular recess. *Source:* Reprinted from *Managing Low Back Pain* by WH Kirkaldy-Willis (Ed) with permission of Churchill Livingstone Inc, © 1983.

DIFFERENTIAL DIAGNOSIS

Herniation of the nucleus pulposus, when the symptoms and signs are slightly atypical, may present as lateral stenosis. The diagnosis is made by the CT scan.

A posterior joint syndrome sometimes presents in a similar way. Indeed, this syndrome may accompany lateral stenosis. In this case, a posterior joint injection with local anesthetic gives the diagnosis and may cure the patient. Reproduction of the pain distribution as the needle reaches the joint and abolition of the pain by the anesthetic confirms the presence of the syndrome. Manipulation of the posterior joint can provide similar evidence.[11]

A sacroiliac syndrome may be confused with lateral stenosis. Clinical tests usually differentiate this condition. When manipulation of this joint or the injection of local anesthetic abolishes the local and the referred pain, then it is a sacroiliac syndrome, not lateral stenosis.[11]

A piriformis syndrome may cause similar confusion. Injection of this muscle with local anesthetic abolishes the pain and provides the diagnosis.[28]

A gluteus medius syndrome can mimic lateral stenosis. The pain of the lesion can be relieved by spraying and stretching the muscle or by injection of local anesthetic.[26]

CONSERVATIVE TREATMENT

Every case of proven lateral stenosis does not require operation. Indeed, it is always wise to try conservative measures first.[17]

1. Attendance at a low back school and an exercise program are of great help to patients with minimal symptoms.[18]
2. A light elastic supporting garment often helps to control the pain.[20]
3. Manipulation by a skilled clinician can be expected to relieve about 50 percent of patients. This is thought to work by shifting the position of the superior facet 1–2 mm.[19]
4. A therapeutic selective nerve block relieves the pain for a period of time in a few patients in whom the symptoms are not severe.[24]
5. When these measures have failed, it is wise to request a psychological assessment of the patient before making the decision to embark on any operative procedure.

OPERATION

General Considerations

The operation should be carried out with such care that damage to nerves is avoided, that bleeding is controlled throughout, and that there is no injury to dura and extradural veins so that postoperative adhesions are reduced to the minimum.[1–6]

The patient is positioned on a modified Hastings or Williams Frame or on a Crock Sausage. These devices leave the abdomen free and so reduce the risk of hemorrhage. The use of a headlight and of magnifying glasses is also of considerable assistance. Bipolar cautery is essential to control bleeding from extradural veins (Figure 27–5).

The Approach

A posterior midline incision is made. The paravertebral muscles are elevated on both sides and the interlaminar space is identified. After excision of the ligamentum flavum, the interlaminar space is widened by excision of the upper and lower laminar edges and spinous processes. The medial third of the inferior articular process on each side is removed with osteotome and mallet passing obliquely forward and outward to expose the cartilage on the superior facet. At this point, the diameter of the lateral canal and foramen is measured using probes or gauges of 2, 3, 4, and 5 mm diameter.[17,29,31]

Identification of Site of Entrapment and Decompression

The most medial site of nerve entrapment is anterior to the superior facet of the lower vertebra, between it and the back of the vertebral body and disc. The size of the subarticular gutter or recess thus formed is easily assessed using the appropriate gauge. The gutter is enlarged by removal of the medial third of this facet with Kerrison forceps, osteotome, sonic tool, or compressed air burr. During this part of the procedure, the nerve is protected with a small retractor. It may also be necessary to remove a part of the anterior surface of the facet. On completion of the decompression, the recess should be at least 5 mm in diameter from front to back (Figures 27–6 and 27–7).

More laterally and at a slightly higher level, between the medial and lateral edges of the pedicle, the exiting nerve can be entrapped between the front of the superior facet and the back of the vertebral body and disc above it. In relieving this entrapment the medial third of the superior facet is removed as described in the preceding paragraph. It is then necessary to enlarge the lateral canal to 5 mm as far as the foramen. This can be done with a curette or burr. Great care should be taken to protect the nerve. The procedure should be slow and time-consuming (Figures 27–8 and 27–9).[1–3]

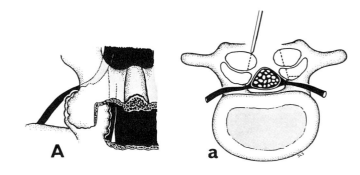

Figure 27–6 (A,a) The medial third of the L5 inferior articular process is osteotomised. *Source:* Reprinted from *Managing Low Back Pain* by WH Kirkaldy-Willis (Ed) with permission of Churchill Livingstone Inc, © 1983.

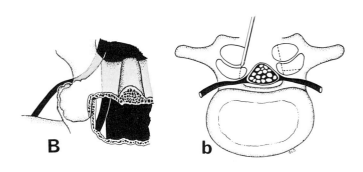

Figure 27–7 (B,b) The medial third of the S1 superior articular process is osteotomised. The nerve root should be retracted and protected. *Source:* Reprinted from *Managing Low Back Pain* by WH Kirkaldy-Willis (Ed) with permission of Churchill Livingstone Inc, © 1983.

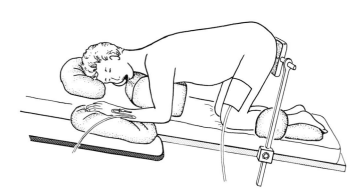

Figure 27–5 Modified Hastings Frame. Take care to prevent injury to the eyes, cervical spine, brachial plexus, ulna, and peronael nerves. *Source:* Reprinted from *Managing Low Back Pain* by WH Kirkaldy-Willis (Ed) with permission of Churchill Livingstone Inc, © 1983.

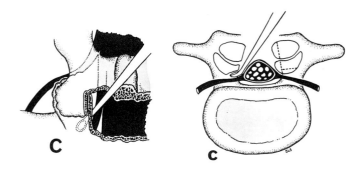

Figure 27–8 (C,c) The anterior surface of the S1 superior articular process (roof of the lateral recess) is shaved with a curette. *Source:* Reprinted from *Managing Low Back Pain* by WH Kirkaldy-Willis (Ed) with permission of Churchill Livingstone Inc, © 1983.

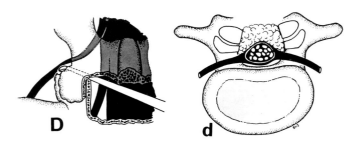

Figure 27–9 (D,d) The tip of the S1 superior articular process is removed to decompress the exiting L5 nerve. A free fat graft is loosely sutured to cover the dura. *Source:* Reprinted from *Managing Low Back Pain* by WH Kirkaldy-Willis (Ed) with permission of Churchill Livingstone Inc, © 1983.

Entrapment at the foramen, the door, is more difficult to assess. If the gauge passes with ease to a point beyond the foramen, it is likely that there is no entrapment by a foraminal ligament. It must be admitted that this point is not yet entirely clear. Ray suggests that foraminal entrapment should be approached by a posterolateral incision. It does not seem that his approach is adequate for more medial types of entrapment. How to diagnose this type of entrapment other than by exclusion is not yet known. It seems reasonable to use Ray's approach in the absence of CT evidence of lateral stenosis when leg pain resulting from other causes has been carefully excluded.[22]

Relief of Wiltse's "far out syndrome" at the L5–S1 level is done through a lateral muscle-splitting approach. The transverse process of L5 is exposed, the site of entrapment between it and the sacral ala is identified, and enough of this transverse process is removed to free the nerve.[27]

Decompression and Stability

In patients with instability demonstrated before the operation, it is wise to follow the decompression by a one-level posterolateral fusion.

When the segment is stable before operation, it is not likely that decompression will render the spine unstable, provided that only the medial third of each of the articular processes is removed. Undoubtedly, in some cases it is necessary to remove so much bone that the segment is rendered unstable. In this case, it is necessary to fuse. Any time the surgeon is in doubt about the stability, fusion is wise. But fusion is not often necessary following decompression for lateral canal stenosis. An exception to this, which does not come within the scope of this paper, is degenerative spondylolisthesis where decompression should usually be followed by fusion.[4,5,6,31]

The Presence of Extradural Fibrosis

When an operation is being done for lateral stenosis following a previous exploration, it is common to encounter a varying degree of extradural and perineural fibrosis. The nerve is often fixed by scar, which makes the dissection difficult and increases the risk of damage to the nerves. It is safer to start the intraspinal exploration far laterally. If the ligamentum flavum is intact, the dissection should be kept lateral to this structure. In this manner, the nerve root and dura are pushed toward the midline by a combination of blunt and sharp dissection. This always takes a considerable amount of time and a great deal of very careful dissection. The use of a headlight and of magnifying glasses is invaluable (Figure 27–10). Upon completion of the dissection and decompression it should be possible to obtain a 1.0 cm excursion of the nerve from side to side.[2,3,30,31]

Recurrence of fibrosis can sometimes be prevented by epidural steroid injections given as soon as the patient complains of leg pain, which can be repeated when the pain recurs again.[17,30,31]

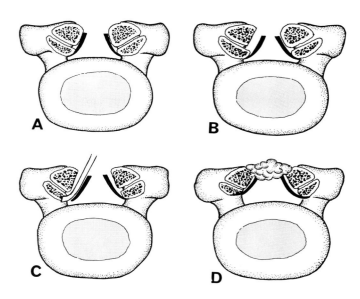

Figure 27–10 Cross sectional diagram of the four steps of our operation to decompress the nerves lateral to the dura and in the lateral canal when fibrosis is present in the multioperated back. (A) Laminectomy performed. (B) On the left the lateral expansion of the ligamentum flavum has been separated from the medial aspect of the inferior articular process and the medial third of this process has been removed. (C) The sonic tool or curette is inserted between the ligamentum flavum and the superior articular process to remove its medial and anterior portions. (D) The lateral canals have been enlarged and a free fat graft placed posterior to the dura. *Source:* Reprinted from *Managing Low Back Pain* by WH Kirkaldy-Willis (Ed) with permission of Churchill Livingstone Inc, © 1983.

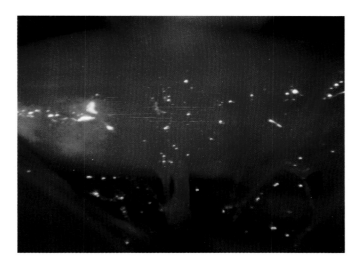

Figure 28–8 Neuroma formation in the cutaneous and subcutaneous tissue layers is not an uncommon etiology of hyperesthetic lumbar wounds. Such lesions may be visible microsurgically and should be suspected when trigger points exist. This photomicrograph shows the typical swirling bundles of nerve fibers with interlacing islands of fibroblastic hyalinized scar tissue. Well-localized minimal skin incisions significantly reduce the possibility of this postsurgical complication.

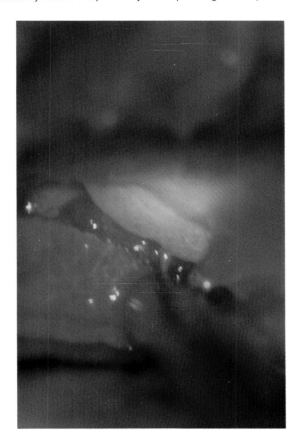

Figure 28–10 Synovial membrane histology can be demonstrated by biopsy of the glistening white fluid-filled sac that protrudes into the microsurgical field when approaching the facet. The histological picture is one of a well-vascularized synovial villus covered by cuboidal epithelium.

Figure 28–4 Neural inflammation following intradiscal enzyme injection. Under high magnification, a lumbar nerve root is viewed to be markedly inflamed following the treatment of a herniated intervertebral disc by intradiscal enzyme injection some eight weeks previously. The patient had experienced rather immediate and severe burning sciatica following the injection. Since decompression of the associated lateral recess and microdiscectomy without intervertebral curettement, the symptoms have slowly subsided over a 12-month period.

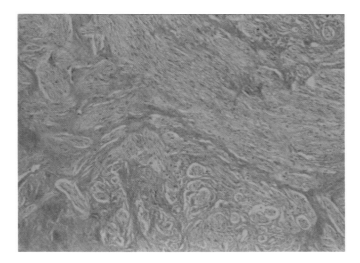

Figure 28–9 Synovial membrane of the facet. With the neural elements retracted downward, the synovial balloon of the facet can be visualized as the most lateral fibers of the ligamentum flavum are removed from the recess. High magnification demonstrates its glistening white appearance. Care should be taken not to injure this structure for fear of initiating a postsurgical facet pain syndrome.

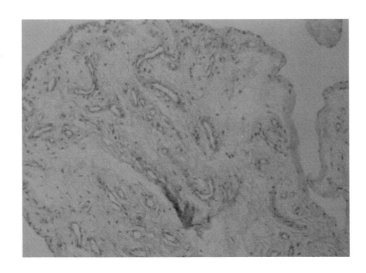

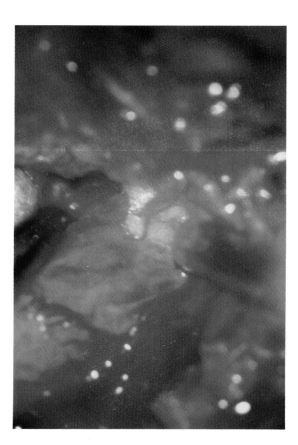

Figure 28–11 Iatrogenic osteophytes are not uncommon as an etiology of continued nerve root irritation following use of the surgical rongeur. Pictured here through the operating microscope, the bony spicule protrudes from the lateral canal some eight weeks following initial surgery for an intervertebral disc herniation. This patient's sciatica was intense upon awakening from first operation. Care must always be taken to smooth bone edges following the use of such instruments.

Figure 28–12 Fat grafts applied over the neural structures with the intent of preventing dense adhesion reactions and reestablishing tissue planes are usually unsuccessful. Most often the transposed fat serves only as a matrix for scar tissue formation. Visualized grossly in this photo is a thick fibrous scar, which has generated in an interlaminar fat graft placed some four months previously.

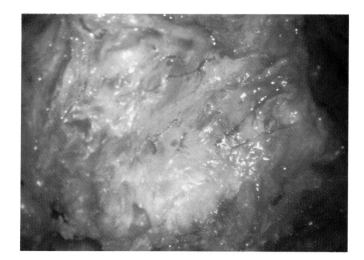

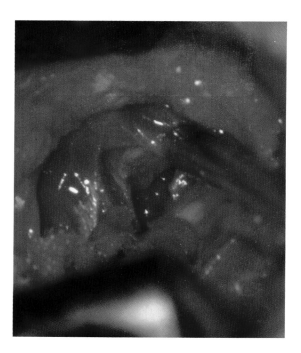

Figure 28–13 Arteriovenous malformations may occasionally be visualized with high magnification in the extradural space in patients with postsurgical sciatic pain syndromes. With the neural elements retracted downward to expose an area of rongeured lateral recess, such a lesion has been photographed. Although the exact mechanism of its formation remains speculative, a major possibility is that of vascular injury secondary to surgical instrumentation.

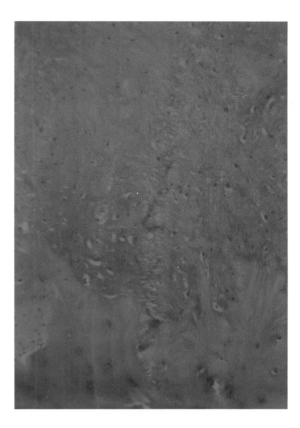

Figure 28–15 A scalpel window in the annulus fibrosis may serve as an easy exit for further herniation of disc material following intervertebral curettement. Such is the case pictured in this photo. Note the neo-vascularization suggested to be arterial that overlies the recurrent protrusion.

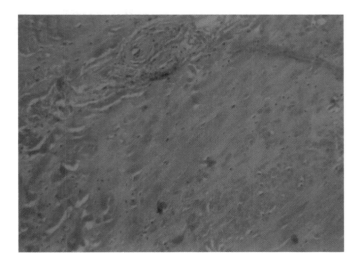

Figure 28–17 Histological study of a three-month-old fat graft demonstrates dense fibroblastic growth within the fat cell matrix. In the photo, some vacuolated fat cells still remain between the bands of fibrous scar. Sacrifice of normal epidural fat tissue during lumbar operations seems to carry a high risk of fibrous tissue formation as a replacement. Such a practice should be strictly avoided if the patient is to have any chance at reestablishing tissue planes.

Figure 28–14 Healing of the annulus fibrosis of the intervertebral disc following scalpel incision is not by primary intention. The fibroelastic tissue of the annulus is replaced only by fibroplastic scar, thus weakening its retaining wall function for the years ahead. Such a phenomenon is demonstrated in this photomicrograph. Disc tissue with its typical chondrocytes appears at the right of the picture restrained only by a thin fibroblastic covering visible to the left. Note the fingers of intervertebral tissue protruding into the fibrous layer. The specimen was obtained from the surface of a large recurrent disc herniation.

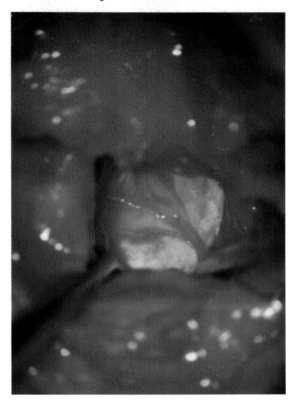

Figure 28–16 Thus far, all densities of epidural scar tissue appear to vary only in their degree of vascularity and number of cell nuclei. Pictured is a fibroblastic scar of six months duration. Note the degree of hyalinization that has already occurred.

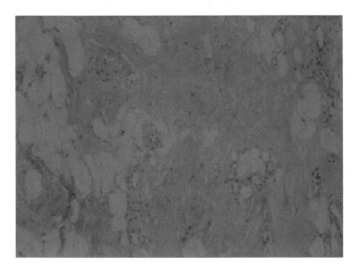

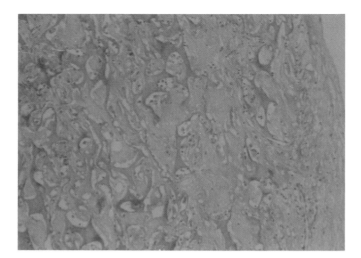

Figure 28–18 Although hemostatic materials foreign to the epidural space may be effective for that purpose, fibroblastic scar tissue growth within the matrix of such substances is usually ravenous. Pictured is a histological study of such a phenomenon. Note the residuals of the foreign body throughout the fibrous scar.

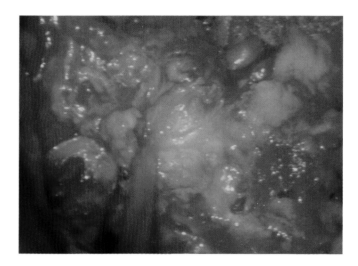

Figure 28–19 Scar tissue formation following the use of electro-coagulation in the epidural space is the most scirrhous of all. On occasion, it has been virtually impossible to successfully mobilize the neural elements from such an entrapment. Pictured here through the surgical microscope, an extremely dense scar is encountered in the lateral recess in a patient who suffered significant hemorrhage at first surgery. The operative dictation relating to the incident described vividly the burning of extradural tissue in an attempt to stop the hemorrhage.

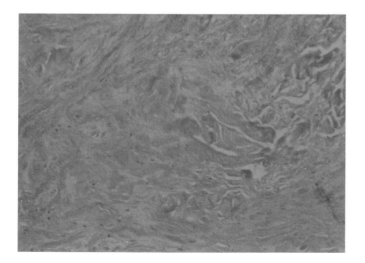

Figure 28–20 The histology of epidural scar tissue following electro-coagulation shows extreme hyalinization and rare cell nuclei. In addition, note the absence of vascularity. Fibroblastic tissue of this type is extremely difficult to neurolyse without somewhat dangerous maneuvers that not infrequently rupture into the subarachnoid space. The use of electrocoagulation in the epidural space carries grave consequences.

Vertebral Body Osteophytes

Toward the end of the decompression it may be necessary to remove projecting osteophytes that are causing nerve entrapment. Of special note are the uncinate spurs that sometimes project from the posterolateral aspect of the lower surface of the vertebral body. Sometimes, it may be necessary to deal in a similar way with osteophytes projecting backward on either side of the disc. The surgeon may also need to remove a hard fibrous ridge of projecting disc material. When a frank definite disc herniation is present, it must be dealt with in the usual manner. Such an additional lesion is more likely to cause nerve entrapment when it is laterally sited.[7,21]

Two Nerves Entrapped at One Intervertebral Level

Two nerves may be entrapped at one spinal level. Before the operation, the surgeon should determine from the CT images what to expect but inspection of both nerves in every case is wise. At the L4–5 level, for example, the exiting L4 nerve must be explored and probed laterally at the more cephalad point. More medially and caudad, the L5 nerve in its subarticular gutter must be probed, explored, and decompressed if necessary.[1,2,3,12]

One Nerve Entrapped at Two Intervertebral Levels

On occasion, one nerve is entrapped at two levels. The presence of the double lesion should be suspected from study of the CT images before operation. The L5 nerve may be compromised in the subarticular recess at the L4–5 intervertebral level, and again as it leaves the spine, between the superior facet of the sacrum and the back of the body of L5 and the L5–S1 disc at the L5–S1 intervertebral level. The L5 nerve must be explored at both sites of entrapment by exploration at both the L4–5 and L5–S1 intervertebral spaces.[1,2,3,12]

Insertion of Free-Fat Grafts

It is essential to place a large free-fat graft posterior to the dura in every case. Experimental work has shown that fibrosis originates from fibroblasts that proliferate on the deep surface of the posterior muscles, and that one large graft survives much better than several small pieces of particulate fat. Often it is possible to harvest a graft of adequate size from beneath the skin at the lower end of the incision. Sometimes, in a thin patient it is necessary to take the graft through a separate more lateral incision. Rarely, it is necessary to take the graft through an incision in the gluteal fold.[2,3,30]

Epidural Morphine

The insertion of 4 mm of morphine in preservative-free solution to the epidural space 3–4 cm above the upper end of the incision, as advocated by Burton and his colleagues, reduces postoperative pain and decreases the amount of analgesics required.[2,3]

Wound Drainage

It is wise to insert a medium-sized polyethylene drain deep to the posterior muscles, and it is essential to insert a small drain deep to the skin at the site from which the fat graft has been taken.[31]

AFTERCARE

The patient is allowed out of bed the day following the operation and should be ready to leave the hospital from 7 to 10 days later. Before the patient leaves he or she is fitted with a light elastic garment to give some support to the low back. Arrangements are made for the patient to reattend the Low Back School and he or she is advised that activity at home should be gradually increased.

The patient is seen for follow-up at one month and thereafter at three monthly intervals. The time at which he or she can return to work varies greatly, largely depending on the type of work. Many surgeons agree that recovery is often slow after surgery for lateral canal stenosis; it will certainly take several months and may take as long as one year.[17,31]

REFERENCES

1. Burton CV, Kirkaldy-Willis WH, Yong-Hing K, Heithoff KB: Causes of failure of surgery on the lumbar spine. *Clin Orthop* 1981;157:191.

2. Burton CV: How to avoid the failed back surgery syndrome, in Cauthen JC (ed): *Lumbar Spine Surgery*, Baltimore, Williams & Wilkins Co, 1983, p 204.

3. Burton CV: Diagnosis and treatment of lateral spinal stenosis, in Genant HK (ed): *Spine Update 1984*. University of California at San Francisco, 1984, p 235.

4. Crock HV: Isolated disc resorption as a cause of nerve root canal stenosis. *Clin Orthop* 1976;115:109.

5. Crock HV: Anterior lumbar interbody fusion: Indications for its use and notes on surgical technique. *Clin Orthop* 1982;165:157.

6. Crock HV: *Management of Failed Spinal Operations in Practice of Spinal Surgery*. New York, Springer-Verlag, 1983, p 245.

7. Dupuis PR, Kirkaldy-Willis WH: The spine, integrated function, and pathophysiology, in Cruess RL, Rennie WJR (eds): *Adult Orthopaedics*. New York, Churchill Livingstone, 1984, p 673.

8. Farfan HF: Biomechanics of the lumbar spine, in Kirkaldy-Willis WH (ed): *Managing Low Back Pain*, New York, Churchill Livingstone, 1983, p 9.

9. Kirkaldy-Willis WH, McIvor GWD: Lumbar spinal stenosis, editorial. *Clin Orthop* 1976;115:2.

10. Kirkaldy-Willis WH, Wedge JH, Yong-Hing K, Reilly J: Pathology and pathogenesis of lumbar spondylosis and stenosis. *Spine* 1978;3,4:319.

11. Kirkaldy-Willis WH, Hill RJ: A more precise diagnosis for low back pain. *Spine* 1979;4,2:102.

12. Kirkaldy-Willis WH, Wedge JH, Yong-Hing K, Tchang S, de Korompay V, Shannon R: Lumbar spinal nerve lateral entrapment. *Clin Orthop* 1982;169:171.

13. Kirkaldy-Willis WH: A comprehensive outline of treatment, in Kirkaldy-Willis WH (ed): *Managing Low Back Pain*. New York, Churchill Livingstone, 1983, p 147.

14. Kirkaldy-Willis WH, Tchang S: Diagnosis, in Kirkaldy-Willis WH (ed): *Managing Low Back Pain*. New York, Churchill Livingstone, 1983, p 109.

15. Kirkaldy-Willis WH, Manipulation, in Kirkaldy-Willis WH (ed): *Managing Low Back Pain*. New York, Churchill Livingstone, 1983, p 175.

16. Kirkaldy-Willis WH: Pathology and pathogenesis of low back pain, in Kirkaldy-Willis, WH (ed): *Managing Low Back Pain*. New York, Churchill Livingstone, 1983, p 23.

17. Kirkaldy-Willis WH: The site and nature of the lesion, in Kirkaldy-Willis WH (ed): *Managing Low Back Pain*. New York, Churchill Livingstone, 1983, p 91.

18. Kirkaldy-Willis WH: Spine education program, in Kirkaldy-Willis WH (ed): *Managing Low Back Pain*. New York, Churchill Livingstone, 1983, p 161.

19. Kirkaldy-Willis WH: Supports and braces, in Kirkaldy-Willis WH (ed): *Managing Low Back Pain*. New York, Churchill Livingstone, 1983, p 185.

20. Kirkaldy-Willis WH: The three phases of degenerative disease, in Kirkaldy-Willis WH (ed): *Managing Low Back Pain*. New York, Churchill Livingstone, 1983, p 75.

21. Kirkaldy-Willis WH, Heithoff KB, Tchang S, Bowen CVA, Cassidy JD, Shannon R: Lumbar spondylosis and stenosis: Correlation of pathological anatomy with high resolution computed tomographic scanning, in Post MJD (ed): *Computed Tomography of the Spine*. Baltimore, Williams & Wilkins Co, 1984, p 546.

22. Ray CD: The paralateral approach to lumbar decompression, in *Proceedings of the American Association of Neurological Surgeons*, 1983, p 191.

23. Simmons EH, Segil CM: An evaluation of discography in the localisation of symptomatic levels in discogenic disease of the spine. *Clin Orthop* 1975;108:57.

24. Tajuma T, Furukawa K, Kuramochi E: Selective lumbosacral radiculography and block. *Spine* 1980;5:68.

25. Wedge JH: The natural history of spinal degeneration, in Kirkaldy-Willis WH (ed): *Managing Low Back Pain*. New York, Churchill Livingstone, 1983, p 3.

26. Wedge JH, Tchang S: Differential diagnosis of low back pain, in Kirkaldy-Willis (ed): *Managing Low Back Pain*. New York, Churchill Livingstone, 1983, p 129.

27. Wiltse LL, Guyer RD, Spencer CW, Glen WV, Porter IS: Alar transverse process impingement of the L5 nerve—The far out syndrome. *Spine* 1984;9:31.

28. Wyant GM: Chronic pain syndromes and their treatment, III The piriformis syndrome. *Can Anaesth Soc J* 1979;26:305.

29. Yong-Hing K, Kirkaldy-Willis WH: Osteotomy of lumbar spinous process to increase surgical exposure. *Clin Orthop* 1978;134:218.

30. Yong-Hing K, Reilly J, de Korompay V, Kirkaldy-Willis WH: Prevention of nerve root adhesions after laminectomy. *Spine* 1980;5:59.

31. Yong-Hing K: Surgical techniques, in Kirkaldy-Willis WH (ed): *Managing Low Back Pain*. New York, Churchill Livingstone, 1983, p 199.

Chapter 28

Postsurgical Lumbar Scarring: A Study of Surgical Morbidity

Robert Warren Williams, M.D., FACS

The mechanical compression of neural structures along the lumbar spinal axis by a wide variety of mechanisms continues to provide an endless reservoir of individuals the world over who are racked by intractable sciatic pain, addicted to narcotics, and totally economically disabled. Years of experience with such clinical problems might suggest to any spine surgeon that the miseries of failed lumbar surgery usually do not resemble the common sciatic syndromes for which an initial operative procedure was performed. Rather, the postoperative tragedy for these patients seems best related to the innocent destruction of normal anatomy critical to lumbar spine function during an attempt to resolve what initially should have been a simple lumbar surgical condition.

Such conclusions are the end result of many years of detailed study of the progressive stages of "failed disc syndrome." Utilizing the operating microscope as an investigative tool, clear correlations are often suggested between specific patterns of chronic postsurgical lumbar and sciatic pain as they relate to the visible surgical morbidity of individual tissue layers following failed lumbar operations. For some patients, new varieties of pain are immediately experienced in the postoperative period indicating that some alteration in previously competent functional lumbar anatomy occurred at the operating table as a direct result of surgical instrumentation and/or technique.

For others, the evolution of new pain patterns is much more insidious, occurring over weeks or months and these are associated with specific lumbar activities, which usually cannot be tested early in the postsurgical state. Characteristically, these patients suffer from sciatica only during weightbearing activities or they may experience severe attacks of acute localized lumbar pain, which can be precipitated by specific kinetic maneuvers. Even more evasive and puzzling in this same group, however, are the nonweightbearing sciaticas which slowly evolve, increase in intensity and neurological deficit, and suggest the postsurgical growth of a new tissue that is foreign to the spinal canal. This tissue progressively entraps the neural elements.

Finally, the most unfortunate of all are a third group of patients who do not experience any resolution of their original symptoms, but experience the addition of pain over new distributions. It must be concluded that this pain is iatrogenic by any degree of scientific reasoning.

So it is—with the scars of lumbar surgery and the patients whose personal, family, and economic lives have been devastated by the process. Perhaps the time has come to take a closer look at the mechanisms of failed surgery and what the spine surgeon cannot afford to do to the lumbar anatomy if operative techniques are to provide any reasonable chance of success for the lumbar disease patient.

PRELIMINARY MECHANISMS FOR THE CREATION OF POSTSURGICAL SCAR TISSUE

Common sense would dictate that the functional anatomy of the lumbar spine is the product of 50 million years of evolution. Although this major region of structural support has its design problems, it is a far better piece of engineering than anything reconstructive surgery can achieve. To think that one

---

Note: Figures 28–4 and 28–8 through 28–19 appear as color plates in the front of the book.

can successfully resolve a lumbar nerve root compression syndrome while destroying anatomy critical to lumbar spine function, is very poor judgment indeed.

For the most part, the alignment and stability of the lumbar spine are major functions of the intervertebral discs and facets. The surgical destruction of one of these structures may occasionally be tolerated with minimal long-term residuum, but rarely can the surgical destruction of both at the same segment be tolerated. Further, the intervertebral disc acts as a spacer between the vertebral bodies. The disc significantly assists the facet joints in maintaining the adequacy of the neural foramina. Surgical resection of a massive amount of intervertebral tissue, in an attempt to prevent future disc reherniations, often leaves the patient with a new sciatic syndrome far more severe than the initial syndrome. If one can develop a sincere respect for such basic scientific facts, it becomes far easier to minimize the possibility of a failed lumbar operation.

The successful spine surgeon must be a relentless student of neuroanatomy and lumbar engineering. Although variations in segmental neurological innervation are few for clinical purposes, orthopedic variations that surround the neural elements are not infrequent. Where do the respective lumbar nerve roots exit in a patient with four or six lumbar vertebrae? The surgeon may not know for sure without some years of experience in the correlation of clinical syndromes with surgical pathology. The surgeon should certainly master a sufficient degree of proficiency in neuroanatomy to strongly suspect the level of nerve root compression before attempting to correlate the more sophisticated radiological studies utilized for the investigation of its possible etiologies. Far too often, the patient proceeds to the operating room with a myriad of radiographic studies, which further confuse an already insecure clinical diagnosis as to the mechanisms and location of symptomatic neural compressive pathology. It is here that the ''failed disc syndrome'' will be created through massive surgical exposures and muscle trauma, widespread destruction of the lamina and facets, and frequent multiple-level disc space curettement. The functional anatomy of the lumbar spine can only be irreversibly devastated by such surgical mayhem.

As one becomes more accurate and secure in the neurological examination, proficiency in the correlation of radiographic studies becomes imperative. Plain spine films not only visualize the number of lumbar vertebrae, suggesting possible variations in neuroanatomy, but also allow one to speculate as to the adequacy of the extradural space that houses the surgical pathology. Similarly, degenerative intervertebral collapse and osteoarthritic facet hypertrophy will predict a continuation of chronic back pain regardless of the operative procedure entertained.

The lumbar computed tomography (CT) scan should include axial, coronal, and sagittal views of all levels implicated by clinical neurological dysfunction. Careful evaluation of the spinal canal diameters, adequacy of the lateral recesses, and suspected pathological elevations of the annulus fibrosis will determine the most accurate surgical approach to be utilized for the conservative treatment of a neural compressive lesion.

The CT scans, however, may be quite misleading in the diagnosis of symptomatic intervertebral disc herniations. Normal elevations of the annulus fibrosis may be judged pathological radiographically in patients with mild degrees of scoliosis, spondylolisthesis, or even clinical pelvic tilt from unilateral muscle spasm. A significant rise in the intervertebral tissue as visualized on the scan, however, often does not accurately predict whether a disc herniation is clinically significant, whether it is soft or stony hard in consistency, or whether extruded disc fragments are to be expected. An expert knowledge of all of these possibilities will ultimately prove crucial for the design of an operative procedure that will allow for a successful resolution of any variety of root compressive etiologies while preserving anatomy critical to future lumbar spine competence.

Finally, myelography is notorious for its positive and negative artifacts. It should always be remembered that myelographic defects reflect only flow patterns of the contrast media within the subarachnoid space and often are not accurate in predicting the nature of existing extradural pathology.

Most radiologists have never had the opportunity to correlate their reading room experiences with living spinal surgical pathology. For this reason, surgeons must become extremely proficient in the interpretation and correlation of all radiographic studies as they relate to the necessity for surgical intervention in their patients. When all modalities of conservative management have failed and surgery is required, a patient should not be allowed to go to the operating room without a meticulous clinical and radiographic recorrelation. The spine surgeon will need all the available knowledge that can be mustered to achieve a successful lumbar operation.

THE SURGICAL MICROSCOPE—A MEANS FOR THE EVALUATION OF TISSUE MORBIDITY FOLLOWING FAILED LUMBAR OPERATIONS

Insecure vision in the operating room during critical technical maneuvers led to the evaluation of alternative mechanisms to provide high-intensity concentrated light into the depths of the surgical wound. By 1970, fiber-optic headlamps were available, which proved far more efficient than the diffuse illumination provided by overhead lights. Similarly, experimentation with magnifying loupes naturally followed in an attempt to visualize more accurately the minute vasculature of the central nervous system so critical to the preservation of neurological function. It became apparent rather immediately, however, that the naked eye, though fully corrected to provide maximum visual acuity, was no match for a magnifying apparatus. In addition, extreme neck fatigue was encountered when custom optics, which provided greater than four magnifications, were added to the visual loupes. As the magnification was increased, the depth of field decreased, requiring the surgeon to hold his or her head almost motionless to maintain focus. The answer to this extremely uncomfortable physical situation was of course, the surgical microscope.

If a surgeon experiments with a concentrated light source and high degrees of magnification for a period of time, it will soon become apparent that what is thought to be seen with the naked eye is often not the case. This is certainly true of spinal anatomy and pathology. Since peripheral vision progressively decreases as magnification increases, anatomical orientation may initially be confusing. The rewards of microsurgery are soon to be realized with continued use of the instrument. The magnitude of surgical exposures, operating time, and tissue morbidities can be drastically reduced. Complications such as cerebral spinal fluid leakage and surgical injury to neural structures can virtually be eliminated.

Finally, the surgeon can record on film or videotape experiences that will prove far more rewarding and retrievable than any mental recording, which is vulnerable to the sands of time. With such an instrument available, the iatrogenic failed disc syndrome is soon to become professionally indefensible.

The operating microscope is very simple to use. For the purposes of lumbar surgery, the patient is usually placed in the prone position, with slight flexion to reduce lumbar lordosis. Greater degrees of flexion, for the purpose of spreading the interlaminar spaces, seem unnecessary during microsurgical procedures and only lead to increased intra-abdominal pressure, which distends the epidural veins. An Olympic VAC-PAC #30 is used as an underbody support to create a vacant space under the abdomen, which will decrease intraspinal venous pressure and minimize respiratory movements that otherwise blur the microsurgical field. This can be accomplished by placing a urological irrigation bag containing three liters of solution between the patient and the VAC-PAC, molding the VAC-PAC to the patient during inspiration, and then draining the fluid from the bag (Figure 28–1). The microscope is equipped with angled binoculars, 12.5 eyepieces, and a 400 mm lens, which allows for a comfortable distance between the operator and patient and minimizes the chance of contamination of the surgical instruments. The microscope should enter the field opposite the surgeon, but must be equipped with sufficient arm extensions to allow the surgeon to change sides during the operative procedure without transporting the instrument (Figure 28–2). The scrub nurse is best positioned opposite the surgeon (Figure 28–3).

MATERIALS AND METHODS FOR THE INVESTIGATION OF POSTSURGICAL TISSUE MORBIDITY

With the exception of closed fractures, scar tissue is never found anywhere in the lumbar anatomy unless the patient has

undergone a surgical procedure previously. Regardless of the condition that necessitated surgical intervention on the lumbar spine, the consequences of surgical scarring must be weighed against what is to be gained through operation. For this reason, the surgeon must always be honest with the patient in order to feel professionally comfortable with those aspects of spinal surgery that deal with benign lumbar nerve root compression syndromes. When the surgeon feels that personal experience, clinical acumen, and surgical expertise may be lacking in the management of such conditions, the patient should be referred to a more qualified surgeon rather than taking the risk of initiating a "failed disc syndrome." Next to individuals with extensive burns and spinal cord injuries, these patients represent the most pathetic and depressed group of individuals in the practice of medicine.

There are basically only two types of surgical lumbar patients, those with virgin and those with nonvirgin lumbar anatomy. The first group includes patients with initial soft disc herniations whose CT scan is otherwise normal in spinal canal dimensions, individuals with lumbar spinal stenosis of any variety, and finally, those patients with the occasional combination of both—all of whom have never had previous lumbar surgery.

The second group consists of patients who have had one or more lumbar operations, again present with sciatica. This can hereafter be referred to as postsurgical sciatic pain syndromes (PSP). In this second group those patients with unsatisfactory results following intradiscal enzyme injection must also be included. Although they will not have a visible scar over the lumbar region, the extradural anatomy may be severely

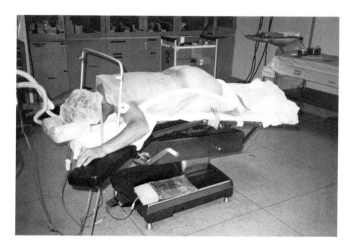

Figure 28–1 Positioning the patient for lumbar surgery. Lumbar operations are carried out with the patient in the prone position. The table is only slightly flexed and a vacant space is created under the abdomen to reduce venous pressure in the epidural space. This is accomplished through the use of a VAC-PAC #30 as an underbody support. In this illustration, the VAC-PAC in its hardened position is visible supporting the patient.

affected by adhesion reactions and inflammation (Figure 28–4). It is the second group of patients with PSP who have supplied the materials for this study in postsurgical tissue morbidity and scarring.

Since 1971, 526 patients with previous lumbar surgery and 23 patients postenzyme injection have been explored utilizing the surgical microscope as an investigative tool and recording device. Detailed observations have been made repeatedly on each layer of the lumbar tissues in an attempt to understand more fully the mechanisms of surgical morbidity that so often seem inflicted on the lumbar anatomy by standard operative techniques. As a by-product of this endeavor, microsurgical approaches have been developed for each type of situation, which will allow for the investigation and treatment of the multiple etiologies of PSP without the additional sacrifice of the residual functional lumbar anatomy.

Having reviewed hundreds of operative reports in reference to these patients, several facts have become apparent. First, the titles given to the former operations rarely describe with any degree of accuracy the actual surgical technique utilized. Second, the operative dictations per se are often grossly inaccurate in their description of the anatomy exposed, extent of tissue dissection performed, and pathology encountered. Such documents provide little help to the surgeon who is faced with treating a failed lumbar patient. It seems reasonable that since surgery should be performed with some degree of scientific accuracy, so should its documents be recorded.

The lumbar operations to be described are microsurgical in type and utilize microsurgical instrumentation. The deeper levels of anatomy requiring exposure are always localized by radiogram before marking the skin incision. Similarly, if any question arises during the procedure as to surgical orientation, a second radiogram is taken for confirmation. For this reason, a lead apron, easily removed from under the surgical gown without contamination, is worn until the surgeon is convinced, through correlation with the CT scan and myelogram, that the right location has been found.

Nomenclature to accurately describe the microsurgical procedures has proved worthwhile. Each vertebral body with its respective lamina and surrounding ligamentum flavum can best be described as a *segment*. The space between two laminae, including the lamina borders and interposed ligamentum flavum, is referred to as an *intersegment*. The terms *symptomatic segmental* and *symptomatic intersegmental* are used to describe the initial operative approach. As the technique utilized is always microsurgical and is being applied to the lumbar anatomy, the word *microlumbar* is then added to the operation title. Finally, patients with previous lumbar surgery require a carefully controlled approach to the neural elements, which will allow for lysis of scar tissue and the treatment of lateral recess osteophytes and stenosis that so often contribute to the pathology. A central approach is used over the neural elements to avoid any possible injury to the facets and is best termed *decompression* for the purposes of nomenclature.

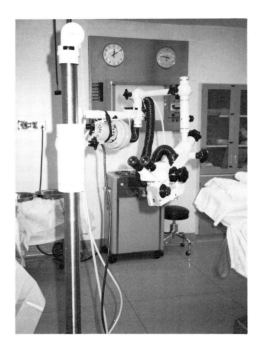

Figure 28–2 The lumbar surgical microscope. Pictured is a Zeiss OPMI #1 operating microscope with 400 mm lens, 12.5 eyepieces, and 100 watt halogen light source necessary for color and video photography. Note the addition of a central arm extension that allows the surgeon to change from one side of the patient to the other during the operative procedure without transporting the instrument. This maneuver proves critical for the safety of the neural elements when surgically treating the lateral recesses.

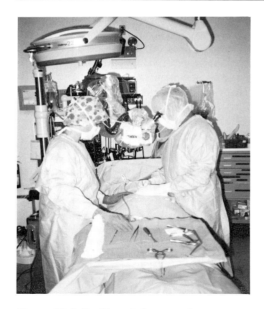

Figure 28–3 Position of the operating room personnel. The scrub nurse can best assist the surgeon when standing on the opposite side of the operating table. During microsurgical procedures, the need for a second physician assistant is eliminated by the minimal wound exposure and ease of hemostasis.

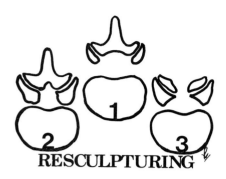

Figure 28–5 Resculpturing procedure for lateral recess collapse or stenosis. This illustration depicts what should be accomplished during lateral recess resculpturing. The technique used requires mobility of the surgeon to microscopically view the recess under treatment from the opposite side of the patient, thus ensuring the safety of the neural elements during resculpturing. The diagram pictures: (1) a spinal canal of normal bony dimensions, (2) that of a patient with lateral recess collapse or stenosis, and (3) the end result following resculpturing. Note that access to the extradural space has been achieved through minimal central laminectomy thus preventing injury to the facet plates.

Finally, the word *resculpturing* is added to the title of the operation if remodeling of the lateral recesses proves necessary (Figure 28–5). Thus, two titles of operation that might be used for the treatment of a failed lumbar patient are as follows:

1. Symptomatic Segmental Microlumbar Decompression and Resculpturing Procedure (SSMDR), (L4–5) (Figure 28–6).
2. Symptomatic Intersegmental Microlumbar Decompression and Resculpturing Procedure (SIMDR), (L4–5) (Figure 28–7).

COMMON POSTSURGICAL TISSUE MORBIDITIES

It would seem logical that there are two basic points crucial to the success of any lumbar operative procedure. Of first importance is the establishment of sound physiological principles, which balance in favor of what can be gained at the operating table as compared with what can be lost. Second, but of no less importance, would be the delayed responses of the individual lumbar tissue layers to the mechanics of surgical insult. Even if the basic theory for the design of a surgical treatment can be clearly established, it will prove of little or no value if the natural processes of wound healing seek to destroy what has been accomplished.

It is for this reason that the failed lumbar patient has been microsurgically studied in order to better understand the possible mechanisms by which postsurgical tissue morbidity can be initiated and the extent to which it may contribute to the

unsuccessful lumbar operation. The most scientific approach to this project was the meticulous recording of scarring reactions in the individual tissue layers, with special attention to those anatomical structures critical to lumbar spine stability. Such observations might well provide a framework for the evaluation of accepted levels of tissue trauma incurred during the treatment of benign surgical lumbar disease.

Skin

The lumbar skin seems abundantly supplied by somatic nerve endings. Just how many of these structures are lacerated by the surgeon's scalpel logically depends on the length of the skin incision. Unless these neural structures can be meticulously anastomosed, which seems a technical impossibility, the regenerative attempts by the axons may occasionally lead to a misdirected swirling growth of fibers proximal to the site of cutaneous nerve laceration. By any definition, this constitutes neuroma formation (Figure 28–8).

Cutaneous neuromas are not uncommon along the healed edges of lumbar skin incisions. At times they can be quite palpable as minute nodules. Pressure upon the neuromas can lead to an extremely disagreeable type of localized burning pain for the patient. In addition, if the pathophysiology of true causalgia is recalled in relation to the type of peripheral nerve injury implicated in its etiology, it seems quite reasonable that dysesthetic healed lumbar skin incisions are clinically fre-

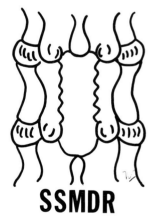

Figure 28–6 Symptomatic segmental microlumbar decompression and resculpturing procedure (SSMDR). Segmental decompression is applied over the central neural elements when root compressive pathology exists beneath a laminar arch associated with ligamentum flavum hypertrophy, both above and below. In the illustration, a total central laminectomy has been performed with complete removal of the surrounding ligament. Care is taken to avoid injury to the facets. Lateral recess neurolysis and resculpturing can be accomplished with a minimal central decompression of this type utilizing the surgical microscope to view the neural gutter under treatment from the opposite side of the patient. The technique is applied only to those levels that are clinically symptomatic.

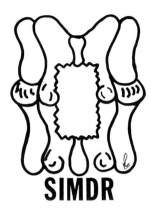

SIMDR

Figure 28–7 Symptomatic intersegmental microlumbar decompression and resculpturing procedure (SIMDR). Intersegmental decompression is utilized to treat intersegmental stenosis and postsurgical pathology that exists between two lamina. The illustration depicts removal of the central portion of two opposing laminar borders along with the interposed ligamentum flavum. Note, again, preservation of the facet plates. Recurrent disc herniation and adhesion reactions can be treated with safety by this limited exposure. The surgical microscope is the key instrument for visualization into the depths of the lateral recesses.

quent. Such a postsurgical tissue morbidity would seem easier avoided than corrected. Repeated observations indicate that, without question, the shorter the length of scalpel incision, the less frequent this miserable complication is encountered. At the risk of initiating such an uncomfortable and intractable situation, the surgeon must accurately localize and minimize skin incisions through the use of preoperative radiograms. The old cliché that skin heals side to side and not end to end, was not meant to condone surgical inaccuracy. In addition, well-placed skin incisions are mandatory if unnecessary surgical trauma is to be eliminated in the deeper tissue layers.

Subcutaneous Tissue

Functionally, the lumbar subcutaneous tissue appears to provide a significant cushion between the skin and underlying bony spinous processes. This layer also is well supplied with somatic nerve fibers, thus allowing for occasional neuroma formation following surgical incision. The most abundant specialized tissue in this layer, however, is fat, which may reach considerable proportions in some individuals. Any significant mechanical manipulation of the subcutaneous layer at surgery will lead to rupture of the fat cells, a release of natural petroleum in the wound, and often a subsequent localized atrophy of the fat cushion along the line of incision. The healed wound will be grooved in appearance and often very hyperesthetic to even the slightest pressure over the deeper spinous

processes. The exact mechanism of this discomfort remains speculative, but it certainly can prove extremely disabling for patients with sitting occupations.

In addition, the use of nonabsorbable sutures to close the subcutaneous tissue layer is still common practice with many spine surgeons. The knots produced by such material are often easily palpable in wounds where fat atrophy has occurred, giving rise to trigger points from which a stabbing type of pain can be elicited with even minimal degrees of pressure over the surrounding area. Here again, an accurate and well-localized incision of this tissue layer would seem worthwhile to minimize the possibility of neuroma formation and liquefaction with subsequent atrophy of subcutaneous fat. Finally, there seems to be no technical reason for the use of nonabsorbable suture material in this tissue layer at wound closure.

Paravertebral Muscle

The paravertebral muscle seems particularly prone to excessive surgical trauma during lumbar operations. Perhaps this is due somewhat to inadequate levels of surgical anesthesia, which permits a low-grade continuous contraction of these longitudinal muscle structures. Under such circumstances, a strong resistance to wound retraction may occur, thus necessitating excessively large exposures and the use of massive surgical instrumentation. Care should be taken to avoid this iatrogenic situation.

The histology of muscle is such that it is highly vascularized and richly supplied with somatic nerve fibers. Lumbar incisions off the midline promote significant bleeding, which seems best controlled through the use of electrocoagulation instruments. The end result will be dense scirrhous scars of electrical burns that most certainly will involve pain-producing end organs. Patients frequently experience intractable muscle spasms on the side of a paramedian incision. When transverse lumbar incisions are used, herniations of muscle tissue through the overlying fascia are not uncommon as a healed residuum. Clinically, these individuals may suffer symptoms similar to those just described.

The transverse fixation of longitudinally contracting paravertebral muscle is still common practice in large wound closures. This is often accomplished with nonabsorbable suture material and apparently is an attempt to eliminate dead space following the removal of several spinous processes. Such a practice would seem unnecessary as postoperative muscle spasm will accomplish the same purpose. Similarly, the transverse fixation of these vertically contracting longitudinal muscle structures with nonabsorbable suture persists as a chronic irritant. Such patients often manifest severe attacks of localized lumbar spasms during specific kinetic maneuvers.

Ligamentum Flavum

The ligamentum flavum provides an interlaminar covering for the dorsum of the neural elements. It appears to be contiguous with the periosteum of the lamina and is suspected to provide some assistance in extension of the spine. The ligament varies greatly in thickness and distribution but always expands laterally into the spinal recesses where it may produce significant mass effect. This is especially true in patients with spinal stenosis. A distinct tissue plane normally exists between the ligament and the deeper neural structures, except in an area of previous lumbar surgery. Occasionally, the structure is extremely thin and offers little protection to the neural elements during surgical approach to the interior of the bony spinal canal. Care must be taken when penetrating this structure as rupture into the subarachnoid space can easily occur.

The ligament appears essentially avascular. Once removed, it does not regenerate by primary intention and will be replaced by a dense fibrous scar, which proliferates downward fixing the neural elements to surrounding structures. During the lysis of such adhesions, minute lacerations of the dura without rupture into the cerebral spinal fluid space can occur, which give rise to the latent onset of pulsatile arachnoid herniations. Recurring seromas and subfacial meningoceles are frequently due to such mechanisms. In addition, a considerable mass effect can be produced by these structures, leading to postsurgical sciatica.

Lamina

The surgical morbidity to the lamina is often extensive when rongeurs are used to increase exposure to the neural elements and intervertebral tissue. For the most part, this appears secondary to regenerative osteoblastic activity along the traumatized bone edges in areas of lateral laminectomy. Such regenerative osteophytes can reach considerable size, projecting downward into the associated lateral recess with subsequent compression of the neural gutter. When combined with the removal of associated ligamentum flavum, fibrous tissue reactions may become intense, giving rise to insidious recurrent sciatica secondary to dense adhesion reactions. Interestingly enough, it is not uncommon to see a considerable hypertrophy of the residuals of ligamentum flavum that remain in the lateral recesses following surgical decompression. Exactly what this means is questionable, but the phenomenon has been observed in many young individuals who otherwise demonstrate no suggestion of similar pathology elsewhere. Repeated microsurgical observations suggest that the lateral regions of the lamina are extremely sensitive to the surgeons' rongeur and are best left undisturbed when at all possible.

Facets

The lumbar facets act to stabilize the lower spine against rotatory dislocations and subluxations. They are abundantly supplied with somatic innervation, as in patients with facet pain syndrome. Attempts to denervate these structures by such procedures as facetectomy and facet rhizotomy, however, have proved generally unsuccessful. It seems, therefore, that the facet joints are critically important to normal lumbar spine physiology and the clinical comfort of the patient.

If one uses the operating microscope to study individuals with postsurgical facet pain syndrome, some interesting facts can be noted. First of all, the facet plates per se lie almost horizontal and are invisible during posterior surgical approach. The synovial membrane, however, will be encountered as the most lateral fibers of the ligamentum flavum are removed from the recess. This structure normally appears as a small white fluid-filled sac that glistens under magnification and seems to pulsate with respiratory movements. For want of a better description, the term *synovial balloon* seems fitting (Figures 28–9 and 28–10).

In patients with iatrogenic facet pain syndrome, however, this structure, as well as the medial border of the facet plate, will often appear destroyed by the surgeons' rongeur. Only hyperemic residuals of the membrane and bony distortions of the medial joint surfaces usually remain. Surgical attempts at denervation, including total unilateral facetectomy, have not been consistently rewarding. Usually, the clinical syndrome is reasonably tolerable if the facet injury is only unilateral, but bilateral involvement has thus far proved intractable to additional surgical treatment. Success with such a disabling condition has been claimed by the proponents of all varieties of spinal fusion with or without total bilateral facetectomy. Such results have not been the experience of all. All such radical treatments are not advised because of the frequency with which progressing and incurable lumbar subluxations occur following bilateral facet removal at the same segment. Although the cure for such an exasperating clinical situation has thus far proved evasive with any degree of consistency in the operating room, decreasing the frequency with which this condition is encountered can be accomplished by eliminating surgical injury to the facet.

Lateral Bony Spinal Canal and Foramen

The smooth surface of the lateral spinal canal commonly becomes severely distorted by osteoblastic regenerative activity following the use of the surgical rongeur. In addition, this instrument frequently produces iatrogenic osteophytes as the jaws close (Figure 28–11). Unless care is taken to smooth these sharp bony spicules at the termination of lateral recess decompression, spurring of the associated nerve root may become the etiology of a rather immediate and intense postsurgical sciatica. The situation usually arises when the surgeon stands on the same side of the patient as the recess under treatment. The potential hazards of this careless error cannot be fully appreciated until magnification is used to view a freshly rongeured lateral recess from the side opposite. Therefore, the surgeon should always remain free to move from one side of the patient to the other during lumbar spine operations. Accuracy in the treatment of lateral recess stenosis can be accomplished only with absolute safety to the neural elements when the mouth of the rongeur remains in full view. In patients with soft initial disc herniations who have no other pathology, the lateral bony spinal canal should remain undisturbed for fear of giving the patient a new disease.

Similarly, the neural foramina in the lumbar region are frequently the recipients of rongeur morbidity during the treatment of sciatica. Whatever the word "foraminotomy" means, it would appear to cover a multiplicity of surgical injuries to the neural window and can be found in the operative reports of all patients with failed disc syndrome.

After years of interrogating many of these patients, it became apparent that the onset of a new perception of radicular pain frequently followed a surgical procedure where the word "foraminotomy" had been used to describe the operative technique. Interest in this phenomenon lead to the observation that the neural foramina react violently to insult by the surgeon's rongeur. Dense adhesion reactions can always be expected, as well as osteoblastic distortions of the nerve root as it passes through the bony tube. Since the passageway lies horizontal and is invisible during posterior surgical approach, such tissue reactions can only be appreciated in patients where partial resection of a foramen roof has occurred as part of the foraminotomy technique. If we assume that true root compressive pathology was present initially, the resulting iatrogenic pathology following decompression of the foramen was surely more severe. Thus far, attempts to surgically resurrect such a situation have proved clinically unrewarding.

Perhaps even more interesting, however, is the treatment of patients with virgin anatomy who appear to have severe osteoarthritic distortions and stenosis of the foramen seemingly well-visualized on high-intensity CT scans. Such individuals, with very few exceptions, have responded dramatically only to the treatment of the neural compressive pathology that exists in the lateral recesses. Most often, this treatment is in the form of hypertrophy of the undersurface of the facet plates and the ligamentum flavum. The exact mechanism by which release of the neural elements in the lateral spinal gutter can resolve sciatica without alteration of the associated neural foramen remains speculative. Consistent results with this conservative surgical approach, however, would lead one to believe that lumbar "foraminotomy" is not only of minimal value in the treatment of sciatica, but may in itself produce grave consequences far more severe than the initial disease the surgeon started out to treat.

The Extradural Space

Fat Tissue

Fat tissue is always present and often abundant in the virgin extradural space. It is usually well vascularized, which would tend to indicate that it is actively involved in metabolic processes. The amount of fat tissue present in the lumbar canal, however, appears to bear no relationship to the patient's general weight or body configuration.

Postsurgical lumbar areas are frequently devoid of extradural fat tissue. The exact mechanisms for such a phenomenon is speculative, but there is no question that it exists. Of further interest is the observation that fat appears to be necessary for the maintenance of tissue planes in the postsurgical patient. Without it, dense adhesions may often occur that totally immobilize the neural elements to the associated surrounding bone. Such adhesions usually do not have a particularly scirrhous quality and frequently can be disrupted with minimal effort. The fact that lysis of this tissue that is foreign to the extradural space can in itself relieve postsurgical sciatic pain is witness to its clinical importance. Perhaps the fat, in effect, lubricates the lateral recesses, allowing for significant mobility of the neural structures under normal circumstances.

Since a peripheral lumbar nerve has minimal elastic qualities and most certainly undergoes lengthening during kinetic activity such as 90-degree straight-leg raises, it seems logical to assume that fixation of the neural elements along the lateral spinal gutter by adhesions of any quality could easily become a viable etiology for postsurgical sciatica. Perhaps it is for this reason that patients who persist with straight-leg raises indefinitely following lumbar operative procedures rarely become afflicted with recurrent sciatica secondary to adhesion reactions.

The presence of extradural lumbar fat in its natural state would, therefore, seem critical for the prevention of postsurgical scar tissue reactions. Thus far, transplanted fat has not produced the same histological barrier in the human patient. Most often, grafted tissue will serve only to provide a matrix within which neovascularization and fibroblastic activity may become ravenous (Figure 28–12). It is for these reasons that extradural fat should be minimally traumatized and never sacrificed at the operating table.

Vascular Tissue

Fortunately for the spine surgeon, *arterial* vasculature is relatively sparse in the lumbar extradural space. When visualized under high magnification, it most often identifies the nerve root in contrast with the annulus fibrosis of the intervertebral disc. This is an extremely valuable anatomical landmark, as both structures otherwise present a glistening white appearance. Caution must be utilized, however, when attempting to identify the nerve in the lateral recess in cases of large, soft disc herniations. In this instance, the upward pressure of the disc mass may stretch and thus blanch the minute arterial vessels on the surface of the root, making it almost impossible to accurately distinguish the nerve from the annulus fibrosis. It is when such conditions exist that the potential for surgical injury to the nerve root by both scalpel and rongeur is at a maximum.

When the surgeon is unsure as to which structure is which, very gentle maneuvers with a blunt microhook will eventually provoke a motor response thus identifying the neural element. Finally, if the surgeon does encounter any significant amount of arterial bleeding in the extradural space, the possibility of an arteriovenous malformation as the cause of sciatica should be considered (Figure 28–13). Otherwise, the most likely etiology for such a terrifying experience will be perforation into the aorta during radical discectomy.

By contrast, *venous* tissue in the extradural space always seems abundant. Whenever a mass effect exists in the spinal canal from a lesion, such as the herniated intervertebral disc, venous distension can pose serious technical problems. The initial positioning of the patient to minimize pressure against the abdomen will prove crucial for the reduction of intraspinal venous pressure.

Massive hemorrhage from large and bulbous extradural veins is always a possibility in even the least complicated lumbar operations. When significant bleeding is encountered, one must take care not to institute techniques of hemostasis that could prove disastrous. An example of such a technique is the use of electrocautery instruments in the extradural space. Other than the surgical rongeur, electrical burns of the neural elements are the most hideous and incurable of all operative complications. Even if the neural tissue is spared in the process, electrocoagulation in the lateral recess will produce the most severe and scirrhous scar tissue reactions of all. One can expect, with almost complete certainty, that postsurgical sciatic pain will eventually evolve.

Such tragedies can be avoided if the surgeon develops expertise in the use of the operating microscope. With such a visual advantage, venous hemorrhage can be accurately localized and arrested by minimal tamponade with microsuction instruments. Once elevated venous pressure has been neutralized by the correction of any mass effect or segmental stenosis, bleeding will subside almost spontaneously. The alternative is to use the naked eye, pack the extradural space with cottonoid sponges, which will only serve to further increase venous engorgement, and hope that a hemorrhagic snowball can be prevented by Mother Nature's spontaneous coagulating mechanisms.

Intervertebral Tissue

The intervertebral disc is crucial to the normal physiology of lumbar spine function. Without its spacer effect, the disc space can progressively narrow often to the extent of partial subluxation of the facet plates. When such a process has taken place, insidious postsurgical sciatica may ensue, as the lateral recesses collapse to eventually entrap the neural elements. Such a sequence of events is not uncommon when relentless attacks utilizing the curettement techniques are made on the intervertebral tissue. When experimental efforts to extract large volumes of *virgin* lumbar disc material are attempted in the autopsy room, it can be demonstrated that even the most radical attack on the disc space will often yield no more than

half of the intervertebral mass. Such a technique, rationalized for the prevention of recurrent disc herniations, however, will ultimately prove ineffective for this purpose and will only serve to destroy the spacer effect and quality of the residual intervertebral tissue. The stage can thus be set for collapse of the intervertebral space and lateral recess.

Annulus Fibrosus

The annulus fibrosus is the retaining wall of the central intervertebral tissue. When it becomes incompetent to intradiscal pressures, the tissue of the nucleus pulposus will migrate toward the surface resulting in disc herniation. It would seem, therefore, that the herniated lumbar disc in reality is a disease of the annulus fibrosus, not the nucleus pulposus.

The histology of the annulus is one of multiple layers of essentially avascular fibroelastic tissue. Once surgically lacerated, it does not heal by primary intention (Figure 28–14). When a scalpel window has been cut in the annulus for the purpose of access to the deeper intervertebral tissue, the end result will be an annulus far more incompetent than that which initially existed (Figure 28–15). It would seem more logical, therefore, to enter the intervertebral space by dilatation of the fibers of the annulus fibrosus, rather than by scalpel incision, to retain wall competence for the years that lie ahead.

Nucleus Pulposus

It is the softer tissue of the central nucleus pulposus that proves critical for the maintenance of an appropriate distance between the vertebral end plates. To unnecessarily destroy the central disc tissue by whatever mechanism is to iatrogenically create a mechanical pathology similar to that of degenerative disc disease. Although occasionally such a withered and collapsed intervertebral space may clinically remain relatively asymptomatic, this will certainly not be the usual case. Most often, the lumbar discogenic pain syndrome insidiously evolves, accompanied by its notorious resistance to medical and surgical treatment. To inflict such a potentially disabling condition upon any patient as the end result of violent disc space curettement, or even intradiscal enzyme injection, is to encourage the latent development of a possibly intractable clinical morbidity.

EPIDURAL SCAR TISSUE AND ARACHNOIDITIS

Although there are a wide variety of conditions that lead the patient with virgin lumbar anatomy to the operating room, the spontaneous generation of fibrous scar tissue in the epidural space is not one of them. For those individuals with postsurgical sciatic pain and failed disc syndrome, however, the growth of this new tissue foreign to the extradural space can be consistently observed leading to mass effect as well as entrapment and fixation of the neural elements to approximating structures. Since remobilization of the affected nerve roots by tedious microsurgical lysis of such adhesions most often results in dramatic relief of postsurgical sciatic pain, it can only be assumed that the nervous system in its normal state must be reasonably mobile within the lumbar bony canal and foramen. Such a thought is not incompatible with the mechanisms of Lasègues' sign and the previously published viewpoint that maintaining the ability to perform 90-degree straight-leg raises indefinitely in the postsurgical lumbar patient is a key factor in the prevention of recurring sciatica secondary to adhesion reactions.

Although grossly epidural scar tissue appears to occur in a variety of colors and densities when viewed tnrough the surgical microscope, histological studies indicate that its basic structure is one of fibroblastic tissue that becomes progressively more hyalinized and devascularized with the passage of time (Figure 28–16). The generation of this often rampant growth appears to begin with the activation of rest cells by any variety of mechanical instrumentation, which leads to the disruption of normal tissue planes, fat necrosis, or hemorrhage. In addition, the utilization of fat grafts and foreign materials, such as Gelfoam for the purpose of preventing adhesion reactions, often seems to provide only a matrix within which intense fibroblastic scar tissue reactions will occur (Figures 28–17 and 28–18).

Although logically each individual's scarring response may vary with the strength of a mechanical stimulus, the burning of epidural tissue by electrocoagulation and laser instruments appears to have no equal. It is here that the most scirrhous and devastating of all epidural scar tissue reactions will be initiated (Figures 28–19 and 28–20).

For years, an additional condition known as arachnoiditis has been a major scapegoat of failed spinal surgery. Since stringy myelographic patterns are not uncommon in patients with postsurgical sciatic pain, microsurgical intradural explorations were carried on as the opportunity presented to confirm or disprove this diagnosis. Interestingly enough, less than 0.3 percent of the patients with this preoperative radiographic diagnosis could be documented to have the disease.

As the failed lumbar patient progresses through multiple operations, the initial mononerve root compression syndrome frequently terminates in a bilateral multilevel radiculopathy, with urinary retention and burning dysesthetic sciatica. Clinically, these patients are most frequently labeled as having "arachnoiditis." Such patients often respond dramatically to tedious microsurgical dissection of epidural scar tissue. The surgical pathology visualized will represent a myriad of anatomical morbidities ranging from osteoblastic masses in the lateral recesses to dense adhesions and vacant wedged disc spaces. Acceptance of a radiographic diagnosis alone as the sole criterion for arachnoiditis should be done cautiously. This is especially true when any degree of spinal stenosis appears on CT scan. True surgically documented arachnoiditis is very rare, but when it does occur, it should never be accepted as the end result of a naturally occurring disease process.

TECHNICAL SUGGESTIONS TO MINIMIZE POSTSURGICAL LUMBAR MORBIDITY AND SCAR TISSUE REACTIONS

It would seem that the microsurgical observations and techniques that have evolved during the investigation and treatment of patients with postsurgical sciatic pain could be put to good use for the design and reevaluation of lumbar surgical operations. If it can be accepted that the intervertebral discs and facet plates are the major stabilizing structures necessary to maintain normal lumbar physiology, and that surgical injury to any lumbar tissue or tissue plane will result in regenerative attempts and fibroblastic scarring, which may ultimately compress and immobilize the neural elements, parameters for spinal surgery can be set beyond which surgical failure will most often result.

Lumbar skin incisions should be minimized by radiographic localization and should always be placed in the midline to avoid cutaneous neuroma formation with resulting hyperesthesia of the healed wound. Similarly, excessive manipulation of the subcutaneous fat by retraction instruments may lead to atrophy of the fat pad with subsequent sinking of the incision and chronic wound tenderness.

Paravertebral muscle structures should be gently retracted along their plane with the spinous processes to avoid excessive bleeding, to avoid the necessity for increasing wound exposure, and to avoid the use of electrocoagulation instruments. Once the bony coverings of the spinal canal have been reached, special consideration must be given to the degree of further exposure necessary to accomplish a purpose.

Even though the laminar arch with its spinous process provides a stabilizing influence between two segmental superior facet plates, it may be resected in its central 75 percent with relative impunity in order to provide wide exposure to the underlying neural elements and approximating intervertebral spaces. This should be done only if absolutely necessary. Any void created over the central neural elements by such a maneuver will be filled postoperatively by a fibroblastic scar tissue reaction, unless the associated ligamentum flavum is allowed to remain.

Scarring over the central dura does not in itself, however, seem sufficient enough to immobilize the lateral neural elements for the production of postsurgical adhesion sciatica. Such a central decompression can, therefore, be applied when access to the lateral recesses proves imperative for the tedious lysis of epidural scar tissue or the resculpturing of the undersurface of the facet joints in cases of lateral recess stenosis. Utilizing this limited approach and a surgical microscope to view from the side opposite the lateral recess under treatment, any surgical injury to the associated facet plates or the synovial membrane can be avoided. Similarly, rongeuring of the lateral vertical bony canal with its subsequent danger of osteoblastic proliferation and further entrapment of the approximating nerve root becomes an unnecessary maneuver to accomplish the resculpturing task.

In cases of initial soft intervertebral disc herniations, injury to the lamina and associated lateral recess and facet can be totally avoided by the use of magnification. Once mastered, postsurgical sciatica secondary to osteoblastic regeneration in the lateral recess, iatrogenic osteophytes, and epidural scar tissue reactions all become extreme rarities. Similarly, the intact facet will provide the postoperative patient with the best chance for a sturdy vertical alignment of the lumbar spine for the years ahead.

Last, but not least, radical attacks on the intervertebral disc and its annular retaining wall may prove disastrous for the lumbar patient. Most certainly, scalpel windows in the annulus serve only to establish a permanent pathway for the reherniation of intervertebral tissue, especially when violent curettement has been applied in an attempt to remove large volumes of disc material during the initial surgery. Experience with microlumbar discectomy over a period of 12 years has proved that dilatation of the annulus fibrosus with a blunt instrument such as a #4 Penfield dissector and the minimal removal of disc material sufficient to eliminate nerve root compression are all that is necessary to achieve an extremely low rate of spontaneous disc reherniations (1.02 percent). Further sacrifice of disc tissue serves only to promote the eventual collapse of the lateral intervertebral space with subsequent overriding of the facet plates and wedging of the associated bony recess. For these patients, attacks of facet pain and recurring sciatica from lateral recess stenosis will often be the end result.

Vast experience in the treatment of patients with postsurgical sciatic pain and a respect for the functional evolution of the lumbar anatomy have set the boundaries for spinal surgery. What is to be gained at the operating table must always be balanced against what is to be lost. It would seem that radically destructive surgical procedures can serve only to increase the rolls of human misery and suffering.

Chapter 29

The Torsional Intervertebral Joint Lesion

Harry F. Farfan, B.Sc., M.D.

To understand the torsional disc lesion, the reader must be able to visualize the pathological anatomy in 3-D because there can be no axial rotation without the forced forward flexion and lateral rotation induced by the facet joints. (See Figure 29–1a and b.)

To permit the deformation to occur, there must be an injury to the disc annulus and injury to the neural arch. During this deformation, the neural arch and vertebral bodies change their position relative to the dural sac and nerve roots not only at the level of the lesion, but also above, and more important, below it.

The symptoms arise because of (1) the injury to the facet joints, (2) the injury to the disc, and (3) from the deformation of intervertebral canal. The symptoms depend partly on the stage of the process. This is particularly true of those arising from the injured disc and from the deformation of the intervertebral canal.

Facet joint symptoms are always part of the torsional injury because with the original injury, the articular cartilages are destroyed on the compressed side. Facet fracture is a common finding at autopsy. The damaged facet gives rise to a unilateral sciatica without neurological deficits. The pain may be described as extending to below the knee as far as the lateral ankle. The distribution of tenderness is characteristically gluteus medius, great trochanter, and iliotibial band to the knee. Other common names for this syndrome are sacroiliac strain, trochanteric bursitis, and dorsal division (ramus) syndrome.

In the later stages, with continued traumatic arthritis of the facet joints, the juxta-articular bone becomes osteoporotic and compression fractures are commonly found in the inferior articular process and in the mamillary process.

Destruction of the facet joint on the other side usually follows and the facet syndrome becomes bilateral.

THE DAMAGED DISC

The disc is distorted by torsion and fails at the posterolateral angles by tearing off from the end plate. The distortion is mainly in the outer layers of the annulus, the disc nucleus remaining intact. Note the possibility of a myelographic defect in the presence of a normal discogram. The distorted bulge of annulus may be large enough to trap the nerve giving rise to sciatica with or without neurological deficit. The tenderness in this instance is midline posterior thigh and calf, in addition to the tenderness from the facet syndrome.

With advancement of the process, the fissuring in the annulus becomes a radial communication between muscles and disc periphery. This provides the venue for typical nuclear material extrusions.

THE DEFORMATION OF THE NEURAL CANAL

Deformation of the neural canal is a common unrecognized cause of persistent postlaminectomy symptoms and because of its special features, it is an explanation for several otherwise incomprehensible problems of disc surgery.

When looking at the spine from behind, try to visualize the dural sac remaining in situ and axial rotation to the patient's left accompanied by forward and left lateral flexion occurring at the L4–5 intervertebral joint. Remember that the axis of

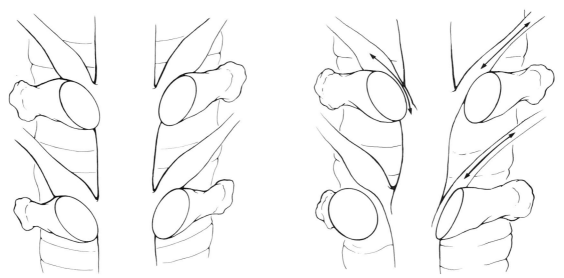

Figure 29–1a and **b** (a) Torsional injury. (b) Note that the nerve content can be stretched tight against the sides of the spinal canal.

rotation is at the center of the disc and the pelvis and L5 is fixed.

The left side of L4 will move backward and the right side will move forward, as the L4 body is rotated and flexed. The left L4 pedicle will pick up the fourth nerve root and pull it tight. The left fifth nerve root will be tightened down across the back of the L4 end plate and the disc. Even without a distorted disc, this may prevent the nerve root sleeve from filling with myelographic contrast.

On the right side, the body and pedicle of L4 move to the right and forward, trapping the fifth nerve root on the back of the upper end plate of L5 and pulling the root tight around the pedicle of L5, again, a filling defect without any disc protrusion. The stretching for nine degrees of rotation may produce twice the physiological 20 percent stretch and may result in neurological deficit.

In the operating room it is difficult to appreciate minor degrees of rotation deformity, especially when the field of vision is necessarily very restricted. Rotation deformity must be suspected when (1) no disc or a small protrusion is found at surgery, especially if there is a large myelographic defect and (2) when the offending disc material has been removed but the root remains tight. The rotation deformity is best detected before surgery.

At surgery the tight nerve root can be slackened in two ways:

1. Removal of the disc will collapse the disc space and reduce the nerve stretch. This is not a likely outcome if the disc has already lost much of its thickness.
2. Correction of the rotational deformity is simply done by forcing the dorsal spine toward the midline. Because of the deformation, we see the possibility of:

   - stretched fourth root—expect transient complaints of thigh weakness, or less commonly, neurological signs

associated normally with an L3–4 lesion. Note stretch of both fifth roots at the level of the lesion. Also, note stretch is greatest on the right side, and on this same side the dorsal root ganglion may be severely squeezed against the pedicle.

- a large myelographic defect without any disc protrusion.

- the myelographic defect appearing to arise also at the joints above and below the level of the lesion.

Note that the dural sac has appeared to move closer to one side at L4–5, but at L5–S1 and at L3–4 it is closer to the other side. The close approximation of dura to neural arch may give the impression at exploration of spinal stenosis. Further, note that the deformity may account for the observation that on occasion after a disc excision, the myelographic defect remains. Exploration at one level for an expected disc protrusion seen in myelogram may be apparently negative with the consequence of unwarranted surgery at the adjacent levels.

The frequency of the torsional injury is quite large. It is the most common problem involving the L4–5 joint. It is less common at the L5–S1 joint, which is often protected from torsion because of the added security of fixation of L5 to the sacrum and pelvis. When the L5 vertebra is high riding, it is not so protected and it also may suffer a torsional injury.

Preoperative assessment for possible torsional injury begins with careful evaluation of AP and lateral x-rays. Laminae of different lengths and abrupt changes in the line of the dorsal spine may be seen on the AP, while on the lateral x-ray changes in pedicle height and in contour of the posterior vertebral body may signify a torsional deformity. Awareness of this problem may affect surgical decision making.

Chapter 30

Summary of Etiologies of Postlaminectomy Syndrome

Robert G. Watkins, M.D.

The postlaminectomy syndrome is defined as residual disabling pain emanating from a prior laminectomized neuromotion segment. It does not imply pain caused by the operation, but rather the residual of a long disease process. The most consistently common cause of patient morbidity in most traumatic conditions is the severity of the initial injury. It may very well be that, despite treatment, the chief prognostic factor is the degree of damage caused by the injury to the disc and its neuromotion segment. A rotational injury may destroy the mechanical properties of the annulus and produce posterior element deformity and facet joint damage. This injury may cause severe disability, regardless of whether a laminectomy is done for nerve root pain. When treatment begins, it must properly address the pathology or it can increase the patient's morbidity. Indeed, total laminectomy done for nerve root pain caused by a dynamic or fixed rotational deformity may fail to relieve the problem by not addressing the pathology and may increase the pain that results from instability.

It is important to understand the natural history of this process. In Chapters 1 and 27, Dupuis and Kirkaldy-Willis have detailed a series of morphologic and symptomatologic changes undergone by the lumbar spine. A patient's lumbar problems follow a natural response to time and injury. The vast majority of people in the dysfunction and instability phases improve with time. Treatment intervention may not affect the natural history of the disease at all but intervention in this natural history is appropriate.

Diagnostic difficulties may contribute to the failure of surgical intervention in lumbar spine disease. For radicular symptoms, the objective of the diagnostic work-up is to determine which nerve is being compressed in which neuromotor segment and what is compressing or irritating the nerve. The diagnostic work-up also determines the pathology present in that neuromotion segment.

The nerve is identified through clinical examination, electromyography (EMG), SEPs, selective nerve root block, or radiographic study. The level and cause are determined through physical examination and radiographic study. When the diagnostic plan fails to identify these things, laminectomy usually fails.

THE WRONG LEVEL

A significant cause of postlaminectomy syndrome is diagnosing and operating on the wrong level. We have emphasized that there are two basic origins that must be considered: (1) the level of the spinal column from which the pain originates and (2) the level of the nervous system from which the spinal pain emanates; this means which neuromotion segment and which spinal nerve. There are distinct exceptions to the frequent patterns. L4–5 herniated nucleus pulposus produces L5 pain and L5–S1 herniated nucleus pulposus produces S1 root pain. Other examples are:

1. A lateral herniated nucleus pulposus at L5–S1 producing pain from the exiting L5 nerve root
2. A prefixed or postfixed lumbosacral plexus that may have a root exiting through a different foramina than usual
3. A conjoined nerve root

4. Lateral foraminal stenosis that produces pain from an exiting nerve root, as an L4–5 foraminal stenosis producing L4 root pain
5. Lateral recess stenosis that produces traversing nerve root pain despite minimal disc pathology such as an L4–5 lateral recess stenosis producing L5 root pain
6. A central disc herniation at L4–5 producing S1 root symptoms
7. A central disc herniation at L3–4 producing a cauda equina syndrome

Decompressive operations done for a clear-cut nerve lesion in which the nerve is specifically identified and can be matched with a specific, appropriate anatomic lesion in the spinal column will produce a good result in relieving the leg pain. Adjuvant tests such as spinal nerve blocks, discography, and excellent foraminal reconstructions on computed tomography (CT) scanning may greatly enhance diagnostic capability.

Another way to avoid the wrong level problem is to use a very specific preoperative and intraoperative routine of identifying the right level: (1) After a thorough review of the x-rays and patient evaluation prior to surgery, the painful leg should be marked on the foot the night before surgery and/or the anesthesiologist should intraoperatively read out the painful leg from the old and current chart, (2) the plain x-rays, the CT scan, and the myelogram should be on the view box in the operating room prior to induction of anesthesia, (3) the level with intraoperative x-rays should always be confirmed by use of the skin marker (for incision level) and the intralaminar marker with a coker after exposure of an intralaminar area with the retractors in place. If there is any question about the pathology found, such as an intervertebral disc that is bulging but reveals no significant fragment of disc, the level should be confirmed with an intraoperative x-ray with a needle in the disc space.

The diagnostic accuracy of each of the tests in determining nerve, level, and pathology is limited. There are false-positives and false-negatives with any test. False-positives, for a clinician, are significant findings in the study that are not causing the patient's problems. False-negatives occur when an anatomic source for the patient's pain is within the scope of a test but the test fails to demonstrate its significance. The testers do not look at it that way but clinicians do. Often the weight of circumstantial data from a number of tests prevails without conclusive proof.

DIAGNOSIS

Proper diagnosis is important for prevention of post-laminectomy syndrome. The preoperative origin of the pain should be diagnosed as specifically as possible. Decompression, that is laminotomy, laminectomy, medial facetectomy, foraminotomy, and/or discectomy may produce excellent

results when the pathology is a herniated disc and/or spinal stenosis. Laminectomy done for predominantly back pain of annular insufficiency and segmental instability produces increased annular insufficiencies, with epidural scar and a high incidence of posterior laminectomy syndrome. A young patient with a long history of severe mechanical back pain, with or without spondylolisthesis, who develops moderate leg pain, cannot expect a pain-free result from laminectomy alone.

Segmental instability is defined as abnormal motion in a neuromotion segment. This is not necessarily hypermobility. The amount of motion has not been related to clinical pain or disability. Abnormal motion produces the mechanical stress that leads to inflammation in the richly innervated annulus or facet capsules. The chief clinical presentation of segmental instability is mechanical back pain with or without leg pain.

The functions of the lamina include support of the ligamentum flavum. The ligamentum flavum is the main stabilizing ligament of the posterior column; resection of this ligament cannot improve stability. As a neuromotion segment rotates, the end point is facet impaction and annular strain. The laminar arch helps dissipate the force of the end point impact of rotation. Without the lamina, the facets and annulus bear more rotational stress. Operative trauma to the facet joint capsule, weakening or removal of the lamina, and cutting a large annular window may increase instability.

As O'Brien points out in Chapter 26, the annulus is richly innervated and injury to the annulus may produce severe incapacitating back and leg pain. Not all leg pain is root pain. It may be referred pain. Discography is the appropriate test for diagnosing annular pain. Laminectomy is an inappropriate treatment for this diagnosis. The progression from annular tear with back and referred leg pain to annular disruption with nuclear herniation and radiculopathy is often observed clinically. Of course, the majority of back and referred leg pain cases do not show this progression. Often they continue on an intermittent basis until the neuromotion segment stabilizes. They may be significantly improved with non-operative rehabilitation—stretching and strengthening exercises, proper body mechanics, and posture correction.

Sciatica, pain along the course of the sciatic nerve, most often results from compressive and inflammatory irritation of a nerve root by herniation of an intervertebral disc. The herniation may be contained within the damaged annulus or fragments of nucleus and annulus may be extruded into the canal. Incapacitating leg pain can result from compression of the inflamed nerve root by the herniated fragments, chemical irritation of the nerve root, and annular pain from distention of the annulus due to contained herniation. Laminectomy and discectomy may result in relief from the nerve root compression and a return to the usually less intense mechanical annular pain. When laminectomy is successful, the neuromotion segment returns to a more natural process of eventual stabilization and response to back rehabilitation. Mechanical stability prevents the postlaminectomy pain of nerve root scar and instability. This, of course, does not mean that primary fusion with laminectomy is indicated to avoid this complication. The key to the successful progression to stability and clinical improvement is decompressing only when there is a compressive problem—when the leg pain of radiculopathy or neurogenic claudication is so incapacitating that decompression offers a significant change of improved spinal mechanics and patient function through rehabilitation.

TECHNIQUE

The foundation of proper technique lies in six areas:

1. Proper training and experience—there is no such thing as a "simple disc." A surgeon doing an occasional back surgery without specialty training in spinal surgery will produce more failures—more postlaminectomy syndromes—than an experienced spinal surgeon.
2. Proper lighting and magnification—fiberoptic headlights, a great variety of magnification glasses, and microscopes can be adapted to fit and improve any surgeon's technique. Proper visualization of the operative field improves with magnification and lighting. The field gets larger not smaller; therefore, less normal tissue is removed to explore the pathology.
3. The proper operative frame—abdominal pressure causes bleeding. The best frame has *nothing* touching the abdomen, not even its sides. Side pressure from long chest and abdominal rolls causes more bleeding than frames with no side pressure. The abdomen should hang free with the hips and knees at 90 degrees.
4. Proper tools—the surgeon must know what tools are available, how to use them, and must understand the least traumatic, most effective method of actually using the instrument.
5. Proper assistance—two pilots flying the same plane at the same time does not work. The assistant must know his or her role, to provide the surgeon with every technical advantage. The assistant can often provide valuable "thinking" during a tense case.
6. Analyze, review, and refine technique—spend hours reviewing each step in a search for facility, ease, effectiveness, and complication presentation.

It is important to avoid totally destabilizing a neuromotion segment through unnecessary removal of uninvolved structures. Too often the exact structure causing the compression is not properly identified, which leads to removal of normal tissue and failure to decompress enough of the pathology.

Failure to appreciate spinal stenosis concomitant with a disc herniation will lead to a high incidence of posterior laminectomy syndrome because of scar under the root, annular bulging, and lateral recess entrapment. Removal of the lamina, instead of medial facet, will fail to relieve lateral stenotic symptoms. Careful evaluation by CT scan for subpedicular

and lateral foraminal stenosis at the level below an operated disc may identify pathologic entrapment of the exiting nerve root at the lower level. The skill of properly decompressing foramina without a total facetectomy requires the ability to cut osteophytes from the posterior body wall or from the under surface of the facet without cutting the nerve. The answer to problems of this kind is proper preoperative diagnostic studies and a controlled, thorough decompression. Laminectomy technique must be immaculate in order to prevent excessive scarring. Every precaution should be taken to avoid unnecessary trauma and pressure on normal tissue while accomplishing a decompression.

The concept of a dynamic stenosis presented by Farfan and Kirkaldy-Willis in Chapters 29 and 27 is chilling to any surgeon obsessed with removal of myelographic defects. The offending pathology may be subtle, mechanical, and totally unappreciated at surgery and also may be uncorrected by discectomy.

Scarring is a source of postlaminectomy syndrome attributable to the treatment. Tissue destruction causes scarring. The most common technical problem with standard laminectomy is "too much destruction getting to the disc" and "not enough decompression of the nerve once you get there." Proper respect for all tissues—the subcutaneous fat, the fascial attachments to the spinous process, the facet joint capsule, and the epidural fat—will decrease postoperative symptoms.

Epidural scarring can have a devastating effect on clinical results. Small amounts of motion may produce pain in an inflamed, scarred nerve. This complex of complications is avoidable through proper technique. Unnecessary removal of epidural fat, leaving raw bone against nerve, unnecessary anticoagulation methods, and leaving a large annular hole under the nerve will produce scar. Subtle mechanical stresses can make a scarred nerve root in a scarred epidural space symptomatic. Improper handling of the nerve can produce direct nerve scarring.

In Chapter 28 Williams brings the spine surgeon back to basics—"Do no harm." If the objective is removal of extruded disc fragment, then do only that. Destroying vital, normal tissue in an attempt to prophylactically affect the natural history of this annular injury is probably inappropriate. Destruction because of inexperience, inability to control bleeding, poor visualization, or a failure to appreciate the anatomy without direct visualization is inappropriate. Williams reminds us to delicately guard every millimeter of tissue like gold.

Philosophically, surgeons differ on immediate and long-term goals in the operative care of disc disease. This difference ranges from microscopic discectomy to standard laminectomy to posterior interbody fusion for disc herniation. There can be future problems with them all. Improvement of clinical results will be through proper diagnosis, thorough decompression of pathologic structures, protection of normal structures during decompression, and proper postoperative rehabilitation.

Index

O

Operating microscope, 219, 254-55, *256*
Operating telescope, 198, *199*
Osteomyelitis, vertebral, 105
Osteopenia, compression fractures, *103*
Osteophytes. *See also* Uncinate spurs
 appearance in restabilization phase, 3, *4*, *197*
 cephalo-caudad stenosis caused by, *56*, *57*, *58*, *60*
 iatrogenic, 259
 removal, *224*, 251
Osteotomes, 175, *199*

P

Pain,
 checklist for radicular, *37*
 delayed onset, 236
 discogenic, 236, *237*
 four symptom complexes, 125, 139
 gateway control theory of, 6
 leg. *See* Leg, pain
 low back. *See* Low back pain
 mechanical, 125, 139
 morbidity classifications, *43*
 nerve root traction tests, 8-11
 neurogenic claudication, 19, 125
 neurotransmitters of, 7
 nonmechanical, 125, 139
 patellar and achilles reflexes, 11-12
 patterns of, 7-8, *236*
 psychic response to, 5
 radicular. *See* Radicular pain
 sciatic. *See* Sciatica, pain
 sensory and motor disturbances with, 12-13
 somatic afferent system, 5-6
 spinal canal innervation, 7
Pain drawing, 38, *39*, *77*
Pantopaque. *See* Iophendylate myelography
Paraspinous fascia incision, 159, *160-61*
Patellar reflex and sciatica, 11-12
Patient(s),
 care. *See* Conservative care;
  Interventional (nonsurgical) care;
  Surgery
 history/examination. *See* Patient history and examination
 pediatric. *See* Children
 position. *See* Patient positioning
 postoperative care, 177, 226, 242, 251
 postoperative complications, 177, 242-43
 response to disc injection, 122
 spinal headaches. *See* Headache, postspinal puncture

symptom complexes of, 125, 139
Patient history and examination, 28, 37-38, 125, 139
 examination form, *31-36*
 final forms of, *40-43*
 history form, *29-30*
 morbidity classification, *43*
 pain drawing, 38, *39*, *77*
Patient positioning, *255*
 to avoid pressure injuries, 152
 for laminotomy, 174
 lateral position for decompression surgery, 179, *180*
 lateral stenosis decompression, 248, *249*
 to lower blood pressure, 151
 paralateral approach, *219*, 220
 posterior approach to the lumbar spine, 159
 for subarticular and far out lateral stenosis surgery, 198
Patrick's F-AB-E-R-E sign, *9*
Pedicle(s),
 at diastematomyelia level, *111*
 removal, and nerve decompression, *207*, *209*, 224
 as a surgical reference point, *164*, 169, *170*, *192*, 195, *196*
Perikarya, 5, 6
Perineural cyst, 89, *92*
Piriformis syndrome, 248
Positioning. *See* Patient positioning
Posterior joint syndrome, 248
Posterior longitudinal ligament,
 calcified, producing suarachnoid block, *93*
 nerves of, 7
Post laminectomy syndrome, 235-44, 267-69. *See also* Failed back surgery syndrome
Postsurgical lumbar scarring, 253-63. *See also* Epidural scarring; Fibrosis
 common morbidities, 257-61
 epidural scarring and arachnoiditis, 261-62
 materials/methods for investigating, 255-57
 preliminary mechanisms for the creation of, 253-54
 suggestions to minimize, 262-63, 269
 surgical microscope evaluation, 254-55
Pressure injuries, avoiding, 152
Pseudoarthrosis, 136, 211

R

Radicular pain, 37, 125
Radiculogram, 109

Radiography. *See* X-rays
Retractor instruments, *154*
Retro-olisthesis,
 degenerative changes and, 3, *4*
 posterior articular facets, 111, *112*
 spinal instability, 50, *51*
Rongeur instruments, *155*, *156*, *157*

S

Sacrohorizontal angle, *47*
Sacroiliac syndrome, 8, 248
Sacrospinalis muscle, 217
Sacrum, tumor of, 119, *120*
SCAPF operation. *See* Simultaneous combined anterior and posterior fusion (SCAPF)
Sciatica, 8-13, 268
 burned out syndrome, 63
 demonstrated by myelography, 110, 115
 motor deficits, 12-13
 pain, 8, 110, 115
 patellar and achilles reflexes, 11-12
 postsurgical, 255
 sensory disturbances, 12
 tests for, 8-11, 140-41
Scoliosis,
 in children, *230*
 degenerative, 206, *209*
 decompression techniques for, *207-8*
 fusion to treat, *238*, 239-43
 produced by sciatica, 8
Sensory disturbances, 12
 neurogenic claudication, 19-20
Sherrington, Charles, 6
Simultaneous combined anterior and posterior fusion (SCAPF) technique, 238, 239-43
 bone graft, 240, 242
 complications, 242-43
 instruments for, 239, *240*
 posterior instrumentation and fusion, 242
 postoperative care, 242
 replacing disc with bone, 241
 results, 243
 surgical procedure, 239
 turning the patient, 241-42
 wound closure, 242
Skin, postsurgical scarring, 257
Soft tissue lesions, *78*, *79*
Somatic afferent system, 5-6, 257
Somatostatin, 7
Sphincter dysfunction, 20
Spinal bifida, 229. *See also* Diastematomyelia